*Progress in
Cancer Research and Therapy
Volume 25*

STEROIDS AND ENDOMETRIAL CANCER

Progress in Cancer Research and Therapy

Progress in
Cancer Research and Therapy
Volume 25

Steroids and Endometrial Cancer

Editors

**Valerio Maria Jasonni,
M.D.**
*Senior Assistant, Department of
Reproductive Pathophysiology
University of Bologna
St. Orsola's General Hospital
Bologna, Italy*

Italo Nenci
*Chief, Department of Pathology
University of Ferrara
Ferrara, Italy*

Carlo Flamigni
*Chief, Department of Reproductive Pathophysiology
University of Bologna
St. Orsola's General Hospital
Bologna, Italy*

Raven Press ■ New York

Raven Press, 1140 Avenue of the Americas, New York, New York 10036

Made in the United States of America

Library of Congress Cataloging in Publication Data
Main entry under title:

Steroids and endometrial cancer.

    (Progress in cancer research and therapy ; v. 25)
    Includes bibliographical references and index.
    1. Endometrium—Cancer—Etiology—Addresses, essays,
lectures. 2. Estrogen—Receptors—Addresses, essays,
lectures. 3. Steroid hormones—Metabolism—Addresses,
essays, lectures. 4. Estrogen—Therapeutic use—Side
effects—Addresses, essays, lectures. I. Jasonni,
Valerio Maria. II. Nenci, Italo. III. Flamigni, C.
IV. Series. [DNLM: 1. Estrogens—Adverse effects.
2. Uterine neoplasms—Etiology. 3. Estrogens—
Therapeutic use. W1 PR667M v.25 / WP 458 S839]
RC280.U8S74   1983   616.99′466   83-17606
ISBN 0-89004-834-7

Preface

This volume presents current research on the interactions of steroid hormones and endometrial cancer. Receptor studies and molecular biology are discussed in order to present the basic aspects of this intriguing problem.

The metabolism of steroid hormones is considered describing the several studies for and against the "estrogen theory" in the etiology of endometrial cancer. The production and peripheral metabolism of androgens and estrogens and their possible involvement in determining endometrial cancer is also presented.

This volume examines estrogen therapy and its possible disposition to endometrial cancer as well as modern trends to evaluate endometrial resistance to exogenous estrogens. The correct approach to the hormonal replacement therapy is very important in preventing endometrial cancer as soon as it appears.

The final section of this volume presents some short communications that review preliminary results of researchers in this field.

This volume will be of interest to clinicians and experimental scientists interested in endometrial cancer, as well as to endocrinologists and gynecologists.

Dr. V. M. Jasonni
Prof. I. Nenci
Prof. C. Flamigni

Acknowledgments

We would like to thank the following for contributing to the success of the meeting of the First International Symposium on Steroids and Endometrial Cancer held at St. Orsola's General Hospital, Bologna, Italy.

The Public Health Department of Regione Emilia, Romagna and the CNR for providing the necessary framework and backup, as well as financial support, and particularly Dr. Ricci, President of the Credito Romagnolo and Dr. A. Simonelli.

Our thanks also go to Drs. C. Bulletti, A. P. Ferraretti, and M. Bonavia who were responsible for the secretarial organization before and during the meeting.

Finally, the editors gratefully acknowledge the expert and efficient assistance of Raven Press for their technical support.

The Editors

Contents

Basic Aspects

Steroids Action on Endometrium

Abnormalities of Steroid Metabolism and Their Effects on Endometrium

Estrogen Therapy and its Possible Effects on Determining Endometrial Cancer

Short Communications

Contributors

M. G. Acampora
Department of Obstetrics and
 Gynecology
Catholic University
Largo Gemelli 8
00168 Rome, Italy

R. Andriesse
Department of Endocrinology
University Hospital
State University of Utrecht
101 Catharisnesingel
Utrecht, The Netherlands

F. Battaglia
Department of Obstetrics and
 Gynecology
Catholic University
Largo Gemelli 8
00168 Rome, Italy

Etienne-Emile Baulieu
INSERM U33 and CNRS ER 125
Lab Hormones
94270 Bicêtre, France

Luisa Belforte
Department of Gynecological
 Endocrinology
St. Anna's Gynecological Hospital
60 Spezia Avenue
10126 Turin, Italy

Paola Belforte
Department of Gynecological
 Endocrinology
St. Anna's Gynecological Hospital
60 Spezia Avenue
10126 Turin, Italy

M. Benedetto
Department of Obstetrics and
 Gynecology
Catholic University
Largo Gemelli 8
00168 Rome, Italy

E. W. Bergink
Scientific Development Group
Organon International B.V.
Oss, The Netherlands

P. Biondani
Department of Obstetrics and
 Gynecology
University of Padua, Verona
 Branch
"B. Roma" Clinical Center
37100 Verona, Italy

G. F. Bolelli
Department of Reproductive
 Physiopathology
St. Orsola's General Hospital
University of Bologna
13 Massarenti Road
40138 Bologna, Italy

A. Bompiani
Department of Obstetrics and
 Gynecology
Catholic University
Largo Gemelli 8
00168 Rome, Italy

M. Bonavia
Department of Reproductive
 Pathophysiology
St. Orsola's General Hospital
University of Bologna
13 Massarenti Road
40138 Bologna, Italy

S. C. Brooks
Department of Biochemistry
Wayne University School of
 Medicine
540 Canfield
Detroit, Michigan 40201

C. Bulletti
*Department of Reproductive
 Pathophysiology*
St. Orsola's General Hospital
University of Bologna
13 Massarenti Road
40138 Bologna, Italy

Carlo Campagnoli
*Department of Gynecological
 Endocrinology*
St. Anna's Gynecological Hospital
60 Spezia Avenue
10126 Turin, Italy

L. Cantafio
*Department of Obstetrics and
 Gynecology*
Catholic University
Largo Gemelli 8
00168 Rome, Italy

L. Castagnetta
Institute of Biochemistry
Faculty of Medicine—Policlinico
90127 Palermo, Italy

R. Cavallina
*Department of Obstetrics and
 Gynecology*
St. Orsola's General Hospital
University of Bologna
13 Massarenti Road
40138 Bologna, Italy

G. Cerruti
*Department of Obstetrics and
 Gynecology*
*University of Padua, Verona
 Branch*
"B. Roma" Clinical Center
37100 Verona, Italy

C. Christensen
Department of Biochemistry
*Wayne University School of
 Medicine*
540 Canfield
Detroit, Michigan 48201

B. Cinque
*Department of Obstetrics and
 Gynecology*
Catholic University
Largo Gemelli 8
00168 Rome, Italy

Gary M. Clark
Department of Medicine
Division of Oncology
*University of Texas Health Science
 Center*
San Antonio, Texas 78284

Giuseppe Conti
Institute of Pharmacology
Faculty of Medicine
University of Turin
30 Raffaello Avenue
10125 Turin, Italy

J. Corombos
Department of Biochemistry
*Wayne University School of
 Medicine*
540 Canfield
Detroit, Michigan 48201

C. Costanzo
*Department of Obstetrics and
 Gynecology*
*University of Padua, Verona
 Branch*
"B. Roma" Clinical Center
37100 Verona, Italy

A. Cunsolo
II Surgical Clinic
St. Orsola's General Hospital
University of Bologna
9 Massarenti Road
40138 Bologna, Italy

G. D'Agostino
Institute of Biochemistry
Faculty of Medicine—Policlinico
90127 Palermo, Italy

E. Dalla Vecchia
*Department of Obstetrics and
 Gynecology*
University of Modena
41100 Modena, Italy

A. D'Angelo
*Department of Obstetrical and
 Gynecological Pathology*
University of Sassari
4 Manzella Street
07100 Sassari, Italy

G. D'Aurizio
Department of Obstetrics and
 Gynecology
Catholic University
Largo Gemelli 8
00168 Rome, Italy

F. De Cicco Nardone
Department of Obstetrics and
 Gynecology
Catholic University
Largo Gemelli 8
00168 Rome, Italy

L. Deligdisch
Division of Reproductive Biology
 and Pathology
Departments of Obstetrics and
 Gynecology
Mount Sinai School of Medicine
New York, New York 10029

S. Dell'Acqua
Department of Obstetrics and
 Gynecology
Catholic University
Largo Gemelli 8
00168 Rome, Italy

D. De Lucia
Institute of General Pathology
I Medical School
University of Naples
S. Andrea delle Dame 2
80138 Naples, Italy

A. D'Errico
Institute of Histopathology
St. Orsola's General Hospital
University of Bologna
9 Massarenti Road
40138 Bologna, Italy

M. S. de Winter
Scientific Development Group
Organon International B.V.
Oss, The Netherlands

Francesco Di Carlo
Institute of Pharmacology
Faculty of Medicine
University of Turin
30 Raffaello Avenue
10125 Turin, Italy

G. C. Di Renzo
Department of Obstetrics and
 Gynecology
University of Modena
41100 Modena, Italy

G. H. Donker
Department of Endocrinology
University Hospital
State University of Utrecht
101 Catharisnesingel
Utrecht, The Netherlands

V. Eusebi
Institute of Histopathology
St. Orsola's General Hospital
University of Bologna
9 Massarenti Road
40138 Bologna, Italy

A. P. Ferraretti
Department of Reproductive
 Physiopathology
St. Orsola's General Hospital
University of Bologna
13 Massarenti Road
40138 Bologna, Italy

C. Flamigni
Department of Reproductive
 Pathophysiology
St. Orsola's General Hospital
University of Bologna
13 Massarenti Road
40138 Bologna, Italy

Elizabeth J. Folkerd
Department of Chemical Pathology
St. Mary's Hospital Medical School
London W2 1PG, England

F. Franceschetti
Department of Reproductive
 Physiopathology
St. Orsola's General Hospital
University of Bologna
13 Massarenti Road
40138 Bologna, Italy

Elena Gallo
Institute of Pharmacology
Faculty of Medicine
University of Turin
30 Raffaello Avenue
10125 Turin, Italy

Joseph C. Gambone
Division of Reproductive
Endocrinology and Gynecologic
Oncology
Department of Obstetrics and
Gynecology
University of California, Los Angeles
Los Angeles, California 90024

M. Gangemi
Obstetric and Gynecological Clinic
University of Padua
3 Giustiniani Street
35100 Padua, Italy

O. M. Granata
Institute of Biochemistry
Faculty of Medicine—Policlinico
90127 Palermo, Italy

A. Grasso
Department of Obstetrics and
Gynecology
University of Modena
41100 Modena, Italy

Hans-Jörg Grill
Department of Experimental
Endocrinology
Johannes Gutenberg
Universität
Langenbeckstrasse 1
6500 Mainz, Federal Republic of
Germany

Matti Grönroos
Department of Obstetrics and
Gynecology
University of Turku
Turku, Finland

E. Gurpide
Division of Reproductive Biology
and Pathology
Department of Obstetrics and
Gynecology
Mount Sinai School of Medicine
New York, New York 10029

C. F. Holinka
Division of Reproductive Biology
and Pathology
Department of Obstetrics and
Gynecology
Mount Sinai School of Medicine
New York, New York 10029

S. Iacobelli
Laboratory of Molecular
Endocrinology
Catholic University of San Cuore
00168 Rome, Italy

V. H. T. James
Department of Chemical Pathology
St. Mary's Hospital Medical School
London W2 1PG, England

V. M. Jasonni
Department of Reproductive
Pathophysiology
St. Orsola's General Hospital
University of Bologna
13 Massarenti Road
40138 Bologna, Italy

Howard L. Judd
Division of Reproductive
Endocrinology and Gynecologic
Oncology
Department of Obstetrics and
Gynecology
University of California, Los
Angeles
Los Angeles, California 90024

Antti Kauppila
Department of Obstetrics and
Gynecology
University of Oulu
SF-90220 Oulu 22, Finland

A. M. Kaye
Department of Hormone Research
The Weizmann Institute of Science
Rehovot, 76100 Israel

R. J. B. King
Hormone Biochemistry Department
Imperial Cancer Research Fund
P.O. Box 123
Lincoln's Inn Fields
London WC2A 3PX, England

H. J. Kloosterboer
Scientific Development Group
Organon International B.V.
Oss, The Netherlands

William A. Knight III
Department of Medicine
Division of Oncology
University of Texas Health Science
Center
San Antonio, Texas 78284

H. Kopera
Institute of Experimental and
Clinical Pharmacology
University of Graz
University-Platz 4
A-8010 Graz, Austria

Leo D. Lagasse
Division of Reproductive
Endocrinology and Gynecologic
Oncology
Department of Obstetrics and
Gynecology
University of California, Los
Angeles
Los Angeles, California 90024

R. E. Leake
Department of Biochemistry
Glasgow University
G. 12–8QQ, Glasgow, United
Kingdom

U. Leone
Department of Obstetrical and
Gynecological Pathology
University of Sassari
4 Manzella Street
07100 Sassari, Italy

Carlos Lévy
Institute of Oncology "Angel H.
Roffo"
Buenos Aires, Argentina

S. Lodi
Department of Reproductive
Pathophysiology
St. Orsola's General Hospital
University of Bologna
13 Massarenti Road
40138 Bologna, Italy

A. Lucisano
Department of Obstetrics and
Gynecology
Catholic University
Largo Gemelli 8
00168 Rome, Italy

William L. McGuire
Department of Medicine
University of Texas Health Science
Center
San Antonio, Texas 78284

David T. MacLaughlin
Vincent Research Laboratory
Department of Gynecology
Massachussetts General Hospital;
and
Department of Obstetrics and
Gynecology
Harvard Medical School
Boston, Massachussetts 02114

T. Maggino
Obstetric and Gynecological Clinic
University of Padua
3 Giustiniani Street
35100 Padua, Italy

D. Mango
Department of Obstetrics and
Gynecology
Catholic University
Largo Gemelli 8
00168 Rome, Italy

E. Maniccia
Department of Obstetrics and
Gynecology
Catholic University
Largo Gemelli 8
00168 Rome, Italy

Bernd Manz
Department of Experimental
Endocrinology
Johannes Gutenberg Universität
Langenbeckstrasse 1
6500 Mainz, Federal Republic of
Germany

D. Marchesoni
Obstetric and Gynecological Clinic
University of Padua
3 Giustiniani Street
35100 Padua, Italy

P. Marchetti
Laboratory of Molecular
Endocrinology
Catholic University of San Cuore
00168 Rome, Italy

Graziella Martoglio
Department of Gynecological
Endocrinology
St. Anna's Gynecological Hospital
60 Spezia Avenue
10126 Turin, Italy

V. Mazza
Department of Obstetrics and
Gynecology
University of Modena
41100 Modena, Italy

N. Medici
Institute of General Pathology
I Medical School
University of Naples
S. Andrea delle Dame 2
80138 Naples, Italy

M. Messeni Leone
Department of Histology and
Embryology
University of Genoa
10 Marsano Street
16100 Genoa, Italy

S. Meyers
Department of Biochemistry
Wayne University School of
Medicine
540 Canfield
Detroit, Michigan 48201

A. M. Molinari
Institute of General Pathology
I Medical School
University of Naples
S. Andrea delle Dame 2
80138 Naples, Italy

A. Montemurro
Department of Obstetrics and
Gynecology
Catholic University
Largo Gemelli 8
00168 Rome, Italy

Rodrigue Mortel
The Milton S. Hershey Medical
Center
The Pennsylvania State University
Hershey, Pennsylvania 17033

B. Mozzanega
Obstetric and Gynecological Clinic
University of Padua
3 Giustiniani Street
35100 Padua, Italy

V. Natoli
Laboratory of Molecular
Endocrinology
Catholic University of San Cuore
00168 Rome, Italy

Usko Nieminen
Department of Obstetrics and
Gynecology
University of Helsinki
Helsinki, Finland

E. Nola
Institute of General Pathology
I Medical School
University of Naples
S. Andrea delle Dame
80138 Naples, Italy

T. Ojasoo
Roussel-Uclaf
35, Boulevard des Invalides
75007 Paris, France

C. Kent Osborne
Department of Medicine
Division of Oncology
University of Texas Health Science
Center
San Antonio, Texas 78284

B. A. Pack
Department of Biochemistry
Wayne University School of
Medicine
540 Canfield
Detroit, Michigan 48201

William M. Pardridge
Division of Endocrinology and
Metabolism
Department of Medicine
University of California, Los
Angeles
Los Angeles, California 90024

E. Parlati
Department of Obstetrics and
  Gynecology
Catholic University
Largo Gemelli 8
00168 Rome. Italy

D. Paternoster
Obstetric and Gynecological Clinic
University of Padua
3 Giustiniani Street
35100 Padua, Italy

G. Pelusi
Department of Obstetrics and
  Gynecology
St. Orsola's General Hospital
University of Bologna
13 Massarenti Road
40138 Bologna, Italy

Kunhard Pollow
Department of Experimental
  Endocrinology
Johannes Gutenberg Universität
Langenbeckstrasse 1
6500 Mainz, Federal Republic of
  Germany

J. Poortman
Department of Endocrinology
University Hospital
State University Of Utrecht
101 Catharisnesingel
Utrecht, The Netherlands

Luisa Prelato Tousijn
Department of Gynecological
  Endocrinology
St. Anna's Gynecological Hospital
60 Spezia Avenue
10126 Turin, Italy

S. Preti
Department of Reproductive
  Pathophysiology
St. Orsola's General Hospital
University of Bologna
13 Massarenti Road
40138 Bologna, Italy

A. M. Previdi
Department of Obstetrics and
  Gynecology
University of Modena
41100 Modena, Italy

G. A. Puca
Institute of General Pathology
I Medical School
University of Naples
S. Andrea delle Dame 2
80138 Naples, Italy

Clemente Pullè
Department of Obstetrics and
  Gynecology
University of Messina
98100 Messina, Italy

Silvia Racca
Institute of Pharmacology
Faculty of Medicine
University of Turin
30 Raffaello Avenue
10125 Turin, Italy

J. P. Raynaud
Roussel-Uclaf
35, Boulevard des Invalides
75007 Paris, France

Camilla Reboani
Institute of Pharmacology
Faculty of Medicine
University of Turin
30 Raffaello Avenue
10125 Turin, Italy

M. J. Reed
Department of Chemical Pathology
St. Mary's Hospital Medical School
London W2 1PG, England

N. A. Reiss
Department of Hormone Research
The Weizmann Institute of Science
Rehovot, 76100 Israel

George S. Richardson
Vincent Research Laboratory
Department of Gynecology
Massachussetts General Hospital;
  and
Department of Obstetrics and
  Surgery
Harvard Medical School
Boston, Massachussetts 02114

Antonio Rigano
Departments of Oncology and
  Obstetrics and Gynecology
University of Messina
98100 Messina, Italy

Paul Robel
INSERM U33 and CNRS ER 125
Lab Hormones
94270 Bicêtre, France

A. Ros
Department of Obstetrics and
 Gynecology
University of Padua, Verona
 Branch
"B. Roma" Clinical Center
37100 Verona, Italy

Gian Paolo Rossini
Department of Biological Chemistry
University of Modena
287 Campi Street
41100 Modena, Italy

N. Russo
Department of Obstetrics and
 Gynecology
Catholic University
Largo Gemelli 8
00168 Rome, Italy

Alessandra Sandzi
Department of Gynecological
 Endocrinology
St. Anna's Gynecological Hospital
60 Spezia Avenue
10126 Turin, Italy

G. Scambia
Laboratory of Molecular
 Endocrinology
Catholic University of San Cuore
00168 Rome, Italy

P. Scirpa
Department of Obstetrics and
 Gynecology
Catholic University
Largo Gemelli 8
00168 Rome, Italy

S. Scirpa
Department of Obstetrics and
 Gynecology
Catholic University
Largo Gemelli 8
00168 Rome, Italy

V. Sica
Institute of General Pathology
I Medical School
University of Naples
S. Andrea delle Dame 2
80138 Naples, Italy

Paul E. Sylvan
Vincent Research Laboratory
Department of Gynecology
Massachusetts General Hospital
Boston, Massachusetts 02114

G. Tanara
The National Center for Research
 on Cancer
University of Genoa
Benedetto XV Avenue
16100 Genoa, Italy

J. H. H. Thijssen
Department of Endocrinology
University Hospital
State University of Utrecht
101 Catharisnesingel
Utrecht, The Netherlands

A. Traina
Cancer Hospital Center "M.
 Ascoli"
Palermo, Italy

W. H. M. van der Velden
St. Josephziekenhuis
Eindhoven, The Netherlands

J. van der Vies
Scientific Development Group
Organon International B.V.
Oss, The Netherlands

A. Volpe
Department of Obstetrics and
 Gynecology
University of Modena
41100 Modena, Italy

M. I. Whitehead
Department of Obstetrics and
 Gynecology
King's College Hospital Medical
 School
Denmark Hill
London SE5 8RX, England

Steroids and Endometrial Cancer,
edited by V. M. Jasonni, et al.
Raven Press, New York © 1983.

Biochemistry and Biology of Estrogen Receptor: Identification of Cytoskeletal Binding Sites for Receptor in a Membrane Model

G. A. Puca, E. Nola, A. M. Molinari, N. Medici,
D. De Lucia, and V. Sica

*Institute of General Pathology, I Medical School, University of Naples,
80138 Naples, Italy*

Within the last few years, extensive data have been published indicating that steroid hormone receptors are associated with particulate fractions of target cells (11,14–20,31) and that the question of intracellular distribution of steroid receptors needs to be reevaluated (22,29,32).

The possible relationship of the soluble "cytosolic" estradiol receptor to complex membranous and cytoskeletal structures of the cell matrix was studied using a model erythrocyte system (26,27). Extraction of erythrocyte ghosts with a nonionic detergent (Triton X-100) under conditions that yield a cytoskeletal matrix reveals the presence of a limited number (fewer than 100) of specific sites having high affinity ($K_D = 10^{-9}$ M) for the estradiol receptor complex. Our data suggest that the estradiol receptor, which generally has been considered freely "soluble" in the cytoplasm, actually may be associated physiologically in an integral manner with a complex cytoskeletal network in the cell cytoplasm.

This chapter provides further information on the estradiol receptor–cytoskeleton interaction, the effect of pretreatment with various enzymes of either the cytoskeleton or the receptor, and the inhibition by specific glycosaminoglycans and nucleic acids of the interaction.

EXPERIMENTAL PROCEDURES

All reagents were of analytical grade: 17 β-estradiol-2,4,6,7,-t_4 (84–110 Ci/mmole) was from Amersham. *Flavobacterium heparinum* crude heparinase (proteolytic activity less than 1 μg papain/mg of protein, specific activity: 1 μl hydrolyzes 10 μg heparin in 30 min at 37°C), dermatan sulfate, hyaluronic acid, and heparan sulfate were generous gifts of Dr. V. Chiarugi, Institute of General Pathology, University of Florence, Italy. Cow blood erythrocyte ghosts and cytoskeletons were prepared as described by Bennet and Branton (4); these were resuspended with phosphate buffer at a protein concentration of 3 to 10 mg/ml, diluted 1:1 (vol/vol) with 99% glycerol and stored at $-70°C$ until used. Calf uterine cytosol was prepared as previously described (24), except that only phosphate buffer (7.5 mM phosphate buffer, pH 7.5) instead of Tris-HCl ethylenediaminetetraacetate (EDTA) and dithiothreitol buffer was used. The assay of specific binding activity of cytosol was performed by the dextran-coated charcoal method (28). The binding of the ^{3}H-estradiol receptor complex to erythrocyte ghosts and cytoskeletons was performed in duplicate. Calf uterine cytosol was preincubated for 10 min at 20°C in a total volume of 0.4 ml phosphate buffer with 2.5 pmoles ^{3}H-estradiol, 12.5 μmoles KCl, and 1.25 μmoles MgCl$_2$. The reaction was started by addition of 0.1 ml cytoskeleton or ghost suspension (0.25 to 2 mg protein) and followed either for 2 hr at 20°C or for 30 min at 30°C. Parallel tests were performed in the presence of 1×10^{-6} M unlabeled estradiol. The reaction was stopped by addition of 10 ml ice-cold phosphate buffer. Samples were centrifuged at $30,000 \times g$ for 20 min at 4°C, and the pellets were washed three times. The final pellet was resuspended with 1 ml phosphate buffer and assayed for radioactivity. The values obtained in the presence of unlabeled hormone were subtracted from the total. Calf uterine cytosol was prepared free of estrogen receptor by adsorption of estradiol receptor on 17-hemisuccinil-17 β-estradiol-ovalbumin-Sepharose 4B prepared as described elsewhere; other methods and procedures were as previously described (23–27).

RESULTS

Erythrocyte ghosts display binding sites for the native 8S estradiol receptor only when most of the lipid bilayer and many of the proteins are removed by the nonionic detergent Triton X-100 (27). The inability of the intact erythrocyte ghosts to bind the estradiol receptor may be due to an internal localization of the binding sites or to their occupancy by other molecules that can be removed by detergent. To distinguish between these two possibilities, erythrocyte ghosts were subjected to other extraction procedures. Treatment of ghosts with high ionic strength (1 M KCl), chaotropic salt (NaSCN, 0.5 M), acetic acid (0.1 M), sodium hydroxide (0.05 M), and EDTA (5 mM) are procedures known to remove nonintegral proteins of the membrane (30) and expose binding sites for the estradiol receptor. Further, incubation at low ionic strength for 60 min at 30°C, which removes most of actin and spectrin (13), also increases the binding. Inside-out vesicles obtained from spectrin- and actin-depleted ghosts also bind estradiol receptor. In all these cases, however, binding is always lower than with shells (cytoskeletons) obtained by detergent extraction.

The receptor's affinity for estradiol does not change when it is bound to cytoskeleton (26), whereas the affinity of the receptor for the cytoskeleton is improved consistently by the presence of the hormone. In the experiment reported (Fig. 1), the affinity increased at least five-fold. In other experiments, Scatchard plots demonstrate only low-affinity unsaturable binding sites in the absence of estradiol.

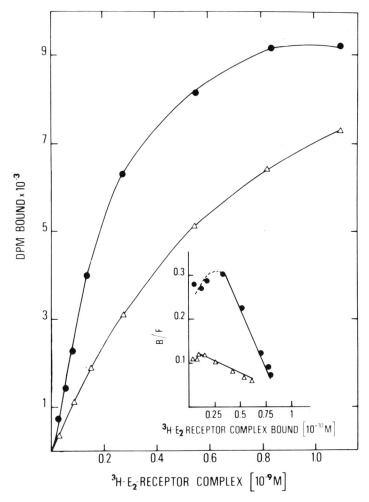

FIG. 1. Binding of estradiol receptor to erythrocyte cytoskeleton in presence and absence of estradiol. Erythrocyte cytoskeleton was incubated with various amounts (5–200 μl) of calf uterine cytosol in presence (●) or absence (△) of 5×10^{-9} M[^{3}H]estradiol. At the end of the incubation, the reaction was stopped by addition of 10 ml ice-cold phosphate buffer. Samples were centrifuged (20 min, 4°C, 30,000 × g) and pellets were washed with 10 ml buffer. After centrifugation (20 min, 4°C, 30,000 × g), erythrocyte cytoskeleton was resuspended in a total volume of 0.5 ml of phosphate buffer, 25 mM KCl, 2.5 mM MgCl$_2$, 5×10^{-9} M estradiol and incubated overnight (16 hr) at 4°C. The reaction was stopped by addition of 10 ml buffer, and erythrocyte cytoskeleton was washed by centrifugation three times. The final pellets were resuspended with 1 ml buffer and radioactivity measured as described. Parallel tests were performed in the presence of 1×10^{-6}M cold estradiol. **Inset:** Data plotted according to Scatchard.

The saturability of the interaction between receptor and cytoskeleton is observed even when partially purified estradiol receptor is used (26) and when the cytosol protein concentration is kept constant by addition of different amounts of estradiol receptor-free uterine cytosol (Fig. 2).

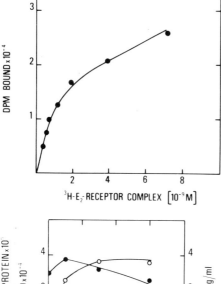

FIG. 2. Binding of estradiol–receptor complex to erythrocyte cytoskeleton as a function of estradiol–receptor complex in presence of the same protein concentration. The indicated concentration of estradiol–receptor complex was incubated with 0.1 ml erythrocyte cytoskeleton in the presence of different amounts of receptor-free calf uterine cytosol in order to maintain the same protein concentration. Bound estradiol–receptor complex was assessed as described in the legend to Fig. 1.

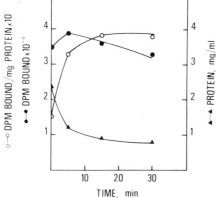

FIG. 3. Effect of mild tryptic digestion of erythrocyte cytoskeleton on estradiol–receptor complex binding. Aliquots of cytoskeleton were incubated at 0°C with 10 μg/ml trypsin. At the indicated time, samples were diluted with phosphate buffer and centrifuged at 39,000 × g. Pellets were washed twice by centrifugation and then resuspended in 0.5 ml phosphate buffer. Aliquots (0.1 ml) of cytoskeleton were incubated with 0.2 ml calf uterine cytosol. Protein concentration (▲); estradiol–receptor complex bound (●); estradiol–receptor complex bound per mg of protein (○).

Limited proteolysis of the estradiol receptor by trypsin or receptor transforming factor (RTF) (25) affects the capacity of the receptor to bind the cytoskeleton (26,27). Further, treatment of cytosol with other enzymes, such as ribonuclease (RNase), deoxyribonuclease (DNase) I, neuraminidase, hyaluronidase, heparinase, or chondroitinase ABC has no effect.

Treatment of erythrocyte cytoskeleton with phospholipase A_2, phospholipase C, chondroitinase ABC, α- and β-glucosidase, β-glucuronidase, α-galactosidase, neuraminidase, dextranase, RNase, DNases I and II, or heparinase has no effect on the estradiol receptor binding to cytoskeleton. On the other hand, an increase in the total binding is observed when cytoskeleton is partially digested with proteases. Figure 3 illustrates the time course at 0° of the effect of the digestion of cytoskeleton by 20 μg of trypsin/ml. Total binding increases slightly after 5 min, but then declines. Protein content drops rapidly and, consequently, specific activity increases. Pronase and papain have similar effects. When digestion of skeletons is continued for long periods, the estradiol receptor binding activity disappears, and cytoskeleton disassembles.

A large number of simple sugars and saccharide compounds were screened for their capacity to inhibit the binding of estradiol receptor to erythrocyte cytoskeletons. None of the following sugars at 5 mM concentration had an effect on the binding: p-aminophenyl-1-thio-β-D-galactopyranoside, p-aminophenyl-β-D-galactopyrano- side, methyl-β-D-thiogalactoside, D(+)raffinose,p-aminophenyl-α-L-glucopyrano- side, O-aminophenyl-β-D-glucuronide, 3-O-methyl-α-D-glucopyranoside, isopropyl- β-D-thiogalactopyranoside, 1-O-methyl-β-D-glucopyranoside, 1-O-methyl-β-D- galactopyranoside, 1-O-methyl-α-D-galactopyranoside, 1-O-methyl-α-D-glucopyr- anoside. Proteins such as albumin, ovalbumin, human immunoglobulin, concana- valin A, and wheat germ agglutinin up to 2 mg/ml have no effect. Gangliosides tested either as a mixture of bovine brain commercial gangliosides (up to 1 mg/ ml), as pure GM_1 gangliosides (up to 0.5 mg/ml), or as gangliosides extracted from erythrocyte skeleton (corresponding to 6 mg cytoskeleton protein) do not inhibit the interaction between the estradiol receptor and cytoskeleton.

It has been shown that the native form of the estradiol receptor interacts with high affinity with heparin but not with other glycosaminoglycans, such as hyaluronic acid and chondroitin sulfate (15). The similarity between estradiol receptor inter- actions with erythrocyte cytoskeleton and heparin suggested the investigation of the effect of glycosaminoglycans. Heparin and heparan sulfate inhibit the binding very strongly, whereas hyaluronic acid and chondroitin sulfate have no effect at a con- centration of 1 mg/ml. Heparin affects mainly the high-affinity type of binding sites. In fact, saturation analysis of estradiol receptor interaction with the erythrocyte cytoskeleton in the presence of 100 μg/ml of heparin shows the selective disap- pearance of the high-affinity binding sites. When binding data obtained in the presence of heparin are subtracted from those obtained in its absence and plotted according to Scatchard, a single class of binding sites with high affinity is evident (Fig. 4). The inhibition of estradiol receptor binding to cytoskeleton when heparin is present in the medium is constant and does not reverse spontaneously. The heparin effect is due to this glycosaminoglycan's occupation of the receptor binding site for the erythrocyte cytoskeleton, as indicated by cytosol preincubation experiments. Pretreatment of cytosol with heparin (1 mg/ml) and dialysis through Sephadex G- 50 to eliminate the free heparin results in 50% inhibition in estradiol receptor binding to cytoskeleton. On the other hand, preincubation of erythrocyte cytoskeleton with heparin determines an increase of the binding. This enhancement of binding activity is due to incorporation in a saturable manner of heparin into cytoskeleton structures as indicated by the incorporation of [^{35}S]heparin in the erythrocyte cytoskeleton. This heparin incorporation, which parallels the enhancement of binding of estradiol receptor, is very similar to that observed with cholera toxin binding in erythrocytes by exogenous gangliosides (8).

RNA and DNA inhibit the binding of the estradiol receptor to erythrocyte cy- toskeletons. DNA is much more effective than RNA (Fig. 5).

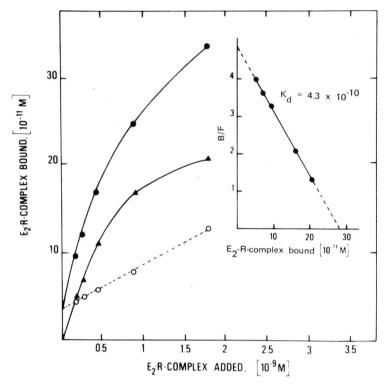

FIG. 4. Binding of estradiol–receptor complex to erythrocyte cytoskeleton in presence and absence of heparin. Erythrocyte cytoskeleton was incubated with the indicated concentration of estradiol-receptor complex in the presence (○) and in the absence (●) of 100 μg of heparin. (▲): Difference between data obtained in the presence of heparin from those obtained in the absence of heparin. **Inset:** Data plotted according to Scatchard.

The observation that heparin, RNA, and DNA inhibit the interaction of the estradiol receptor to erythrocyte cytoskeleton suggested the possibility that addition of these substances to the medium might be capable of reversing the binding. Figure 6 illustrates that among the substances used, heparin is the most effective in dissociating the receptor–cytoskeleton complex. Chondroitin sulfate, which does not inhibit the receptor-cytoskeleton interaction, has no effect. DNA and RNA, which are able to inhibit the receptor–cytoskeleton interaction, have a limited effect. The heparin-eluted cytoskeletal bound radioactivity, analyzed on linear sucrose gradient in low and high ionic strength, shows the same sedimentation as the native cytosol receptor (23).

Attempts to solubilize the cytoskeletal binding site for the estradiol receptor were partially unsuccessful. These attempts included: (a) low-salt incubation of ghosts and cytoskeletons; (b) cytoskeleton disassembly in 4 M guanidine-HCl; (c) EDTA, acetic acid, $HClO_4$, and sodium hydroxide extraction; (d) sonication. In all cases,

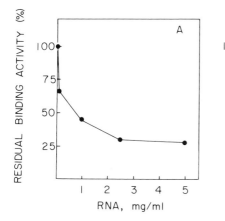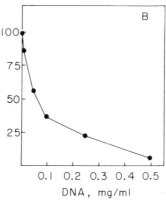

FIG. 5. Effect of nucleic acids on the binding of estradiol–receptor complex to erythrocyte cytoskeleton. Erythrocyte cytoskeleton was incubated for 30 min at 30°C with 0.2 ml of calf uterine cytosol in the presence of the indicated concentration of RNA **(A)** and DNA **(B)**.

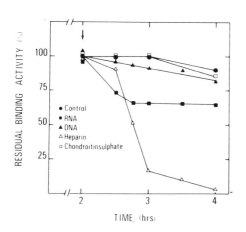

FIG. 6. Effect of DNA, RNA, heparin, and chondroitin sulfate on the dissociation of the estradiol–receptor complex from erythrocyte cytoskeleton. Aliquots of erythrocyte cytoskeleton were incubated 2 hr at 20°C with 2 ml calf uterine cytosol in a total volume of 5 ml phosphate buffer containing 2.5 mM MgCl₂ and 25 mM KCl. At the end of the incubation, samples were centrifuged, washed three times with the same buffer, and resuspended at a final volume of 1 ml. Heparin (1 mg/ml final concentration), chondroitin sulfate (1 mg/ml final concentration), RNA (10 mg/ml final concentration), DNA (0.5 mg/ml final concentration) were added to the samples and the incubation was continued at 20°C. At the indicated time periods, aliquots of the incubation mixture were withdrawn, centrifuged (15 min, 4°C, 38,000 × g), washed with phosphate buffer, and assessed for residual estradiol–receptor complex bound.

the solubilized material was either minimally or not at all effective in the inhibition of the estradiol receptor–cytoskeleton interaction.

DISCUSSION

The inability of erythrocyte ghosts to bind the estradiol receptor does not seem due to the localization of estradiol receptor binding sites on the internal side of the membrane, but is most probably due to their steric inaccessibility. Removal of the lipid bilayer and proteins by Triton X-100, as well as removal of proteins with EDTA, acetic acid, KCl, or heating in hypotonic buffer causes an increase of the number of the binding sites.

Analysis of the receptor–cytoskeleton interaction reveals the presence of a limited number of high-affinity binding sites. The consequent saturability clearly distinguishes this *in vitro* system from that described by Clark and Gorski, which is linearly related to the concentrations of uterine cytoplasmic fraction (6). Further, experiments in which protein concentration is kept constant with receptor-free cytosol (Fig. 2) indicate that the observed high affinity of the interaction is not an artefact consequent to the increase of some cytosol component, as described by Chamness et al. (5) for other systems.

The affinity of the estradiol receptor for the erythrocyte cytoskeleton is increased by the presence of estradiol. This fact may be of great importance in explaining why in target cells the receptor estradiol complex formed after hormone administration is found in a nonsoluble form. Only the "native" form of the estradiol receptor binds to cytoskeleton. When the receptor is partially hydrolyzed either by the Ca^{2+}-dependent RTF or by mild tryptic digestion, the binding disappears (26). On the other hand, the treatment of receptor with nucleases, neuraminidase, heparinase, hyaluronidase, or chondroitinase ABC does not influence its subsequent binding of cytoskeleton. Therefore, the receptor domain for the binding to the cytoskeleton appears to be proteinaceous.

The investigation of the nature of the erythrocyte cytoskeleton binding site for estrogen receptor has been approached either by treating erythrocyte cytoskeleton with various enzymes or by studying the effect of the addition of various compounds on the estradiol receptor–cytoskeleton interaction. Among the various enzymes used, the only ones affecting the binding were proteases. Mild proteolytic digestion caused an increase of the binding. This enhancement resembles the increase of binding to erythrocyte ghosts when proteins are removed with different methods. Otherwise, the lack of inhibition of the binding after mild proteolytic treatment, together with the reported (26) very low number of sites, rules out the participation of the major accessible proteins of the erythrocyte cytoskeleton in the binding of estradiol receptor. However, this does not exclude the proteinaceous nature of this binding. The susceptible bonds can be masked by phospholipids or other compounds not removed by Triton X-100 (7,9). Another possibility is that the erythrocyte binding sites are proteins highly resistant to protease treatment, as described by Bennet (3) for periodic acid-Schiff (PAS)-positive proteins of erythrocyte inside-out vesicles. Extensive proteolytic digestion of cytoskeleton dissolves this structure and makes measurement of the binding by the centrifugation assay method impossible. Therefore, the results of the enzymatic digestion of the cytoskeleton do not provide an answer to the question of the nature of the erythrocyte cytoskeleton binding sites for estrogen receptor.

Several compounds have been tested for their capacity to affect the binding of the estradiol-receptor complex to the erythrocyte cytoskeleton. Only glycosaminoglycans and nucleic acids demonstrate competition for binding. Glycosaminoglycans can be ruled out as cytoskeleton binding sites for the estradiol receptor, mainly because heparinase treatment of cytoskeleton has no effect, and no glycosaminoglycans are found in erythrocyte cytoskeleton. Further, solubilization experiments with guanidine-HCl and sodium hydroxide indicate a great instability of the cytoskeleton site, although glycosaminoglycans are very resistant to strong denaturating conditions.

The possibility that nucleic acids are the cytoskeleton binding site for the estradiol receptor cannot be excluded. DNA and RNA, both able to bind the estradiol receptor (12,33), have been found to be associated with membranes (10) in a way resistant to a variety of conditions, including treatment with detergents, chelating agents, and high and low salt concentrations (9). The lack of susceptibility to nuclease degradation might be due to the close association with the membranes, or, in the case of RNA, to the double-stranded structure.

CONCLUSIONS

Findings presented in this chapter are consistent with the presence of specific binding sites for the estrogen receptors in the cytoskeletal matrix of the erythrocyte membrane. Similar systems do exist in target cells (Sica et al., *in preparation*), which could in part explain data apparently contradicting the general model of action of steroid hormones (2,18,19,31). The water-soluble nature of the estradiol receptor found in cytosol might be an artefact of tissue homogenization and preparation, as recently demonstrated by Pietras and Szego (21,22), and the membrane receptor described by Parikh et al. (19) and by others (1,18) might be that fraction of receptor that has not been released during the cell fractionation.

ACKNOWLEDGMENTS

The authors thank Dr. Pedro Cuatrecasas for his continuous encouragement and critical suggestions and Dr. Marvin Siegel for the revision of the manuscript. This work was supported by the Progetto Finalizzato: "Controllo della Crescita Neoplastica," by a grant from the Wellcome Research Laboratories, Research Triangle Park, North Carolina and the National Institute of Health Contract NO1-CB-64074.

REFERENCES

1. Barrack, E. R., and Coffey, D. S. (1980): The specific binding of estrogens and androgens to the nuclear matrix of sex hormone responsive tissues. *J. Biol. Chem.*, 255:7265–7275.
2. Baulieu, E. E., Godeau, F., Schorderet, M., and Schorderet-Slatkine, S. (1978): Steroid-induced meiotic division in *Xenopus laevis* oocytes: Surface and calcium. *Nature (Lond.)*, 275:593–598.
3. Bennet, V. (1978): Purification of an active proteolytic fragment of the membrane attachment site for human erythrocyte spectrin. *J. Biol. Chem.*, 253:2292–2299.
4. Bennett, V., and Branton, D. (1977): Selective association of spectrin with cytoplasmic surface of human erythrocyte plasma membranes. *J. Biol. Chem.*, 252:2753–2763.
5. Chamness, G. C., Jennings, A. W., and McGuire, W. L. (1974): Estrogen receptor binding to isolated nuclei. A nonsaturable process. *Biochemistry*, 13:327–333.
6. Clark, J. H., and Gorski, J. (1969): Estrogen-receptors: An evolution of cytoplasmic nuclear interactions in a cell free system and a method for assay. *Biochim. Biophys. Acta*, 192:508–515.
7. Cooper, M. B., Craft, J. A., Estall, M. R., and Robin, B. R. (1980): Asymmetric distribution of cytochrome P-450 and NADPH-cytochrome P-450 (cytochrome c) reductase in vescicles from smooth endoplasmic reticulum of rat liver. *Biochemistry*, 190:737–746.
8. Cuatrecasas, P. (1973): Gangliosides and membrane receptors for cholera toxin. *Biochemistry*, 12:3558–3566.

9. Franke, W. W. (1974): Structure, biochemistry and function of the nuclear envelope. *Int. Rev. Cytol. (Suppl.)*, 4:71–236.
10. Herman, R., Zieve, G., Williams, J., Leuk, R., and Penman, S. (1976): Cellular skeletons and RNA messangers. *Prog. Nucleic Acid Res. Mol. Biol.*, 19:379–401.
11. Jackson, V., and Chalkley, R. (1974): The binding of estradiol 17β to the bovine endometrial nuclear membrane. *J. Biol. Chem.*, 249:1615–1626.
12. Liao, S., Smythe, S., Tymoczko, J. L., Rossini, G. P., Chen, C., and Hiipakka, R. A. (1980): RNA-dependent release of androgen and other steroid–receptor complexes from DNA. *J. Biol. Chem.*, 255:5545–5551.
13. Marchesi, V. T. (1979): Functional proteins of the human red blood cell membrane. *Semin. Hematol.*, 16:3–20.
14. Milgrom, E., Atger, N., and Baulieu, E. E. (1973): Studies on estrogen entry into uterine cells and an estradiol–receptor complex attachment to the nucleus. Is the entry of estrogen into uterine cells a protein mediated process? *Biochim. Biophys. Acta*, 320:267–283.
15. Molinari, A. M., Medici, N., Moncharmont, B., and Puca, G. A. (1977): Estradiol receptor of calf uterus: Interaction with heparin agarose and purification. *Proc. Natl. Acad. Sci. USA*, 74:4886–4890.
16. Munck, A., and Brinck-Johnson, T. (1968): Specific and nonspecific physiochemical interactions of glucocorticoids and related steroids with rat thymus cells *in vitro*. *J. Biol. Chem.*, 243:5556–5565.
17. Nenci, I., Fabris, G., Marchetti, E., and Mazzola, A. (1980): Intracellular flow of particulate steroid-receptor complexes in steroid target cells. *Virchows Arch. [Cell Pathol.]*, 32:139–145.
18. Noteboon, W. D., and Gorski, J. (1965): Stereospecific binding of estrogens in the rat uterus. *Arch. Biochem. Biophys.*, 111:559–568.
19. Parikh, I., Lee Anderson, W., and Neame, P. (1980): Identification of high affinity estrogen binding sites in calf uterine microsomial membranes. *J. Biol. Chem.*, 255:10266–10270.
20. Pietras, R. J., and Szego, C. N. (1977): Specific binding sites for oestrogen at the outer surfaces of isolated endometrial cells. *Nature (Lond.)*, 265:69–72.
21. Pietras, R. J., and Szego, C. N. (1979): Estrogen receptors in uterine plasma membrane. *J. Steroid Biochem.*, 11:1471–1483.
22. Pietras, R. J., and Szego, C. N. (1980): Partial purification and characterization of estrogen receptors in subfractions of hepatocyte plasma membranes. *Biochem. J.*, 191:743–760.
23. Puca, G. A., Nola, E., Sica, V., and Bresciani, F. (1971): Estrogen binding proteins of calf uterus. Partial purification and preliminary characterization of two cytoplasmic proteins. *Biochemistry*, 10:3769–3780.
24. Puca, G. A., Nola, E., Sica, V., and Bresciani, F. (1972): Estrogen binding proteins of calf uterus. Interrelationship between various forms and identification of a Receptor Transforming Factor. *Biochemistry*, 11:4157–4165.
25. Puca, G. A., Nola, E., Sica, V., and Bresciani, F. (1977): Estrogen binding proteins of calf uterus. Molecular and functional characterization of the Receptor Transforming Factor: a Ca⁺⁺ activated protease. *J. Biol. Chem.*, 252:1358–1366.
26. Puca, G. A., Nola, E., Molinari, A. M., Armetta, I., and Sica, V. (1981): Interaction of calf uterus estradiol receptor with erythrocyte cytoskeleton. *J. Steroid Biochem.*, 15:307–312.
27. Puca, G. A., and Sica, V. (1981): Identification of specific high affinity sites for the estradiol receptor in the erythrocyte cytoskeleton. *Biochem. Biophys. Res. Comm.*, 103:682–689.
28. Sanborn, B. M., Rao, R. B., and Koreman, S. G. (1971): Interaction of 17β-estradiol and its specific uterine receptor. Evidence for complex kinetic and equilibrium behavior. *Biochemistry*, 10:4955–4965.
29. Sheridan, P. J., Buchanan, J. M., Anselmo, V. C., and Martin, P. M. (1979): Equilibrium: the intracellular distribution of the steroid receptors. *Nature (Lond.)*, 282:579–582.
30. Steck, T. L. (1974): The organization of proteins in the human red blood cell membrane. *J. Cell. Biol.*, 62:1–19.
31. Suyemitsu, T., and Terayama, H. (1975): Specific binding sites for natural glucocorticoids in plasma membranes of rats liver. *Endocrinology*, 96:1499–1508.
32. Szego, C. M., and Pietras, R. J. (1981): Membrane recognition and effector sites in steroid hormone action. *Biochem. Actions Horm.*, 8:307–463.
33. Yamamoto, K. R., and Alberts, B. M. (1972): *In vitro* conversion of estradiol receptor protein to its nuclear form: Dependence on hormone and DNA. *Proc. Natl. Acad. Sci. USA*, 69:2105–2110.

Steroids and Endometrial Cancer,
edited by V. M. Jasonni, et al.
Raven Press, New York © 1983.

Receptor Binding Profiles of Progestins

T. Ojasoo and J. P. Raynaud

Roussel-Uclaf, 75007 Paris, France

Renewed interest in synthetic progestins for sequential therapy of hormone-dependent cancers (e.g., endometrial cancer) has been generated primarily because of their antiestrogenic potency. However, the chemical substitutions that engender resistance to inactivation by liver and gastrointestinal enzymes, and thereby confer oral activity, also modify interactions with steroid receptor binding sites. Many progestins can bind to receptors other than the progesterone receptor and give rise to secondary effects such as androgenic and/or glucocorticoid activity. It is therefore necessary, when choosing a progestin for therapy, to inspect its biochemical and pharmacological profile. In this chapter, we report the rationale of a routine screening system for determining the receptor binding profiles of steroids and describe the results obtained for a few selected progestins.

STEROID-RECEPTOR COUPLING

According to X-ray crystallography studies, many steroids are flexible molecules whose functional groups can span a considerable area (16,33,47) and therefore presumably come into contact with one or more binding sites on receptor proteins. The snugness of fit between receptor and protein will depend on steric hindrance from neighboring substituents, van der Waals interactions, etc. The receptor protein, which also has some flexibility, can adjust to accommodate different steroids.

Because many synthetic steroids show affinity for the binding sites of several classes of endogenous hormone (progestin, androgen, glucocorticoid, mineralocorticoid) (16,37,49), it is tempting to deduce that there is a close similarity among these binding sites. For instance, RU 2999 (17β-hydroxy-17α-methyl-2-oxa-estra-4,9,11-trien-3-one), with four identified crystalline conformations (Fig. 1), has on incubation with cytosol for 2 hr at 0°C a relative binding affinity (RBA) of 260 for the progestin receptor in rabbit uterus (compared with 100 for progesterone) and an RBA of 160 for the androgen receptor in rat prostate (compared with 100 for testosterone). It also interacts, although much less markedly and with lower stability (see below), with the mineralocorticoid and glucocorticoid receptors, but it does not interact with the estrogen receptor. In pharmacology tests, RU 2999 is a potent androgen, 10 times more active subcutaneously than testosterone in increasing castrated rat prostate weight (3,29,48), and a progestin that induces a significant endometrial response in the estrogen-primed rabbit at a daily oral dose of 10 to 50

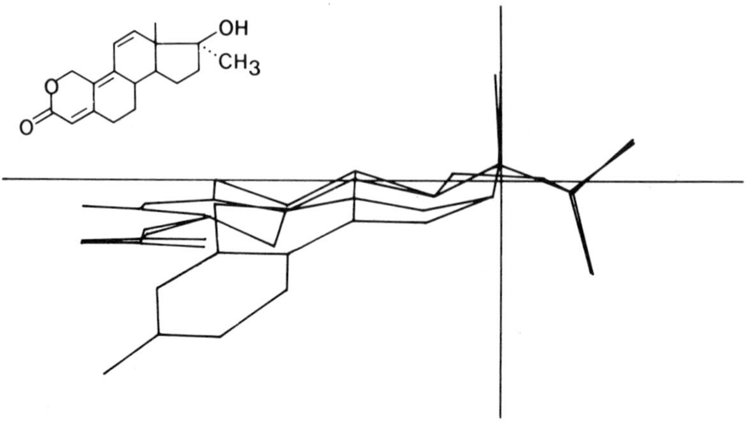

FIG. 1. Conformations of RU 2999 in the crystal. Superimposition of crystalline conformations using a D-ring reference system (16,33). (J. P. Mornon, *personal communication.*)

μg. It has virtually no glucocorticoid activity on tyrosine aminotransferase (TAT) induction in hepatoma tissue cells (HTC) in culture but can counteract the action of a glucocorticoid (45,48,50). Thus, routine binding studies suggest and biological activity tests confirm that RU 2999 can be termed an androgen, a progestin, or an antiglucocorticoid. Together with similar evidence on a large number of steroids (16,37,49), this suggests that the receptor binding sites of the endogenous 3-keto-Δ 4 steroids possess common features (47). Several studies have already confirmed similarities among the receptor proteins (58). For instance, three classes of steroid hormones have been shown to form remarkably similar, large, asymmetric complexes in buffers containing molybdate and KCl (36). On the other hand, evidence of binding of an antibody against a highly purified preparation of glucocorticoid receptor from rat liver to the androgen, estrogen, or progestin receptors was not seen (38).

ROUTINE SCREENING SYSTEM

To determine the receptor binding profile of a steroid, we currently measure its interaction with five hormone receptors (estrogen, progestin, androgen, mineralocorticoid, and glucocorticoid) (37,49; Table 2). The system is based on competition between the steroid and the natural hormone labeled with high specific activity (or of a radiolabeled highly potent synthetic analog) for binding to the receptor during incubation with high-speed supernatant (cytosol) from target organ homogenates from the species routinely used to assess biological activity. For example, competition for the progestin receptor is measured against the binding of a highly potent labeled progestin (promegestone, RU 5020) (41) in uterine cytosol from estrogen-primed rabbits, as progestomimetic activity is often estimated by the endometrial proliferation induced in the rabbit. Further, labeled RU 5020 is stable during incubation and does not bind to any contaminating plasma proteins in the cytosol

(39,51). Binding profiles have been determined in this way for over 1,000 steroids (37,49).

KINETICS OF THE RECEPTOR INTERACTION

Under standardized routine screening conditions *in vitro*, the kinetic stabilities of complexes formed between a given steroid and the receptor binding sites of different hormone classes vary. *In vivo*, kinetic stabilities may be further influenced by factors such as cell type, medium, etc. The stability of the complexes can be assessed *in vitro* by measurement of their rates of association and dissociation as illustrated in Fig. 2 for the potent androgen RU 1881 (metribolone, methyltrieno-lone, 17β-hydroxy-17α-methyl-estra-4,9,11-trien-3-one) (i.e., RU 2999 without the oxygen atom in ring A). The rates were measured on rat prostate cytosol, which contains neither detectable progestin receptor to which RU 1881 can bind (49) nor contaminating sex steroid binding protein (SBP), to which RU 1881 binds only minimally (7,51). RU 1881 associates with the androgen receptor at about the same rate as testosterone ($k_{+1} = 4.2 \times 10^4 M^{-1} sec^{-1}$ and $5 \times 10^4 M^{-1} sec^{-1}$, respectively, at 0°C), but the RU 1881 complex dissociates far slower than the testosterone complex ($t_{1/2} = 5$ hr and 2 hr at 15°C).

Radiolabeled compound for the measurement of rate constants is not always available. It is now generally accepted that the kinetic stability of a steroid–receptor complex can be evaluated by following the evolution of RBAs with increasing incubation time. The more slowly the complex dissociates in comparison with the rate of dissociation of the endogenous hormone, the greater the increase in RBA (2,8,42,53). This has been demonstrated for several steroid estrogens (44), glu-cocorticoids (59,64), and androgens (43,45). Thus, the RBA of RU 1881 increases with incubation time when measured against labeled testosterone (unpublished observation), confirming the slower dissociation rate observed in Fig. 2. The competition of a series of steroids and nonsteroids known to interfere with androgen receptor binding versus labeled RU 1881 shows important variations in RBA on increasing incubation time (Fig. 3). In the case of RU 1881 itself, the concentration that inhibits binding by 50% (IC_{50}) at 5 min is about twice that recorded between 15 min and 2 hr, probably because, at 5 min, association is still the predominant event; all binding sites present in the cytosol are not necessarily yet occupied by labeled RU 1881. At later times, the influence of the rate of dissociation is over-riding. With respect to RU 1881, the competitors cyproterone acetate and RU 2956 (the 2-gem dimethyl derivative of RU 1881) have IC_{50}s that vary little between 5 min and 30 min incubation, but at 2 hr a noticeable increase is recorded. The flutamide curve with an IC_{50} of about 50 nM at 5 min moves systematically to the right with increasing incubation time, crossing the IC_{50} axis at 10 μM after 15 min and well beyond this concentration after longer incubation times. The competition curves for hydroxyflutamide (reputedly the active metabolite of flutamide) and RU 23908 show similar behavior moving toward the right but according to slightly different time schedules. This difference may not be significant, as Fig. 3 represents

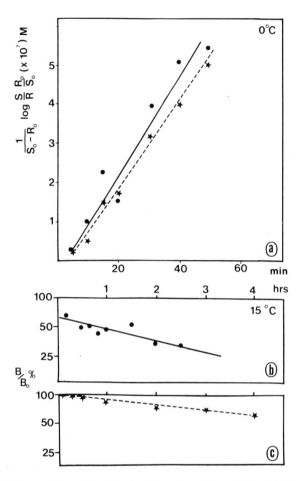

FIG. 2. Association and dissociation kinetics. The rates of association (**a**) of testosterone (●) and RU 1881 (★) with the androgen receptor were measured by incubating 5 nM tritiated substance with cytosol from castrated rat prostate for 5 to 60 min at 0°C. The dissociation rates (**b** and **c**) of the androgen receptor complexes were measured by incubating 25 nM of radioligand with cytosol for 14 hr at 0°C, then adding 2,500 nM cold steroid and incubating at 15°C. Bound steroid was measured in each case by a DCC adsorption technique.

the results of a single experiment that compares the relative effects of the six test compounds simultaneously and therefore could not include more than two or three competing concentrations per substance. However, these results have been fully confirmed at two incubation times (30 min and 24 hr) using six-point competition curves (43). The mean RBAs deduced from these curves and others are given in

FIG. 3. Time-dependence of competition. Two or three concentrations of unlabeled steroid were allowed to compete with [³H]RU 1881 for binding to castrated rat prostate cytosol incubated at 15°C for the indicated times. The bound fraction was separated by a DCC adsorption technique. All determinations were performed in the same experiment.

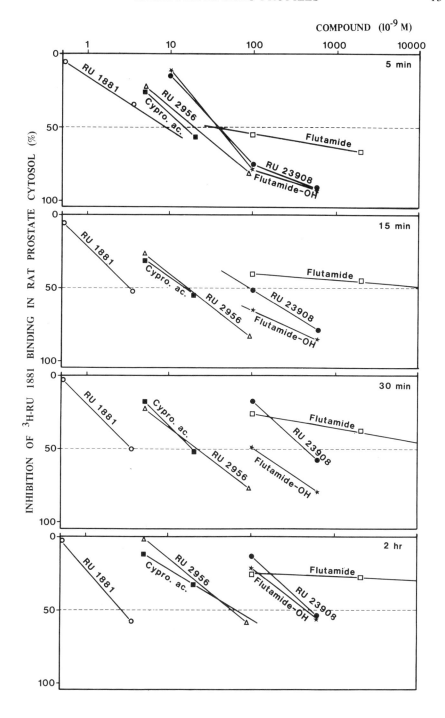

TABLE 1. *Relative binding affinities for the cytosol androgen receptor in rat prostate in a routine screening system*[a]

	30 min, 0°C	2 hr, 0°C	24 hr, 0°C
RU 1881	160	205	295
5α-Dihydrotestosterone	95	120	180
Testosterone	100	100	100
RU 2956	55	15	3.5
Cyproterone acetate	50	15	5.5
Hydroxyflutamide	8	1	0.2
RU 23908	9	1	0.4

[a]See footnote to Table 2 for methodology. Competition was measured versus labeled RU 1881 but expressed in relation to testosterone (RBA = 100) by performing a rule of three.

Table 1 and clearly show an increase with incubation time for RU 1881 and 5α-dihydrotestosterone (5α-DHT), which are both potent androgens (3,4,37,60) and a decrease for the remaining four compounds which can all antagonize the effects of androgens (35,43,45). The rapid dissociation of these compounds from the receptor could contribute toward their antihormonal activity. If they transiently occupy available binding sites without inducing a full response, the endogenous hormone will have difficulty in gaining adequate access to these sites and a decrease in the expected action will ensue (5,15,42,46).

INFLUENCE OF *IN VITRO* DEGRADATION

The above experiments were performed on cytosol that contains no contaminating specific plasma binder (SBP) and no interfering receptor (progestin receptor), but the possibility of metabolic degradation also has to be envisaged. Because the trienic structure of RU 1881 renders it relatively resistant to degradation, it is a good marker for the androgen receptor (51). Testosterone also undergoes little degradation in rat prostate cytosol, but 5α-DHT is readily converted to androstanediols (7,51). Possible interference by metabolism is illustrated in Fig. 4, which shows correlations among the RBAs of 44 test substances for the dexamethasone-labeled glucocorticoid receptor in rat HTC, thymus, and liver cytosols. There is an excellent correlation between RBAs in cytosols from HTC cells and thymus after 4 hr and 24 hr incubation at 0°C (Fig. 4a and b) indicating either that there is little degradation under these conditions or that any degradation that may occur is strikingly similar in both systems. On the other hand, the wide scatter of points in Fig. 4c and d suggests that many of the test substances undergo extensive degradation by the liver (40) and/or interact with more than one binding protein (18). Any comparison of RBA values obtained in this organ must therefore be treated with the greatest circumspection and presumed kinetic effects deduced from decreasing RBA values with increasing incubation time may just reflect the rate of conversion of the test substance to low-affinity degradation products.

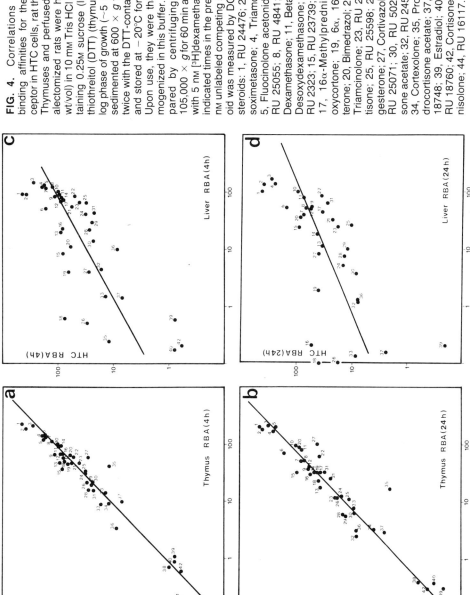

FIG. 4. Correlations between relative binding affinities for the glucocorticoid receptor in HTC cells, rat thymus, and rat liver. Thymuses and perfused livers from adrenalectomized rats were homogenized (1/10, wt/vol) in 10 mm Tris HCl buffer (pH 7.4) containing 0.25m sucrose (livers) and 2 nm dithiothreitol (DTT) (thymus). HTC cells in the log phase of growth (~5 × 10⁵ cells/ml) were sedimented at 600 × *g* for 10 min, washed twice with the DTT-containing buffer, frozen, and stored at −20°C for less than 15 days. Upon use, they were thawed and then homogenized in this buffer. Cytosols were prepared by centrifuging homogenates at 105,000 × *g* for 60 min at 4°C and incubated with 5 nm [³H]dexamethasone at 0°C for the indicated times in the presence of 0 to 2,500 nm unlabeled competing steroid. Bound steroid was measured by DCC adsorption. Test steroids: 1, RU 24476; 2, RU 25113; 3, Desoximetasone; 4, Triamcinolone acetonide; 5, Fluocinolone acetonide; 6, RU 25253; 7, RU 25055; 8, RU 4841; 9, RU 25593; 10, Dexamethasone; 11, Betamethasone; 12, 21-Desoxydexamethasone; 13, RU 25340; 14, RU 2323; 15, RU 23739; 16, Corticosterone; 17, 16α-Methylprednisolone; 18, Desoxycortone; 19, 6α, 16α-Dimethyl-progesterone; 20, Bimedrazol; 21, Prednisolone; 22, Triamcinolone; 23, RU 2999; 24, Hydrocortisone; 25, RU 25598; 26, 16α-Methyl progesterone; 27, Cortivazol; 28, RU 23747; 29, RU 25071; 30, RU 5020; 31, Dexamethasone acetate; 32, RU 2453; 33, Aldosterone; 34, Cortexolone; 35, Progesterone; 36, Hydrocortisone acetate; 37, RU 22779; 38, RU 18748; 39, Estradiol; 40, Testosterone; 41, RU 18760; 42, Cortisone; 43, 1-Methyl prednisolone; 44, RU 16117.

IMPLICATIONS FOR BIOLOGICAL ACTIVITY

In a routine screening system, one needs to standardize the nature and concentration of radioactive ligand, the nature of the cytosol (species, organ, protein concentration), the incubation conditions, etc. (37,49). The screening system will thus indicate if a particular steroid can interact with a given receptor, as well as the stability of the interaction under a specific set of circumstances. From this, one can expect to deduce if a steroid with the same mechanism of action as the endogenous hormone is likely to act as a powerful or weak agonist, and if, by virtue of its partial agonist activity, it may not exert an antihormonal action. The final biological response will depend on its relative concentration at the target site compared with the endogenous hormone and on the number of available binding sites for each hormone class.

An attempt to correlate the biological response of several steroids with the kinetics of the steroid–receptor interaction is shown in Fig. 5. The parallelism in binding values obtained in HTC cells and thymus (Fig. 4) justified correlating a response recorded in HTC cells (TAT induction) with RBAs measured on thymus cytosol, especially in the same species (22). Further, HTC cells apparently lack 11β-hydroxylase and dehydrogenase metabolic activity (57). However, no allowance could be made for interference by a putative progestin receptor possibly present in thymus cytosol. The ratio of the RBAs of corticosterone measured at 1 hr and 24 hr was taken to be equal to 1 by definition. Regardless of extraneous factors influencing response in this system (e.g., binding of steroids to calf serum present in the cell cultures, continuous presence of added steroid failing to mimic pharmacodynamic conditions), compounds with an RBA ratio greater than 1, i.e., dissociating slowly from the receptor, were all well known for their glucocorticoid activity. All the remaining steroids with an RBA ratio of about 0.5, primarily progestins, had considerably lower inducing potential and were for the most part partial agonists/antagonists. No strict relationship between binding and response could be deduced within each group.

BINDING AND ACTIVITY OF A FEW SELECTED PROGESTINS

The RBAs of a few progestins for the progestin, androgen, and glucocorticoid receptors are given in Table 2. Most form stable high-affinity complexes with the progesterone receptor as indicated by high and increasing RBA values. Measurement of the dissociation rates of medroxyprogesterone acetate (MPA) and promegestone have confirmed that they dissociate more slowly from the rabbit uterus cytosol receptor than progesterone (21,39). A comparison of the capacity to induce endometrial proliferation in the estrogen-primed rabbit has shown that most are potent progestins (45,65). The compound with both the lowest RBA and activity (gestrinone) is an impeded progestin and can in certain circumstances counteract the effects of progesterone (56).

Four of the progestins listed in Table 2 are able to form stable complexes with the androgen receptor: norgestrel, RU 2999, MPA, and gestrinone. As mentioned

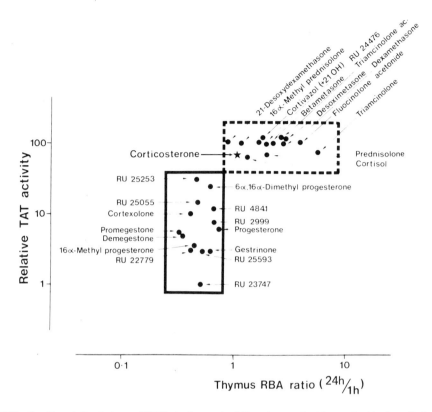

FIG. 5. Correlation between TAT induction and relative glucocorticoid receptor binding affinity: Cultured rat hepatoma tissue (HTC) cells were grown at 37°C as suspensions in modified SWIM's S₇₇ medium containing 10% calf serum as previously described (23,45). Test steroids were added in a 10 μl solution of ethanol per 10 ml of culture (density ~2 × 10⁵ cells/ml); equivalent amounts of ethanol were added to controls. Tyrosine aminotransferase was assayed at 37°C according to Diamondstone (17) as previously described (23,45). One unit of activity represents the formation of 1 μmole of *p*-OH-phenyl-pyruvate/min. Enzyme-specific activity is expressed as milliunits of TAT/mg of cell protein. Relative binding affinities (RBA) for the cytosol glucocorticoid receptor were determined after incubation for 1 hr and 24 hr as described in the legend to Fig. 4, and their ratio was calculated.

above, RU 2999 is a potent androgen (3,29); norgestrel, MPA, and gestrinone have known androgenic properties (12,45,65,69). They all increase prostate weight in the castrated rat. MPA inhibits the nuclear uptake of labeled testosterone in mouse kidney minces (10). The reduced nuclear uptake recorded in androgen-insensitive mice with testicular feminization indicates that its action is dependent on the presence of an androgen receptor (10–12) as demonstrated in other tissues (31). Norgestrel and MPA are able to decrease luteinizing hormone (LH) released by LH-RH in rat pituitary cells in culture to a level equivalent to that observed with the endogenous androgens, testosterone and 5α-dihydrotestosterone, but not with progesterone (27). Such androgenic effects are not found with compounds that bind weakly and with decreasing RBA values to the androgen receptor such as pro-

TABLE 2. *Relative binding affinities in a routine screening system[a]*

	PG[b]		AND[c]		GLU[d]	
	2 hr, 0°C	24 hr, 0°C	30 min, 0°C	2 hr, 0°C	1 hr, 0°C	24 hr, 0°C
Progesterone	100	100	20	5.5	115	75
Norgestrel	170	905	110	85	210	40
Promegestone (RU 5020)	220	535	10	1.5	100	30
Demegestone (RU 2453)	230	420	7.5	1	40	10
Chlormadinone acetate	175	320	80	20	215	35
RU 2999	260	305	205	160	85	55
Medroxyprogesterone acetate	125	305	40	50	470	215
6α, 16α-dimethylprogesterone	50	155	5	8	395	220
16α-methylprogesterone	65	60	10	1	160	55
Gestrinone (RU 2323)	75	50	95	85	265	150
Testosterone	~1	~1	100	100	3	0.5
Corticosterone	5	3	—	0.5	100	100
Cortivazol–21OH	<0.1	—	—	<0.1	305	530
Dexamethasone	0.5	<0.1	—	<0.1	165	455
Cortexolone	1	0.5	<0.1	0.3	40	15

[a]The RBAs of progesterone, testosterone and corticosterone for their receptor were taken to be 100. Results are expressed as the means of 3 or more determinations. The following organs were homogenized in 10 mM Tris-HCl (pH 7.4), 0.25M sucrose buffer: estradiol-primed rabbit uteri (1/50, wt/vol), castrated rat prostates (1/5, wt/vol), and adrenalectomized rat thymuses (1/10, wt/vol). The Tris-sucrose homogenates were centrifuged at 105,000 × g for 60 min at 0–4°C to obtain cytosols that were incubated as indicated with [³H]RU 5020, [³H]RU 1881, and [³H]–dexamethasone respectively in the presence or absence of 0 to 2,500 nM unlabeled steroid. Bound radioactivity was measured by a DCC adsorption technique.
[b]PG = progestin receptor.
[c]AND = androgen receptor.
[d]GLU = glucocorticoid receptor.

megestone, demegestone, and chlormadinone acetate. On the contrary, these compounds can inhibit the testosterone propionate-induced prostate weight increase in the castrated rat by 20 to 30% at daily doses of 1 to 3 mg (50).

An antiandrogenic effect has been reported in the case of MPA but is not necessarily mediated directly via the receptor. It appears to be explained by the induction of hepatic testosterone reductase activity, which in turn increases the catabolism of the hormone, leading to its lower plasma concentration and consequently to a lower target tissue uptake of testosterone (1). Indeed, *in vivo* actions of progestins are known to involve alterations in androgen biosynthesis and clearance from the blood. A further reported action of MPA is its so-called synandrogenic action, i.e., its ability to enhance androgen stimulation of mouse kidney β-glucuronidase (11,12).

The RBAs of these progestins, unlike those of well-known glucocorticoids for the glucocorticoid receptor in rat thymus (Table 2, Fig. 5), do not increase but rather decrease with incubation time. The highest values, either at 1 hr or 24 hr, are recorded with MPA and 6α, 16α-dimethylprogesterone, implying that these

TABLE 3. *ACTH release in rat anterior pituitary cells in culture and induction of tyrosine-amino-transferase (TAT) in hepatoma tissue cells (HTC) in culture*[a]

	ACTH[b] release		TAT induction			
				Antagonism vs 100 nM DXM		
	Agonism ED_{50} (nM)	Antagonism vs 10 nM DXM Kd (nM)	Agonism at 1 μM	% inhibition at		
				10^{-5}M	10^{-6}M	10^{-7}M
Triamcinolone acetonide	0.3	0	127			
Cortivazol-21 OH (Bimedrazol)	0.5	0	130			
Dexamethasone (DXM)	3.0	0	100			
Corticosterone	10	0	71			
Cortisol	—	—	66			
6α,16α-dimethylprogesterone	80	0	25	—	50	—
Cortexolone	80	400	11	—	40	—
Medroxyprogesterone acetate	100	>300	—	—	—	—
Progesterone	300	>1,000	6	50	0	0
Demegestone (RU 2453)	>1,000	>300	3	65	34	20
Promegestone (RU 5020)	0	400	6	70	24	0
Gestrinone (RU 2323)	0	300	3	38	34	16
RU 2999	0	300	8	88	56	8
16α-methyl progesterone	0	200	3.5	60	36	34

[a]Steroid was preincubated with primary cultures of anterior pituitary cells from adult female rats for 4 hr at 37°C under an atmosphere of 95% air–5% CO_2 in 1.0 ml DMEM containing 2% DCC-adsorbed sera. This was followed by a 4–hr incubation in DMEM with 2% sera in the presence of steroid and "CRF extract" [obtained from the median eminence homogenized in 2 N acetic acid as previously described (50)]. ACTH was determined by radioimmunoassay. Antagonist activity was measured in the presence of 10 nM dexamethasone. TAT induction was measured as described in the legend to Fig. 5. Data for agonist activity are taken from ref. 23 and for antagonist activity from ref. 45.
[b]ACTH = adrenocorticotropic hormone.

compounds manifestly have affinity for the glucocorticoid receptor from which they dissociate faster than corticosterone but nevertheless relatively slower than certain other progestins. They are therefore most likely to give rise to agonist glucocorticoid-receptor mediated effects. A similar reasoning applies to gestrinone and even to progesterone, which has an RBA equivalent to that of corticosterone at 1 hr but slightly lower at 24 hr. Jones and Bell (5,25) have shown that the dissociation rate constant for progesterone from the glucocorticoid receptor in rat thymus cytosol at 0°C is considerably greater than that for dexamethasone. Demegestone, promegestone, and cortexolone (the latter is not a progestin) reach the lowest RBA values at 24 hr and should, as a result, demonstrate low intrinsic glucocorticoid activity. However, since the RBAs of all these compounds decrease, under appropriate conditions each may exert some antiglucocorticoid activity.

Certain compounds with high RBAs for the progestin receptor also possess the additional property of increasing the dissociation rate of glucocorticoids from the cytosol glucocorticoid receptor (25,32,61–63). It has been suggested that this enhanced dissociation results from a cooperative effect due to interaction with a binding

TABLE 4. [³H]uridine incorporation into RNA in mouse thymocytes at 37°C[a]

	Agonism Relative activity (ratio of $ED_{50}s$)	Antagonism 1 µM steroid vs 50 nM DXM (% control without DXM)
Dexamethasone (DXM)	100	40.4 ± 1.7
+ 6α,16α-dimethylprogesterone	<1	1.2 ± 2.0
+ Progesterone	<1	21.7 ± 2.0
+ Demegestone	<1	23.5 ± 2.2
+ RU 2999	<1	25.4 ± 1.8
+ Cortexolone	<2	27.8 ± 1.7

[a]Mouse thymocytes (6 × 10⁶ cells/ml in minimal essential medium) were prepared as previously described (14). Aliquots of the cell suspension were incubated at 37°C for 3 hr in the presence of steroid. [³H]uridine (1 µCi) was then added to each sample, which was incubated at 37°C for another hour. Samples were chilled and centrifuged (10 min at 3,000 × g) and the pellets were resuspended in tracer-free medium and precipitated with cold 5% (wt/vol) trichloroacetic acid. The radioactivity of the precipitates was measured by liquid scintillation spectrometry. The antagonist activity of 1 µM steroid was measured vs 50 nM dexamethasone.
Data are from ref. 14.

TABLE 5. Relative effective dose (ED_{50}) inhibiting estrogen receptor (ER) replenishment and uterine growth

	[ER]	Uterine weight
Progesterone	100	100
Promegestone (RU 5020)	3	5
Megestrol acetate	3	50
Demegestone (RU 2453)	10	8
Norgestrel	10	10
Medroxyprogesterone acetate	10	100
RU 2999	20	3
Chlormadinone acetate	30	120
Gestrinone (RU 2323)	40	10

Data for inhibition of ER replenishment and estradiol-induced uterine growth in immature mice are derived from ref. 44.

site with progestin-like specificity. A recent report (32) shows that RU 2999, promegestone, norgestrel, and demegestone, compounds with comparable RBAs for the progestin receptor after 2 hr incubation at 0°C, increased the dissociation rate of dexamethasone by 46 to 60% when preincubated with cytosol. This cooperative effect between the progestin and glucocorticoid receptors may thus also constitute a mechanism for the antiglucocorticoid activity of progestins and lead to further antagonism. The final antagonist response will depend on the relative concentrations of glucocorticoid and progestin binding sites present in the medium and on the ability of the test steroid to stabilize preferential receptor conformations.

From the in vitro biological results on three tests (uridine incorporation into RNA in mouse thymocytes, TAT induction in HTC cells, and ACTH release in rat anterior pituitary cells in culture) taken from previous publications (14,23,45,50), a few tentative conclusions can be drawn. As expected from the RBA values, MPA, 6α, 16α-dimethylprogesterone and progesterone had the greatest agonist potential (Table 3). Progesterone and 6α, 16α-dimethylprogesterone could be described as partial agonists/antagonists: 6α, 16α-dimethylprogesterone was the most powerful antagonist on uridine incorporation (Table 4), a result that requires confirmation, and a good antagonist of TAT-induction at 10^{-6}M (Table 3); progesterone could also antagonize uridine incorporation and TAT induction. Some glucocorticoid activity would be expected for gestrinone, but the compound was a pure antagonist on ACTH and TAT. Cortexolone was likewise a partial agonist/antagonist, as evidenced by the results obtained both on ACTH and TAT (Table 3). Demegestone and promegestone, which have low RBAs for the glucocorticoid receptor, were either inactive or antagonists in these tests.

No strict concordance is thus found between binding kinetics and activity, although high RBA values for the glucocorticoid receptor in general favor agonist activity (55). Nevertheless, it is possible to conclude that these compounds with decreasing RBAs are all partial agonists/antagonists. It would seem that a continuous spectrum of activities exists between the two extremes of optimal agonist and optimal antagonist activities and that, depending on the conditions, one may prevail upon the other. Duncan and Duncan (19) have remarked on the low-dose antagonist activities of progesterone and high-dose glucocorticoid activity ("the biphasic action of progesterone"). This observation lends support to our interpretation, as it has been established that flooding of the receptor with high doses (or repeated low doses) of a partial agonist can lead to a full biological response (9,13,28).

Reports of antiglucocorticoid activity *in vitro* largely outweigh observations *in vivo* (19,24,34,68). Several teams have demonstrated *in vivo* glucocorticoid properties of MPA in animals (19,24,68). Guthrie and John (24), however, also observed an antiglucocorticoid action of MPA on dexamethasone-stimulated plasma glucose and hepatic glycogen content. On a battery of *in vivo* tests involving determination of thymus weight, ACTH, and corticosterone levels, Duncan and Duncan (19) demonstrated glucocorticoid-like effects of MPA and nonthymotrophic antiglucocorticoid activity of 16α-methylprogesterone. Regression of the thymus can be induced by 6α,16α-dimethylprogesterone. Indeed, under physiological conditions, the situation is complicated by the existence of glucocorticoid receptors in both central and peripheral target cells that are not independently regulated. This lends enhanced interest to the different sensitivities recorded above in the dexamethasone-induced pituitary-ACTH release test and in the tests on thymus and liver cells. As elegantly expressed by Bohus and de Kloet (6), a fine-tuned regulation of receptor-mediated glucocorticoid actions may exist that is based on the interplay of the agonist corticosterone and the various endogenous antagonists.

None of the compounds in Table 2 compete for binding to the estrogen receptor; however, many are potent antiestrogens (Table 5). A previous study (44) has established that in the case of progestins with little or no androgen binding the inhibition of the estradiol-induced uterine weight increase and of estrogen receptor replenishment is well-correlated with affinity for the progestin receptor. High-affinity pure progestins such as promegestone, demegestone, and megestrol acetate are indeed potent antiestrogens (44,45), as potent as, if not more so, than compounds such as norgestrel and MPA.

CONCLUSIONS

Routine screening of steroids for binding to five classes of hormone receptors (estrogen, progestin, androgen, mineralocorticoid, and glucocorticoid) can yield much valuable information. First of all, it enables the specificity profile of a steroid to be established. Second, a comparison of the relative binding affinities recorded after short or prolonged incubation gives an indication of the interaction kinetics between the steroid and receptor binding site as long as the effects of degradation within the cytosol are minimized. Third, structure/affinity correlations on large numbers of highly diversely substituted compounds reveal similarities and dissimilarities among the recognition sites of these receptor proteins (16,47).

Interpretation of the data in terms of biological activity requires caution, as the standardized experimental conditions used in a routine screening system cannot take into account all parameters influencing activity, e.g., species, tissue, and cell differences, receptor–receptor interactions, etc. Nevertheless, if the aim of the screening system is to select suitable compounds for hormone replacement therapy, the RBA data will indicate whether the compound is likely to give rise to any undesirable endocrine side effects due to binding to more than one class of receptor and whether the cytosol interaction kinetics favor long-lived complexes which, as demonstrated by several authors, induce sustained biological effects (13). In general, for compounds simulating the natural hormones, increasing RBAs on prolonging incubation imply high agonist activity, and low and decreasing RBAs are associated with either partial agonist or antagonist activity, depending on the experimental conditions (46,66).

When attempting to correct a hormone imbalance by the administration of synthetic steroids, it is essential that the selected compounds possess similar regulatory properties to the natural hormones and do not disrupt the normal molecular sequence of events leading to biological activity. The agonists (full or partial) should compensate for the impaired workings of the organism, and the dose and administration schedule should be chosen as a function of the interaction kinetics with the receptor.

Although the screening system can distinguish between compounds with low and high affinity, it cannot yet distinguish between high-affinity compounds that form receptor complexes with a conformation similar to that of the natural hormone complexes, able to bind successfully to DNA and trigger the subsequent events leading to a potent hormonal response and high-affinity compounds that block receptor-mediated events and are antagonists (52). At present, such a distinction can be extrapolated only indirectly from a knowledge of the effect of substitutions at various points of the steroid skeleton on steroid conformation, etc. For further insight, thermodynamic studies involving an analysis of the effects of temperature, pH, ions etc. are needed (54). Several authors have shown differences in interaction kinetics and RBAs with temperature (20,26,30,64,67), but inclusion of the additional parameter of temperature in the routine screening to account for "receptor activation" does not seem to be a sufficient criterion. More detailed studies are called for, not with crude cytosols but with highly purified receptor preparations, and in which interference from enzymes and other binding proteins has been eliminated. This will open up the era of a new category of compounds designed no longer to regulate but disrupt, and whose applications will needfully be restricted to crisis situations (e.g., hormone-dependent cancers).

ACKNOWLEDGMENTS

The studies reported in this chapter were performed with the collaboration of G. Beck (CNRS, Strasbourg), C. Bonne, M. M. Bouton, M. Fortin (Roussel-Uclaf), F. Labrie (Molecular Endocrinology Laboratory, University Laval, Quebec), P. Meyer (INSERM U7 Paris), J. P. Mornon (University Paris VII).

REFERENCES

1. Albin, J., Vittek, J., Gordon, G. G., Altman, K., Olivo, J., and Southren, A. L. (1973): On the mechanism of the anti-androgenic effect of medroxyprogesterone acetate. *Endocrinology*, 93:417–422.
2. Arányi, P. (1980): Kinetics of the hormone-receptor interaction. Competition experiments with slowly equilibrating ligands. *Biochim. Biophys. Acta*, 628:220–227.
3. Azadian-Boulanger, G., Bucourt, R., Nédélec, L., and Nominé, G. (1975): Stéroïdes triéniques androgènes et anabolisants. *Eur. J. Med. Chem.*, 10:353–359.
4. Baum, M. J. (1979): A comparison of the effects of methyltrienolone (R 1881) and 5α-dihydro-testosterone on sexual behavior of castrated male rats. *Horm. Behav.*, 13:165–174.
5. Bell, P. A., and Jones, T. R. (1979): Interactions of glucocorticoid agonists and antagonists with cellular receptors. In: *Anti-Hormones*, edited by M. K. Agarwal, pp. 35–50. Elsevier/North-Holland Biomedical Press, Amsterdam.
6. Bohus, B., and de Kloet, E. R. (1981): Adrenal steroids and extinction behavior: Antagonism by progesterone, deoxycorticosterone and dexamethasone of a specific effect of corticosterone. *Life Sci.*, 28:433–440.
7. Bonne, C., and Raynaud, J. P. (1976): Assay of androgen binding sites by exchange with methyltrienolone (R 1881). *Steroids*, 27:497–507.
8. Bouton, M. M., and Raynaud, J. P. (1978): The relevance of interaction kinetics in the determination of specific binding to the estrogen receptor. *J. Steroid Biochem.*, 9:9–15.
9. Bouton, M. M., and Raynaud, J. P. (1979): The relevance of interaction kinetics in determining biological response to estrogens. *Endocrinology*, 105:509–515.
10. Brown, T. R., Bullock, L., and Bardin, C. W. (1979): *In vitro* and *in vivo* binding of progestins to the androgen receptor of mouse kidney: Correlation with biological activities. *Endocrinology*, 105:1281–1287.
11. Bullock, L. P., Bardin, C. W., and Sherman, M. R. (1978): Androgenic, antiandrogenic, and synandrogenic actions of progestins: Role of steric and allosteric interactions with androgen receptors. *Endocrinology*, 103:1768–1782.
12. Bullock, L. P., and Bardin, C. W. (1979): Factors regulating the androgenic actions of progestins in mouse kidney. *Adv. Exp. Med. Biol.*, 117:281–295.
13. Clark, J. H., Paszko, Z., and Peck, E. J. Jr. (1977): Nuclear binding and retention of the receptor estrogen complex: Relation to the agonistic and antagonistic properties of estriol. *Endocrinology*, 100:91–96.
14. Dausse, J. P., Duval, D., Meyer, P., Gaignault, J. C., Marchandeau, C., and Raynaud, J. P. (1977): The relationship between glucocorticoid structure and effects upon thymocytes. *Mol. Pharmacol.*, 13:948–955.

15. Degelaen, J., Lareau, S., Brasseur, N., and Rousseau, G. G. (1981): Differences between the molecular interactions of agonists and antagonists with the glucocorticoid receptor. *Ann. Endocrinol. (Paris)*, 42:282–283.
16. Delettré, J., Mornon, J. P., Lepicard, G., Ojasoo, T., and Raynaud, J. P. (1980): Steroid flexibility and receptor specificity. *J. Steroid Biochem.*, 13:45–59.
17. Diamondstone, T. I. (1966): Assay of tyrosine transaminase activity by conversion of *p*-hydroxyphenylpyruvate to *p*-hydroxybenzaldehyde. *Anal. Biochem.*, 16:395–401.
18. Disorbo, D., Rosen, F., McPartland, R. P., and Milholland, R. J. (1977): Glucocorticoid activity of various progesterone analogs: Correlation between specific binding in thymus and liver and biologic activity. *Ann. N.Y. Acad. Sci.*, 286:355–368.
19. Duncan, M. R., and Duncan, G. R. (1979): An *in vivo* study of the action of antiglucocorticoids on thymus weight ratio, antibody titre and the adrenal pituitary-hypothalamus axis. *J. Steroid Biochem.*, 10:245–259.
20. Duval, D., and Simon, J. (1977): Temperature dependent changes in specificity of glucocorticoid receptors in mouse thymocytes. In: *Multiple Molecular Forms of Steroid Hormone Receptors*, edited by M. K. Agarwal, pp. 229–243. Elsevier/North-Holland Biomedical Press, Amsterdam.
21. Feil, P. D., and Bardin, C. W. (1979): The use of medroxyprogesterone acetate to study progestin receptors in immature, pregnant and adult rabbit uterus. *Adv. Exp. Med. Biol.*, 117:241–254.
22. Giannopoulos, G., and Keichline, D. (1981): Species-related differences in steroid-binding specificity of glucocorticoid receptors in lung. *Endocrinology*, 108:1414–1419.
23. Giesen, E. M., Bollack, C., and Beck, G. (1981): Relations between steroid-cell contact, steroid-binding and induction of tyrosine aminotransferase. *Mol. Cell. Endocrinol.*, 22:153–168.
24. Guthrie, G. P. Jr., and John, W. J. (1980): The *in vivo* glucocorticoid and antiglucocorticoid actions of medroxyprogesterone acetate. *Endocrinology*, 107:1393–1396.
25. Jones, T. R., and Bell, P. A. (1980): Glucocorticoid-receptor interactions. Studies of the negative co-operativity induced by steroid interactions with a secondary, hydrophobic, binding site. *Biochem. J.*, 188:237–245.
26. Jones, T. R., Sloman, J. C., and Bell, P. A. (1979): Competitive binding studies with glucocorticoid receptors from rat-thymus cells: Differential temperature-dependence of steroid binding. *Mol. Cell. Endocrinol.*, 13:83–92.
27. Labrie, F., Ferland, L., Lagacé, L., Drouin, J., Asselin, J., Azadian-Boulanger, G., and Raynaud, J. P. (1977): High inhibitory activity of R 5020, a pure progestin, at the hypothalamo-adenohypophyseal level on gonadotropin secretion. *Fertil. Steril.*, 28:1104–1112.
28. Lan, N. C., and Katzenellenbogen, B. S. (1976): Temporal relationships between hormone receptor binding and biological responses in the uterus: Studies with short- and long-acting derivatives of estriol. *Endocrinology*, 98:220–227.
29. Liao, S., Liang, T., Fang, S., Castañeda, E., and Shao, T. C. (1973): Steroid structure and androgenic activity. Specificities involved in the receptor binding and nuclear retention of various androgens. *J. Biol. Chem.*, 248:6154–6162.
30. MacDonald, R. G., and Cidlowski, J. A. (1979): Alterations in specificity of the glucocorticoid receptor with temperature in rat splenic lymphocytes. *J. Steroid Biochem.*, 10:21–29.
31. Mainwaring, W. I. P. (1977): *The Mechanism of Action of Androgens*. Springer Verlag, New York.
32. Moguilewsky, M., and Deraedt, R. (1981): Interrelations between glucocorticoid and progestin receptors. *J. Steroid Biochem.*, 15:329–335.
33. Mornon, J. P., Delettré, J., Lepicard, G., Bally, R., Surcouf, E., and Bondot, P. (1977): Interactions of hormonal steroids: progestogens. *J. Steroid Biochem.*, 8:51–62.
34. Naylor, P. H., Gilani, S. S., Milholland, R. J., Ip, M., and Rosen, F. (1981): *In vivo* antiglucocorticoids: Comparison between *in vivo* activity and *in vitro* competition of progestins for the glucocorticoid receptor. *J. Steroid Biochem.*, 14:1303–1309.
35. Neri, R. O. (1977): Studies on the biology and mechanism of action of nonsteroidal antiandrogens. In: *Androgens and Antiandrogens*, edited by L. Martini and M. Motta, p. 179. Raven Press, New York.
36. Niu, E. M., Neal, R. M., Pierce, V. K., and Sherman, M. R. (1981): Structural similarity of molybdate-stabilized steroid receptors in human breast tumors, uteri and leukocytes. *J. Steroid Biochem.*, 15:1–10.
37. Ojasoo, T., and Raynaud, J. P. (1978): Unique steroid congeners for receptor studies. *Cancer Res.*, 38:4186–4198.

38. Okret, S., Carlstedt-Duke, J., Wrange, Ö., Carlström, K., and Gustafsson, J. Å. (1981): Characterisation of an antiserum against the glucocorticoid receptor. *Biochim. Biophys. Acta*, 677:205–219.
39. Philibert, D., Ojasoo, T., and Raynaud, J. P. (1977): Properties of the cytoplasmic progestin-binding protein in the rabbit uterus. *Endocrinology*, 101:1850–1861.
40. Philibert, D., and Raynaud, J. P. (1978): Properties of the glucocorticoid receptor in rat tissues and in HTC cells. *J. Steroid Biochem.*, 9:835–836.
41. Raynaud, J. P. (1977): R 5020, a tag for the progestin receptor. In: *Progesterone Receptors in Normal and Neoplastic Tissues*, edited by W. L. McGuire, J. P. Raynaud, and E. E. Baulieu, pp. 9–21. Raven Press, New York.
42. Raynaud, J. P. (1979): The mechanism of action of anti-hormones. In: *Advances in Pharmacology and Therapeutics, Vol. 1, Receptors*, edited by J. Jacob, pp. 259–278. Pergamon Press, Oxford.
43. Raynaud, J. P., Bonne, C., Bouton, M. M., Lagacé, L., and Labrie, F. (1979): Action of a non-steroid anti-androgen, RU 23908, in peripheral and central tissues. *J. Steroid Biochem.*, 11:93–99.
44. Raynaud, J. P., and Bouton, M. M. (1980): The design of estrogens and/or anti-estrogens on the basis of receptor binding. In: *Cytotoxic Estrogens in Hormone Receptive Tumors*, edited by J. Raus, H. Martens, and G. Leclercq, pp. 49–70. Academic Press, New York.
45. Raynaud, J. P., Bouton, M. M., Moguilewsky, M., Ojasoo, T., Philibert, D., Beck, G., Labrie, F., and Mornon, J. P. (1980): Steroid hormone receptors and pharmacology. *J. Steroid Biochem.*, 12:143–157.
46. Raynaud, J. P., Bouton, M. M., and Ojasoo, T. (1980): The use of interaction kinetics to distinguish potential antagonists from agonists. *Tips*, 1:324–327.
47. Raynaud, J. P., Delettré, J., Ojasoo, T., Lepicard, G., and Mornon, J. P. (1981): Steps towards mapping of steroid hormone receptors. In: *Physiopathology of Endocrine Diseases and Mechanisms of Hormone Action*, edited by R. J. Soto, A. de Nicola, and J. Blaquier, pp. 461–476. A. R. Liss, New York.
48. Raynaud, J. P., Fortin, M., and Tournemine, C. (1980): Les antihormones. *Actual. Chimie Thérapeut.*, 7:293–318.
49. Raynaud, J. P., Ojasoo, T., Bouton, M. M., and Philibert, D. (1979): Receptor binding as a tool in the development of new bioactive steroids. In: *Drug Design, Vol. 8*, edited by E. J. Ariëns, pp. 169–214. Academic Press, New York.
50. Raynaud, J. P., Ojasoo, T., and Labrie, F. (1981): Steroid hormones—agonists and antagonists. In: *Mechanisms of Steroid Action*, edited by G. P. Lewis and M. Ginsburg, pp. 145–158. Macmillan Publishers LTD, England.
51. Raynaud, J. P., Ojasoo, T., and Vaché, V. (1979): Unusual steroids in measuring steroid receptors. In: *Steroid Receptors and the Management of Cancer*, edited by E. B. Thompson and M. E. Lippman, pp. 215–232. CRC Press, Inc., Boca Raton.
52. Rochefort, H., and Borgna, J. L. (1981): Differences between oestrogen receptor activation by oestrogen and antioestrogen. *Nature*, 292:257–259.
53. Rochefort, H., and Capony, F. (1977): Estradiol dependent decrease of binding inhibition by anti-estrogens (a possible test of receptor activation). *Biochem. Biophys. Res. Commun.*, 75:277–285.
54. Rousseau, G. G. (1980): Thermodynamics of steroid binding of the glucocorticoid receptor. In: *Abstracts, 6th Int. Congress of Endocrinology*, 849, p. 634.
55. Rousseau, G. G., Baxter, J. D., and Tomkins, G. M. (1972): Glucocorticoid receptors: Relations between steroid binding and biological effects. *J. Mol. Biol.*, 67:99–115.
56. Sakiz, E., Azadian-Boulanger, G., and Raynaud, J. P. (1974): Antiestrogens, antiprogesterones. *Proc. VI Intern. Congr. Endocrinol., Washington 1971, ICS 273*: 988–994.
57. Samuels, H. H., and Tomkins, G. M. (1970): Relation of steroid structure to enzyme induction in hepatoma tissue culture cells. *J. Mol. Biol.*, 52:57–74.
58. Schrader, W. T., and O'Malley, B. W. (1979): Similarities of structure among steroid receptor proteins. In: *Receptors in Human Disease; Report of Macy Conference*, edited by A. G. Bearn and P. W. Choppin, pp. 183–196. Josiah Macy, New York.
59. Simons, S. S., Jr., Thompson, E. B., and Johnson, D. F. (1979): Antiinflammatory pyrazolo-steroids: Potent glucocorticoids containing bulky a-ring substituents and no C_3-carbonyl. *Biochem. Biophys. Res. Commun.*, 86:793–800.
60. Södersten, P., and Gustafsson, J. Å. (1980): Activation of sexual behaviour in castrated rats with

the synthetic androgen 17β-hydroxy-17α-methyl-estra-4,9,11-triene-3-one (R 1881). *J. Endocrinol.*, 87:279–283.

61. Suthers, M. B., Pressley, L. A., and Funder, J. W. (1976): Glucocorticoid receptors: Evidence for a second, non-glucocorticoid binding site. *Endocrinology*, 99:260–269.

62. Svec, F., and Rudis, M. (1981): Progestin-induced enhancement of dexamethasone dissociation from glucocorticoid hormone receptors. *Arch. Biochem. Biophys.*, 212:417–423.

63. Svec, F., Yeakley, J., and Harrison, R. W. III (1980): Progesterone enhances glucocorticoid dissociation from the AtT-20 cell glucocorticoid receptor. *Endocrinology*, 107:566–572.

64. Svec, F., Yeakley, J., and Harrison, R. W. III (1980): The effect of temperature and binding kinetics on the competitive binding assay of steroid potency in intact AtT-20 cells and cytosol. *J. Biol. Chem.*, 255:8573–8578.

65. Tausk, M., and de Visser, J. (1972): Pharmacology of orally active progestational compounds: animal studies. In: *Pharmacology of the Endocrine System and Related Drugs: Progesterone, Progestational Drugs and Antifertility Agents*, edited by M. Tausk, pp. 35–216. Pergamon Press, Oxford.

66. Weichman, B. M., and Notides, A. C. (1980): Estrogen receptor activation and the dissociation kinetics of estradiol, estriol and estrone. *Endocrinology*, 106:434–439.

67. Weisz, A., Hutchens, T. W., and Markland, F. S. (1982): Competitive binding assay for glucocorticoids. Influence of experimental conditions on measurement of the affinity of competitive steroids for the receptor. *J. Steroid Biochem.*, 16:515–520.

68. Winneker, R. C., and Parsons, J. A. (1981): Glucocorticoid-like actions of medroxyprogesterone actetate upon MtTW15 rat mammosomatotropic pituitary tumors. *Endocrinology*, 109:99–105.

69. Worgul, T., Baker, H. W. G., Murray, F. T., Jefferson, L. S., and Bardin, C. W. (1979): Direct effects of medroxyprogesterone acetate on testis: Possible mechanisms examined by testicular perfusion. *Int. J. Androl.*, 2:408–418.

Steroids and Endometrial Cancer,
edited by V. M. Jasonni, et al.
Raven Press, New York © 1983.

Hormone Receptors and Breast Cancer

William L. McGuire, C. Kent Osborne, Gary M. Clark, and William A. Knight III

*Department of Medicine, Division of Oncology, University of Texas
Health Science Center, San Antonio, Texas 78284*

Over the past 10 years the clinician's approach to the treatment of breast cancer has changed due to the development and widespread use of estrogen receptor assays to predict the endocrine dependence of a patient's tumor. When basic researchers discovered that the cytoplasmic estrogen receptor (ER) was responsible for the uptake of estrogen into target cells and necessary for estrogen action, they reasoned that it might be useful in determining the endocrine responsiveness of breast cancers in patients with metastatic disease. This hypothesis has been confirmed, and it is now generally accepted that tumors lacking ER rarely respond to endocrine therapy, whereas ER positive tumors frequently regress with endocrine therapy. Thus, the physician is now better able to tailor specific therapy for his patients. Determination of the tumor ER status is now standard practice in this country.

Over the past several years, additional research on the usefulness of estrogen receptor assays has led to refinements in technique, to improved precision in selecting patients for hormone therapies, and to answers for additional questions regarding the clinical application of the assay. These questions include: (a) What is the value of an ER assay performed on the primary breast tumor at the time of mastectomy? (b) Is tumor ER concentration (quantitative ER) important? (c) What is the role of progesterone receptor (PgR) in determining tumor endocrine dependence? and (d) Is PgR equivalent to quantitative ER in selecting hormone dependent tumors? We will present data from our own laboratory addressing these important questions.

ESTROGEN RECEPTORS IN PRIMARY BREAST CANCER

In clinical practice it is not always possible to obtain sufficient tumor biopsy material to perform an ER assay in women with advanced breast cancer. An invasive procedure with a high risk of morbidity in a sick patient may be unacceptable. Thus, it is important to determine whether or not an ER assay done on the primary tumor at the time of mastectomy will predict endocrine dependence at the time of a future recurrence. Most primary tumors are sufficiently large to permit adequate histopathologic studies and an ER assay. However, since a change in the ER status of a breast cancer could occur with time, the ER status of a primary tumor might not reflect the hormone dependence of the tumor years later when metastatic disease has become clinically evident. Data from our own laboratory, however, suggests that an ER assay on the primary tumor does predict for response to subsequent endocrine therapy for metastatic disease (Table 1). In 50 trials of endocrine therapy for advanced disease, only one of six patients with an ER negative (−) primary tumor responded objectively in contrast to 22 of 44 patients with ER positive (+) tumors. This compares favorably with clinical correlations based on the direct ER assay of a metastatic specimen. Similar data have been reported by Block et al. (3). These studies suggest that an ER assay should be performed on all mastectomy specimens to help guide later therapy of advanced disease in the event that the patient suffers a recurrence of tumor.

Studies of ER in patients with primary operable breast cancer have led to another important clinical application: the receptor status of the primary tumor appears to be an important prognostic variable. Our laboratory originally measured ER in primary breast tumors in order to predict endocrine responsiveness later at the time of recurrence. During analysis of this data an interesting trend became apparent; patients with ER − tumors seemed to recur more frequently and to have a shorter disease-free interval than patients with ER + tumors. More formal analysis of these findings was striking (7). Regardless of age, menopausal status, size of the tumor, or its location in the breast, the rate of recurrence of ER − tumors was significantly worse than for ER + tumors. More important, the status of the axillary lymph nodes, which is considered to be the most important prognostic indicator in patients with primary breast cancer, did not alter these findings. These data are shown in Table 2. Within every subset of patients, those with ER − tumors had a higher rate of recurrence than those with ER + tumors. Furthermore, and perhaps even more important, we have now shown that the ER − patients have significantly worse survival rates than the ER + group (8). Similar data have been obtained by several other investigators (1,5,9,12).

These data have obvious therapeutic implications for the patient with primary breast cancer. First, patients can be categorized according to their relative risk of developing recurrent breast cancer after treatment of the primary tumor. ER − , axillary node positive patients have a very high rate of recurrence and poor survival indicating the need for adjuvant systemic therapy to eradicate micrometastases. ER − , node negative patients might also be considered for adjuvant therapy because

TABLE 1. *Tumor ER and response to*
endocrine therapy

	Objective response	
Biopsy site	ER −	ER +
Primary	1/6 (17%)	22/44 (50%)
Metastatic	4/47 (8%)	48/101 (48%)

TABLE 2. *Estrogen receptor and prognosis in 281 patients with primary breast cancer[a]*

	% Recurrence at 2 years	
	ER −	ER +
Total patients	35	18
Menopausal status		
Pre	35	18
Post	38	15
Axillary nodes		
0	26	8
1–3	43	16
≥4	68	40
Tumor location		
Outer	32	12
Inner + central	50	12

[a]Modified from Knight et al. (7).

of their relatively high rate of recurrence despite the absence of detectable spread to regional nodes. In contrast, ER +, node negative patients have the lowest risk for recurrence and should not be subjected to adjuvant therapy. Second, the ER status of the primary tumor may help in designing the most effective treatment program. Patients with ER + tumors may benefit from adjuvant endocrine therapy alone or combined with chemotherapy, while patients with ER − tumors are not likely to benefit from endocrine therapy and should be treated with aggressive chemotherapy because of their poor prognosis.

QUANTITATIVE ER IN ADVANCED BREAST CANCER

It is clear that the ER assay is most helpful when the tumor is ER −. These patients rarely respond to endocrine therapy. On the other hand, a positive ER does not guarantee a response to endocrine therapy, as about 40% of patients fail to respond despite a positive assay. We have attempted to improve the accuracy in this group by quantitating tumor ER content, rationalizing that tumors with a higher ER level might contain a higher proportion of ER + cells resulting in a larger reduction in tumor burden with endocrine therapy. Our first analysis in 1975 (11) with limited numbers of patients suggested that this hypothesis was correct. Tumors with the highest ER content had the highest regression rates with endocrine therapy. Our most recent analysis of nearly 200 clinical trials of endocrine therapy for advanced breast cancer confirms this observation (Table 3). Tumors with undetectable or very low ER levels had a low response rate to endocrine therapy, whereas tumors with high ER content displayed the highest response rate. Whether the ER assay was performed on the original primary tumor or on a metastatic lesion did not significantly alter these results. These findings have been observed by other

TABLE 3. *Quantitative ER and the response to endocrine therapy*

ER fmoles/mg	Objective response	
	Primary biopsy	Metastatic biopsy
0–3	1/6 (17%)	4/47 (8%)
3–100	17/38 (45%)	26/65 (40%)
>100	5/6 (83%)	22/36 (61%)

TABLE 4. *ER and PgR in 1366 human breast tumors*

Receptor status	Premenopausal (%)	Postmenopausal (%)
ER − PgR−	30	19
ER − PgR+	9	3
ER + PgR−	12	23
ER + PgR+	49	55

investigators (1,4). Thus, quantitative ER improves the clinician's ability to accurately select patients for endocrine therapy.

PROGESTERONE RECEPTOR IN ADVANCED BREAST CANCER

Another method devised to improve the accuracy of predicting response to endocrine therapy is the assay for progesterone receptor (PgR). The rationale behind the use of PgR assays to predict tumor endocrine dependence came from the observation that PgR is induced by estrogen in normal reproductive tissues and in human breast cancer cells in culture (6). Our laboratory hypothesized that certain ER+ tumors do not regress with endocrine manipulation because of a defect in the estrogen response pathway distal to the binding step leading to autonomous growth. PgR, therefore, might be a better marker than ER for an intact estrogen response pathway as it is an end product of estrogen action. The distribution of ER and PgR in a large number of human breast tumor specimens is shown in Table 4. Not surprisingly, ER−, PgR+ tumors are uncommon, as one might have predicted if PgR synthesis is an estrogen-dependent process. About one-half of the specimens contain both receptors and would be expected to respond to endocrine therapy. About 40% of the tumors lack PgR, and by the above hypothesis should not regress with hormonal manipulation, whether or not ER is present.

Clinical responses to endocrine therapy according to receptor status are shown in Table 5. Data from our own laboratory, as well as cumulative data from several other series, are similar and demonstrate the value of the PgR assay. As predicted, tumors lacking both receptors are usually endocrine independent and regress infrequently with endocrine therapy. ER−, PgR+ tumors are rare, but responses to

TABLE 5. *Response to endocrine therapy as a function of ER and PgR*

	ER − PgR−	ER − PgR+	ER + PgR−	ER + PgR+
San Antonio	3/20	—	14/45	16/20
Other series[a]	9/91	6/13	19/76	71/93
Totals	12/111 (11%)	6/13 (46%)	33/121 (27%)	(87/113) (77%)

[a] *Personal communication;* Degenshein and Bloom; King, Redgrave, Rubens, Millis and Hayward; Leclercq and Heuson; Nomura, Takotani, Sugano and Matsumoto; Singhakowinta; DeSombre and Jensen; Skinner, Barnes and Ribeiro; Young, Einhorn, Ehrlich and Cleary.

TABLE 6. *PgR as a function of ER concentration*

ER fmoles/mg	PgR positive tumors (%)
0–3	5
3–100	43
>100	82

endocrine therapy have been observed. The highest response rate (77% overall) is observed in the group of tumors containing both ER and PgR, lending validity to the hypothesis that PgR may be a good marker for endocrine dependence. However, the ER +, PgR − group of tumors should have failed to regress with endocrine therapy, and yet 27% did respond. Perhaps the hypothesis is imperfect, and PgR synthesis may not be linked sufficiently closely to the pathway of tumor growth to be an accurate predictor in all cases. Alternatively, the PgR in some of these cases could be "falsely" negative due to receptor occupancy by high endogenous progesterone levels in the luteal phase of the menstrual cycle in premenopausal women (13), or due to lack of sufficient circulating estrogens to stimulate PgR synthesis in postmenopausal women. In any event, the PgR assay improves our ability to select patients likely to respond to endocrine therapy.

QUANTITATIVE ER VERSUS PgR ASSAYS

The studies noted above suggest that by quantitating ER and by adding PgR assays one can significantly improve the accuracy of predicting tumor endocrine dependence. However, an important question is whether or not the time and expense required for both assays is necessary. It is possible that the two assays are selecting the same set of patients, as tumors with high levels of ER are more likely to contain PgR (Table 6) (10). Thus, a positive PgR might simply be a marker for those tumors with a high ER content. We have recently studied the clinical response to endocrine therapy in 65 ER + patients for which quantitative ER and PgR data were available. In a very preliminary analysis of this limited number of patients, the presence of PgR appears to be a somewhat better discriminant for objective

TABLE 7. *Response to endocrine therapy quantitative ER vs PgR*

	Objective response
ER (fmoles/mg)	
3–100	13/38 (34%)
>100	17/27 (63%)
PgR	
Negative	14/45 (31%)
Positive	16/20 (80%)

response than quantitative ER alone (Table 7). Eighty percent of ER +, PgR + patients responded objectively in contrast to only 63% of those patients with tumor ER content (greater than 100 fmoles/mg protein). These data do not address the question of whether the two assays together could identify a subset of patients (i.e., ER > 100 fmoles/mg and PgR +) with even higher response rates. We are currently investigating this and other related questions in a larger series of patients. The preliminary data, however, suggest that the PgR assay may be an important addition to the armamentarium of the physician treating patients with breast cancer.

SUMMARY

The ER assay has become a standard practice in the management of advanced breast cancer. Tumors lacking ER respond infrequently to endocrine therapy, whereas response rates of 50 to 60% are observed in ER + tumors. Recent studies indicate that the ER status of the primary tumor is a good predictor of the endocrine dependence of metastatic tumors at the time of clinical relapse. Furthermore, the absence of ER in the primary tumor is an important independent prognostic indicator of higher rate of recurrence and shorter survival. Quantitative analysis of ER and an assay for PgR are two methods for increasing the accuracy of selecting or rejecting patients for hormonal therapy; tumors with a high quantitative ER content or those with a positive PgR display the highest objective response rates. Preliminary analysis suggests that the presence of PgR may be a better marker of tumor hormone dependence than quantitative ER.

ACKNOWLEDGMENTS

This work was supported in part by The National Cancer Institute and the American Cancer Society.

REFERENCES

1. Allegra, J. C., Lippman, M. E., Simon, R., Thompson, E. B., Barlock, A., Green, L., Huff, K. K., Do, H. M. T., Aitken, S. C., and Warren, R. (1979): The association between steroid hormone receptor status and disease free interval in breast cancer. *Cancer Treat. Rep.*, 63:1271–1278.
2. Allegra, J. C., Lippman, M. E., Thompson, E. B., Simon, R., Barlock, A., Green, L., Huff,

K. K., Do, H. M. T., Aitken, S. C., and Warren, R. (1981): Estrogen receptor status is the most important prognostic variable in predicting response to endocrine therapy in metastatic breast cancer. *Eur. J. Cancer*, 16:323–331.

3. Block, G. E., Ellis, R. S., DeSombre, E., and Jensen, E. (1978): Correlation of estrophilin content of primary mammary cancer to eventual endocrine treatment. *Ann. Surg.*, 188:372–376.
4. DeSombre, E. R., Green, G. L., and Jensen, E. V. (1978): Estrophilin and endocrine responsiveness of breast cancer. In: *Hormones, Receptors, and Breast Cancer*, edited by W. L. McGuire, pp. 1–14. Raven Press, New York.
5. Hahnel, R., Woodings, T., and Vivian, A. B. (1979): Prognostic value of estrogen receptors in primary breast cancer. *Cancer*, 44:671–675.
6. Horwitz, K. B., McGuire, W. L., Pearson, O. H., Segaloff, A. (1975): Predicting response to endocrine therapy in human breast cancer: a hypothesis. *Science*, 189:726–727.
7. Knight, W. A. III, Livingston, R. B., Gregory, E. J., and McGuire, W. L. (1977): Estrogen receptor is an independent prognostic factor for early recurrence in breast cancer. *Cancer Res.*, 37:4669–4671.
8. Knight, W. A. III, Livingston, R. B., Gregory, E. J., Walder, A. I., and McGuire, W. L. (1978): Absent estrogen receptor and decreased survival in human breast cancer. *Proc. Am. Soc. Clin. Oncol.*, 19:392.
9. Maynard, P. V., Blomey, R. W., Elston, C. W., Haybittle, J. L., and Griffiths, K. (1978): Estrogen receptor assay in primary breast cancer and early recurrence of the disease. *Cancer Res.*, 38:4292–4295.
10. McGuire, W. L., Horwitz, K. B., Pearson, O. H., and Segaloff, A. (1977): Current status of estrogen and progesterone receptors in breast cancer. *Cancer*, 39:2934–2947.
11. McGuire, W. L., Pearson, O. H., and Segaloff, A. (1975): Predicting hormone responsiveness in human breast cancer. In: *Estrogen Receptors in Human Breast Cancer*, edited by W. L. McGuire, Carbone, P. P., and Vollmer, E. P., pp. 17–30. Raven Press, New York.
12. Rich, M. A., Furmanski, P., and Brooks, S. C. (1978): Prognostic value of estrogen receptor determinations in patients with breast cancer. *Cancer Res.*, 38:4296–4298.
13. Saez, S., Martin, P. M., and Chouvet, C. D. (1978): Estradiol and progesterone receptor levels in human breast adenocarcinoma in relation to plasma estrogen and progesterone levels. *Cancer Res.*, 38:3468–3473.

Steroids and Endometrial Cancer,
edited by V. M. Jasonni, et al.
Raven Press, New York © 1983.

Estrogen and Progesterone Receptors in Endometrial Cancer

Kunhard Pollow, Bernd Manz, and Hans-Jörg Grill

*Department of Experimental Endocrinology, Johannes Gutenberg University,
6500 Mainz, Federal Republic of Germany*

Gestagen therapy has been shown to be of objective benefit for about 30% of patients with advanced endometrial cancer (2,21,22,35). If the same sex hormone receptor mechanism is involved in the action of steroid hormones on the endometrial carcinoma cells as detected in normal endometrial tissue, it would be reasonable to assume that the steroid hormone-receptor system is a critical factor in the effectiveness of hormone therapy against endometrial carcinoma cells. Tumor cells that possess the progesterone receptor would respond to gestagen therapy by regressing, whereas tumor cells that have lost their complex endocrine regulatory system would be immune to the hormone. A series of studies on sex hormone receptors in normal and neoplastic human endometrium indicate that this hypothesis is plausible (32). The following investigation was undertaken in an attempt to present a comparison of biochemical and physical properties of estradiol and progesterone receptor in normal and neoplastic endometrium, as well as between endometrial adenocarcinomas with various degrees of differentiation.

MATERIALS AND METHODS

Materials

By thin-layer chromatography, [6,7-^{3}H]estradiol (51 Ci/mmole), [17α-methyl-^{3}H]-R5020 (87 Ci/mmole), [4-^{14}C]estradiol (56 mCi/mmole), [6,7-^{3}H]cortisol (40 Ci/mmole), obtained from New England Nuclear [6,7-^{3}H]-Org.2058 (60 Ci/mmole) obtained from Amersham Buchler, were checked regularly for radiochemical purity.

Unlabeled steroids were purchased from Schering AG (Berlin, Germany). Norit A was obtained from Serva, Dextran T70 from Pharmacia Fine Chemicals, bovine serum albumin and DNA (calf thymus) from Sigma Chemical Company.

Buffer Systems

Buffer A: 10 mmoles/liter Tris-HCl (pH 7.4), 1.5 mmoles/liter Na$_2$-EDTA, 1 mmoles/liter dithiothreitol, 20% glycerol (vol/vol).

Buffer B: 10 mmoles/liter Tris-HCl (pH 7.4), 0.1 moles/liter NaCl, 5 mmoles/liter KCl, 3 mmoles/liter $MgCl_2$, 1.5 mmoles/liter $CaCl_2$, 0.25 moles/liter sucrose.

Buffer C: 10 mmoles/liter Tris-HCl (pH 7.4), 1.5 mmoles/liter Na_2-EDTA.

Tissues

Normal human endometrium from normally menstruating patients and tissue from patients with endometrial carcinoma were obtained after hysterectomy or diagnostic curretage. Immediately after hysterectomy, the endometrium was scraped from the uterine cavity. Adequate samples were taken for histological examination and the rest for determination of steroid binding components as well as 17β-hydroxysteroid dehydrogenase (17β-HSD) activity. Wet tissue was dipped into ice-cold isotonic saline to remove mucus and blood clots. Further processing of the samples was initiated within 30 min. The menstrual age of the mucosa was based on a 28-day cycle according to the method of Noyes et al. (23).

Preparation of Subcellular Fractions

All subsequent operations were made at 4°C. The specimens were homogenized in six volumes (wt/vol) of buffer A by using a motor-driven Potter-Elvehjem-type homogenizer at low speed (1,000 rpm) by five 20-sec bursts with alternate cooling in an ice bath. The homogenate was filtered through four layers of cheese-cloth and centrifuged for 20 min at 800 × g to obtain the crude nuclear pellet. The 800 × g supernatant was diluted 1:1 with buffer A, and centrifuged at 105,000 × g for 90 min. The resulting supernatant fluid was designated cytosol and used for the measurement of cytoplasmic receptors; the 105,000 × g pellet (after two washings with buffer B) was designated "microsomal fraction" and used for determination of 17β-HSD activity.

The 800 × g "nuclear" pellet was resuspended in buffer A and washed in the same buffer three times. Washing is accomplished by adding ice-cold buffer A to the pellet, vortexing thoroughly, and centrifuging at 800 × g for 10 min.

Highly "purified nuclei" were prepared by resuspending the crude 800 × g nuclear pellet in buffer C containing 2.4 moles/liter sucrose. The nuclear suspension was then layered on a cushion of 2.4 moles/liter sucrose buffer C and centrifuged at 60,000 × g for 60 min at 4°C (rotor SW 25.2, Beckman ultracentrifuge L2-65B).

Assay of Cytoplasmic Steroid-Hormone Receptors

Determination of [³H]estradiol binding.   Duplicate aliquots (0.1 ml) of the diluted cytosol (2–6 mg protein/ml buffer A) were incubated for 16 hr at 4°C, followed by 2 hr at 25°C with [³H]estradiol over a 15-fold concentration range (0.5–8 nmoles/liter). Tubes containing 10^{-6} moles/liter diethylstilbestrol (DES) were used to correct for nonspecific binding. Total incubation volume was 0.2 ml. Binding was then measured using the charcoal adsorption technique. Incubation of cytosol for

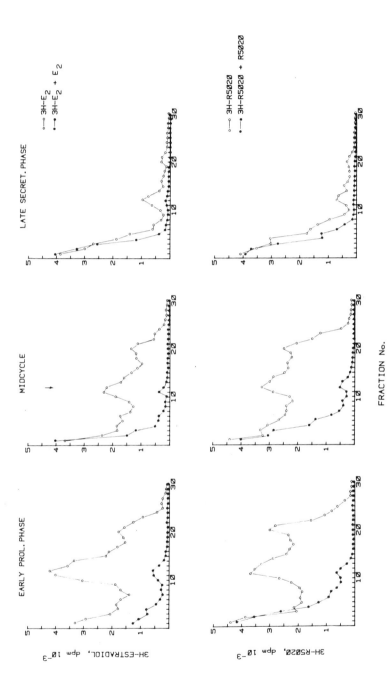

FIG. 1. Sucrose density profiles in the absence of KCl of cytosol estradiol or R5020 binding components of normal human endometrium exposed *in vitro* to [³H]estradiol or [³H]R5020. *Arrow* indicates the fraction where bovine serum albumin sedimented.

estradiol receptor assay was determined by addition to each sample of 0.5 ml ice-cold dextran-coated charcoal solution in buffer A (1 g charcoal, 0.05 g dextran in 100 ml of buffer A), followed by a 20 min incubation at 4°C with vigorous shaking. After centrifugation at 2,500 × g for 10 min, the radioactivity in 0.5 ml samples of the supernatant was measured. The equilibrium association constant (K_a) and the concentration of binding sites were calculated according to Scatchard (36).

Determination of [³H]R5020 binding. Duplicate aliquots (0.1 ml) of the diluted cytosols were incubated with increasing concentrations of [³H]R5020 varying from 0.5 to 15 nmoles/liter. Nonradioactive R5020 was used in an excess of 100-fold that of labeled ligand to correct for nonspecific binding. The incubation was carried out at 4°C for 16 hr. Binding was then measured using the charcoal adsorption technique.

Sucrose Density Gradient Centrifugation of Cytoplasmic Steroid–Hormone Receptors

The cytosol (prepared in buffer A with 10% glycerol) was incubated with 4 nmoles/liter [³H]estradiol or 16 nmoles/liter [³H]R5020 with or without excess unlabeled steroids 200-fold excess relative to ³H-labeled steroids for 4 hr at 4°C followed by the dextran-coated charcoal treatment. Next, 0.2 ml was layered on a linear sucrose gradient (5–20% sucrose in buffer A with or without 0.4 moles/liter KCl and 10% glycerol, vol/vol) and centrifuged for 16 hr at 234,000 × g (rotor SW 50.1, Beckman). Bovine serum albumin was run simultaneously as the reference protein in the estimation of sedimentation coefficients. Fractions were collected from the top of the gradient by means of the Isco piercing unit and drop counter. Radioactivity was determined in 0.1-ml aliquots of undiluted fractions. Quenching of radioactivity by sucrose did not vary significantly.

Assay of Nuclear Steroid–Hormone Receptors

Triplicate aliquots of the nuclear suspension (0.1 ml) in buffer A were incubated using 10 nmoles/liter [³H]estradiol with or without 1 μmole/liter DES at 30°C for 240 min with occasional vortexing. Exchange was determined by the addition of 1 ml of ice-cold buffer A to each tube followed by centrifugation at 800 × g for 10 min. The nuclear pellets were washed three times in buffer A by resuspending the pellet in 2 ml ice-cold buffer A, vortexing, and sedimentation at 800 × g for 10 min. Finally, 1 ml chloroform/ethanol (3:1) was added to the washed nuclear pellets, the samples were stirred for 30 min at room temperature and then centrifuged at 800 × g for 10 min. The total extract of each sample was added to 10 ml scintillation cocktail (Quickszint 501, Zinsser) and counted for radioactivity. The measurement of the nuclear progesterone binding sites by steroid exchange differed slightly from the procedure employed for estrogen receptors.

The final concentration of [³H]R5020 was 20 nmoles/liter with or without 2 μmoles/liter nonradioactive R5020. Incubations were carried out with shaking at 4°C for 16 hr.

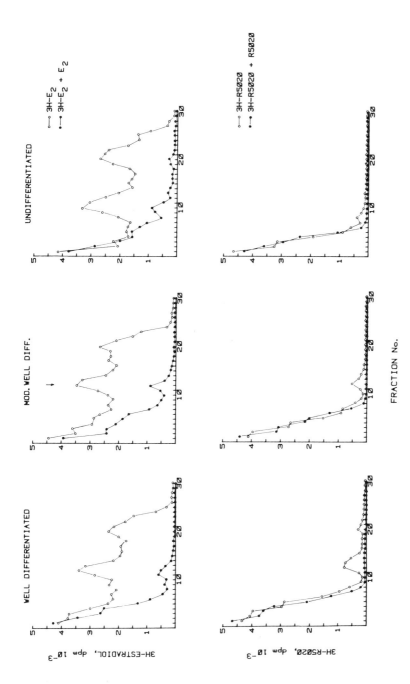

FIG. 2. Sedimentation properties of [3H]estradiol and [3H]R5020 binding proteins in endometrial carcinomas in relation to the degree of tumor differentiation. *Arrow* indicates the fraction where bovine serum albumin sedimented.

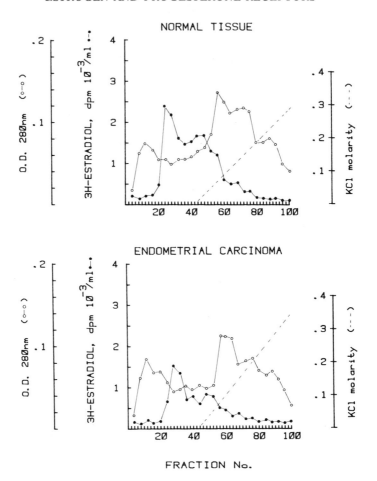

FIG. 3. Elution profiles of labeled cytosol from proliferative endometrium or undifferentiated endometrial carcinomas on DEAE-cellulose. Five ml of [³H]estradiol labeled cytosol, prepared in 10 mmoles/liter KH₂PO₄ buffer, pH 7.4, were applied (after removal of free or loosely bound [³H]estradiol by charcoal-dextran treatment) to a DEAE-cellulose column equilibrated in the phosphate buffer. Elution was carried out with a linear gradient to 0.4 moles/liter KCl. Fractions (0.6 ml) were collected and aliquots were counted for radioactivity.

Glycerol density gradient centrifugation.   Endometrial tissue slices were incubated in Eagle's medium (without vitamins and amino acids) at 4°C for 10 min with 10 nmoles/liter [³H]estradiol (in the presence of 20 nmoles/liter androstanolone) or 20 nmoles/liter [³H]R5020 (in the presence of 2 μmoles/liter cortisol) then rinsed and transferred to fresh Eagle's medium and incubated for various periods at 37°C.

After incubation, cytosol and highly purified nuclei were prepared in buffer A without glycerol as described above. Nuclear pellets were extracted with 0.3 moles/ liter KCl in buffer A without glycerol at 4°C for 30 min. Then aliquots of labeled cytosol or nuclear extracts were layered on top of the glycerol gradient (5–35%)

and centrifuged at 105,000 × g for 18 hr in a SW 50 rotor (Beckman) at 4°C. Bovine serum albumin was used as a marker. Fractions were collected from the top of the gradient by means of the Isco piercing unit and drop counter. Radioactivity was measured in each fraction.

DEAE-Cellulose Ion-Exchange Chromatography

DEAE-cellulose (Whatman DE 52) was equilibrated in 10 mmoles/liter KH_2PO_4 buffer, pH 7.4. Labeled cytosol samples prepared in this buffer (5 ml cytosol incubated with 4 nmoles/liter [^{3}H]estradiol for 4 hr at 4°C followed by the dextran-coated charcoal treatment) were applied to packed columns (bed volume 8 ml) followed by a wash with the same buffer. A linear gradient to 0.4 moles/liter KCl was then introduced. Aliquots from collected fractions were withdrawn for radio-activity measurement. Protein elution profiles were traced from optical density

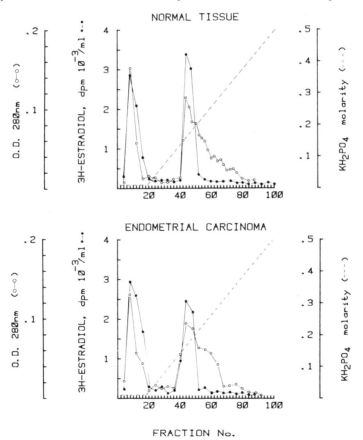

FIG. 4. Elution profiles of labeled cytosol from proliferative endometrium or undifferentiated endometrial carcinoma on a hydroxylapatite. For details, see Materials and Methods.

measurements at 280 nm. The KCl concentration of the effluent was determined conductimetrically.

Hydroxylapatite Chromatography

Columns with a bed volume of 50 ml were prepared with 15 g of hydroxylapatite (BIO RAD) equilibrated in 10 mmoles/liter KH_2PO_4 buffer, pH 7.4. Samples (5 ml) containing [^{3}H]estradiol-receptor complexes, prepared in 10 mmoles/liter KH_2PO_4 buffer, pH 7.4, were applied to hydroxylapatite columns and, after a 100 ml wash with the phosphate buffer, the adsorbed proteins were eluted with a linear gradient to 0.5 moles/liter KH_2PO_4 buffer adjusted to pH 7.4 with 1 moles/liter NaOH.

Competitive Process Experiments

Cytosol (0.2 ml) was incubated with 0.5 nmoles/liter [^{3}H]estradiol or 8 nmoles/ liter [^{3}H]R5020 and increasing amounts of unlabeled steroids for 16 hr at 4°C. Separation of unbound and bound steroid was achieved by the charcoal adsorption technique. Each incubation was carried out in duplicate.

Chemical Analysis

The DNA content of the tissue homogenates and nuclear suspensions was measured by using the method of Burton (4).

Protein concentration was measured by the method of Lowry et al. (16) using bovine serum albumin as standard.

RESULTS

Sucrose Density Centrifugation

Initial evidence for estrogen and gestagen binding in the cytosol of normal and neoplastic endometrium was provided by sucrose density gradient centrifugation (in the absence of KCl). Representative examples of the binding characteristics of normal and neoplastic endometrial samples are shown in Figs. 1 and 2. Each cytosol sample contained two binding components with sedimentation rates of about 4–5S and 8S. The 4–5S estradiol or R5020-binding macromolecule was only partially specific for [^{3}H]estradiol or [^{3}H]R5020, which was demonstrated by the inability of nonlabeled steroids to displace [^{3}H]R5020 or [^{3}H]estradiol completely from the 4–5S region. The sedimentation profiles revealed a striking similarity between the estrogen and gestagen binding components of normal endometrium and neoplastic tissue; however, the absolute amount of radioactivity per fraction varied significantly, suggesting different amounts of steroid binding activity per preparation.

Chromatographic Techniques

The elution profiles presented in Fig. 3 were obtained when [^{3}H]estradiol labeled cytosols of normal and neoplastic endometrium were chromatographed on dieth-

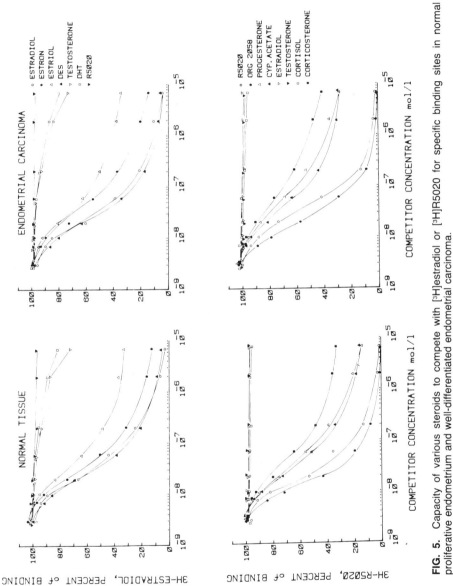

FIG. 5. Capacity of various steroids to compete with [3H]estradiol or [3H]R5020 for specific binding sites in normal proliferative endometrium and well-differentiated endometrial carcinoma.

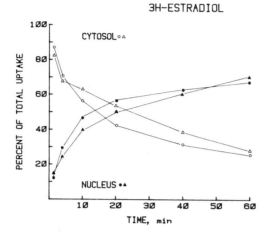

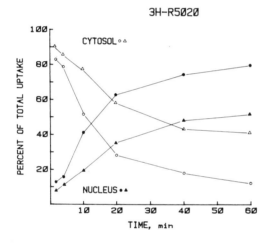

FIG. 6. Transfer of [³H]estradiol or [³H]R5020 from cytosol to nucleus in proliferative human endometrium (○, ●; six cases) and undifferentiated endometrial carcinoma (△, ▲; four cases) during *in vitro* incubation. Tissue slices were incubated in Eagle's medium for 10 min at 4°C with 20 nmoles/liter [³H]R5020, then rinsed and transferred to fresh Eagle's medium and incubated for various periods as indicated at 30°C. After incubation, the tissue was washed three times in buffer A, homogenized, and fractionated as described under Materials and Methods. Nuclear pellet was purified by passing through 2.4 moles/liter sucrose. Cytoplasmic fraction and purified nuclei were then extracted with chloroform/ethanol (3:1). The total extract of each sample was processed for liquid scintillation counting.

ylaminoethyl-(DEAE)cellulose. The [³H]estradiol binding components were repeatedly eluted from these columns over the whole extent of the linear KCl gradient used as elution medium. The KCl elution molarities were zero for the major peak. The elution profile obtained with endometrial carcinoma was similar to that of normal endometrium.

FIG. 7. Distribution of bound [³H]estradiol in the nuclear (●) and cytosplasmic (○) fractions of normal proliferative endometrium and undifferentiated carcinoma. Tissue slices were incubated in Eagle's medium for 10 min at 4°C with 8 nmoles/liter [³H]estradiol, then rinsed and transferred to fresh Eagle's medium and incubated for various periods as indicated at 30°C. Bound [³H]estradiol was measured in the cytosol and nuclear fractions by glycerol density gradient centrifugation (0.3 moles/liter KCl). For detail see Materials and Methods. *Arrow:* serum bovine albumin.

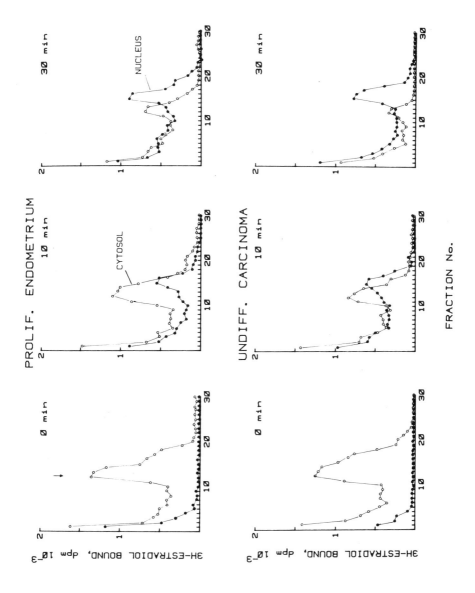

Fractionation of [³H]estradiol labeled cytosol from normal and neoplastic endometrium on hydroxyapatite was also of interest (Fig. 4). By elution with a linear KH_2PO_4 gradient, two peaks of radioactivity were produced, both of which were accompanied by 280 nm absorbing material. No differences in elution profiles could be found between normal and neoplastic endometrial tissue.

Competition Studies

Figure 5 illustrates the ability of various concentrations of unlabeled steroids to compete with [³H]estradiol or [³H]R5020 for specific binding. As anticipated for [³H]estradiol binding, estradiol and diethylstilbestrol both competed well. Estrone and estriol also both compete, although less potently than estradiol; testosterone and dihydrotestosterone competed less effectively; R5020 did not compete. There was no difference between the ligand specificity of the estradiol binding components of normal and neoplastic endometrium. The competition between various progestational and nonprogestational steroids for the [³H]R5020 binding sites at the cytoplasmic progesterone receptor of normal and neoplastic human endometrium demonstrates that R5020 and Org.2058, and to a lesser extent progesterone, cyproterone acetate, and corticosterone, competed effectively with [³H]R5020 for the binding sites on the endometrial receptor protein; however, the binding of [³H]R5020 was unchanged in the presence of testosterone, cortisol and estradiol. There was no difference between the specificity of the [³H]R5020 binding components of normal and neoplastic endometrium.

Measurement of Estradiol and R5020 Receptors
in Nuclei by Exchange Assay

Endometrial tissue slices were preincubated for 10 min at 4°C to allow passive diffusion of the ³H-labeled estradiol or R5020 into the cell, and the tissue was then incubated at 30°C for various periods as indicated in Fig. 6. The relative ³H contents of cytosol and purified nuclei were then determined. Initially, the tritium was located almost completely in the cytosol fraction, but relatively little was present in the purified nuclear pellet. Upon continued incubation, there was an increase in nuclear ³H binding and progressive decrease in ³H binding in the cytoplasm, suggesting that the hormone was sequentially transferred to the nucleus. The transfer mechanism in undifferentiated tumor is comparable to that in normal proliferative endometrium.

To determine whether the shift of [³H]estradiol or [³H]R5020 from the cytoplasmic to the nuclear compartment of the endometrial tissue *in vitro* requires and involves the progesterone receptor protein, the incubation procedure was repeated in the

FIG. 8. Distribution of bound [³H]R5020 in the nuclear (●) and cytoplasmic (○) fractions of normal proliferative endometrium and undifferentiated carcinoma. Tissue slices were incubated in Eagle's medium for 10 min at 4°C with 20 nmoles/liter [³H]R5020, then rinsed and transferred to fresh Eagle's medium and incubated for various periods as indicated at 30°C. Bound [³H]R5020 was measured in the cytosol and nuclear fractions by glycerol density gradient centrifugation (0.3 moles/liter KCl). For detail, see Materials and Methods. *Arrow:* Serum bovine albumin.

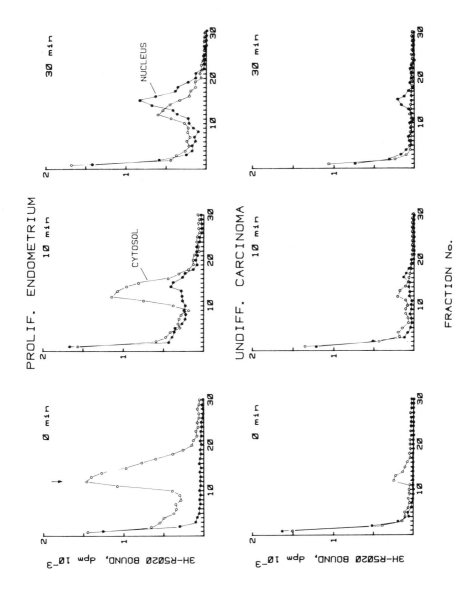

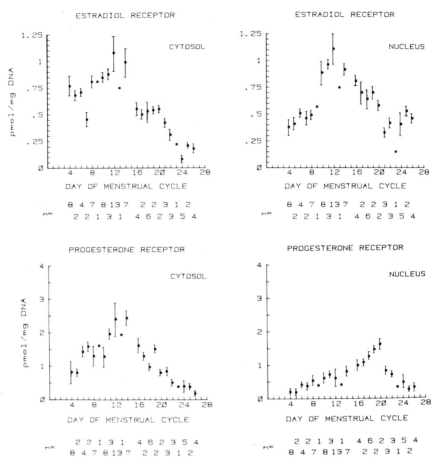

FIG. 9. Variation of the binding capacity for *in vitro* cytoplasmic and nuclear receptor binding to [³H]estradiol and [³H]R5020 of normal human endometrium as a function of menstrual cycle.

same manner; but now the ³H-labeled binding components for estradiol or R5020 in the cytoplasmic and nuclear fractions were characterized using glycerol gradient centrifugation. Figures 7 and 8 contain the results of these experiments. At zero time, the absence of [³H]estradiol and [³H]R5020 nuclear binding during preincubation of the tissue at 4°C for 10 min under conditions of cytoplasmic saturation with ³H-labeled steroid could be interpreted as evidence against artifactual adsorption of cytoplasmic components to the nuclei. At subsequent incubation times at 30°C, the quantity of salt extractable 4–5S [³H]estradiol and [³H]R5020 receptor complexes in the purified nuclear fraction increases.

Variations in Receptor Content During the Menstrual Cycle

Nuclei and cytosol were incubated from normal human endometrial tissue collected at various phases of the menstrual cycle and assayed for *in vitro* [³H]estradiol

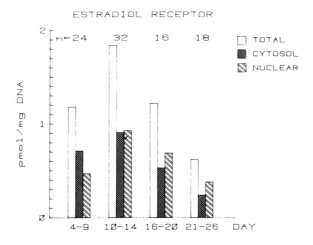

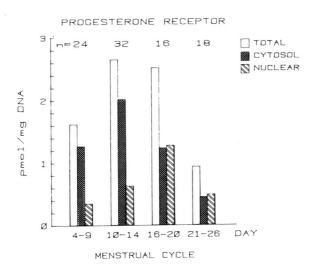

MENSTRUAL CYCLE

FIG. 10. Relationship between total, cytoplasmic, and nuclear receptor concentration for [³H]estradiol and [³H]R5020 in human endometrium during normal menstrual cycle.

and [³H]R5020 binding in cytoplasmic and nuclear fractions. The results, summarized in Fig. 9, show that estradiol and progesterone receptor levels in cytosol and nuclear fractions of normal endometrium are directly dependent on the phase of the menstrual cycle. The level of the [³H]estradiol cytoplasmic and nuclear binding sites was highest in the proliferative phase, with a tendency to increase in the late proliferative phase and decline sharply during the secretory phase. This increase was more than double for the nuclear receptor sites. The ratio of cytoplasmic receptor over nuclear receptor decreased (Fig. 10). Cytoplasmic and nuclear receptors for progesterone also were quantitated in all tissues. The number of cytoplasmic sites for progesterone paralleled those of available estradiol binding sites, whereas the concentration of nuclear progesterone binding sites increased towards the 20th day of the menstrual cycle.

Receptor Levels in Endometrial Carcinomas

No significant correlation was noted between the number of estradiol binding sites and the degree of tumor differentiation. The levels are high but with a tendency to decrease in the undifferentiated tumors. In 5 of 41 tissue samples of undifferentiated tumors, estradiol receptors were not measurable. In contrast, the progesterone data indicated that the number of progesterone binding sites in the carcinomas were related to the degree of tumor differentiation. Progesterone binding was lowest

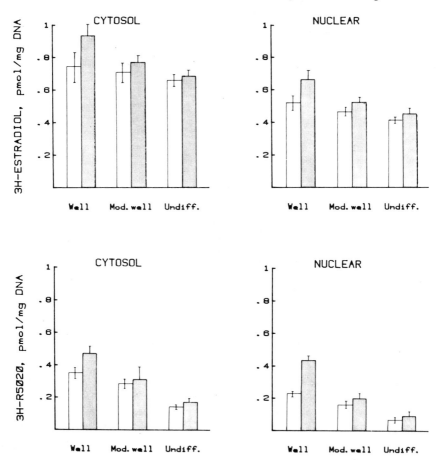

FIG. 11. [³H]Estradiol and [³H]R5020 receptor levels in the cytosol and nuclear fractions of endometrial carcinomas of 19 patients before (□) and after (▨) estrogen treatment. Administered dose of ethinylestradiol was 0.6 to 1.4 mg/day for 5 to 7 days. Well differentiated (five patients), moderately well differentiated (six patients), undifferentiated endometrial carcinoma (eight patients). Median values ± SD.

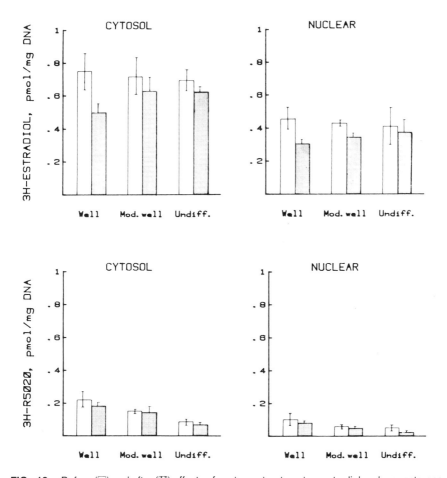

FIG. 12. Before (□) and after (▦) effects of gestagen treatment on estradiol and progesterone receptor levels of endometrial carcinomas of 22 patients. Gestagen used for oral treatment was medroxyprogesterone acetate (doses 100–500 mg/day for 1–2 weeks). Well differentiated (seven patients), moderately well differentiated (five patients), undifferentiated endometrial carcinoma (ten patients). Median values ± SD.

in undifferentiated carcinomas, comparable to the binding in the late secretory phase of a normal endometrium. In 17 of 41 tumor specimens of undifferentiated carcinomas, progesterone binding sites could not be detected (Table 1). Furthermore, it was evident that the specific activity of 17β-HSD decreases with decreasing differentiation of the tumor. It has been known for many years that estradiol-17β can be converted to estrone by human endometrium. Recently, the detailed studies of Gurpide and coworkers (7–10,39–41), including our own (25–32), showed that estradiol is oxidized about 10 times more rapidly in secretory than in proliferative human endometrium. This indicates that 17β-HSD functions as a regulator of estradiol activity in the endometrial target cell. Such comparisons may reveal dif-

TABLE 1. *Cytoplasmic and nuclear steroid receptors and 17β-hydroxysteroid dehydrogenase activity in human endometrial carcinoma dependent on the degree of tumor differentiation*

Degree of tumor differentiation[a]	Estradiol-receptor (fmoles/mg DNA)			Progesterone-receptor (fmoles/mg DNA)			Microsomal 17β-HSD-activity (nmoles E_1/mg protein/30 min)
	Total	Cytosol	Nuclear	Total	Cytosol	Nuclear	
Well-differentiated (56)	1,276 ± 286	712	564	700 ± 98 n = 43	413	287	4.99 ± 0.92 n = 40
Moderately well-differentiated (48)	1,151 ± 152	588	563	202 ± 58 n = 5 n.m.	111	91	1.5 ± 0.52 n = 8 n.m.
Undifferentiated (41)	n = 36 943 ± 168 n = 5 n.m.	491	452	n = 24 98 ± 46 n = 17 n.m.	61	37	n = 20 0.31 ± 0.13 n = 21 n.m.

[a]Numbers in parentheses represent number of cases.
n.m. = Not measurable.

TABLE 2. *Correlation between progesterone receptor capacity and responses after gestagen treatment of recurrent endometrial cancers*

Patient	PRC (fmoles/mg protein)	Degree of tumor-differentiation	Recurrence site	Treatment	Administered total dose (mg)	Response duration (months)
1	11	Undifferentiated	Vulva	MPA	5,700	0
2	n.m.	Undifferentiated	Lung	MPA	3,800	0
3	24	Undifferentiated	Lung	MPA	6,500	0
4	48	Moderately well differentiated	Liver	MPA	2,400	0
5	n.m.	Undifferentiated	Liver	MPA	3,000	0
6	8	Undifferentiated	Abdomen	MPA	5,000	0
7	32	Moderately well differentiated	Vagina	MPA	3,800	0
8	n.m.	Moderately well differentiated	Vagina	MPA	6,000	0
9	n.m.	Undifferentiated	Lung	MPA	6,200	0
10	21	Moderately well differentiated	Lung	MPA	5,700	0
11	n.m.	Undifferentiated	Brain	MPA	3,800	0
12	n.m.	Moderately well differentiated	Vagina	MPA	4,200	0
13	51	Well differentiated	Vulva	MPA	3,100	0
14	96	Moderately well differentiated	Lung	MPA	2,800	11
15	165	Well differentiated	Lung	MPA	5,600	18
16	63	Moderately well differentiated	Brain	MPA	4,200	24
17	712	Well differentiated	Abdomen	MPA	3,800	6
18	78	Moderately well differentiated	Abdominal wall	MPA	5,700	30
19	112	Well differentiated	Vulva	MPA	6,200	8
20	108	Well differentiated	Vagina	MPA	2,000	16
21	1,125	Well differentiated	Lung	MPA	2,000	12
22	248	Well differentiated	Liver	MPA	3,400	11

n.m. = Not measurable; PRC = progesterone receptor concentration; MPA = medroxy progesterone acetate.

ferences between normal and neoplastic cells that can be used for an *in vitro* test to identify hormone-responsive tumors, with the aim of selecting patients for therapy. The idea that there are two fundamentally different types of tumor cells, one of which contains steroid hormone receptors and/or 17β-HSD activity, leads to the possibility that the two tumor types can be distinguished. In 8 of 48 moderately well-differentiated, as well as in 21 of 41 undifferentiated tumor specimens, 17β-HSD activity could be detected.

A comparison of the receptor pattern in endometrial carcinoma demonstrated that 100% of well-differentiated carcinomas and 84% of moderately well-differentiated carcinomas were estradiol receptor and progesterone receptor-positive, whereas only 58% of undifferentiated endometrial carcinomas contained both estradiol and progesterone receptors. An estradiol receptor-negative and progesterone-receptor-positive tumor sample did emerge in any type of tissue.

Influence of Hormonal Treatment on Receptor Levels and 17β-HSD Activity

The estradiol and progesterone receptor levels in cytoplasmic and nuclear compartments of anaplastic carcinomas and more highly differentiated tumor forms, analyzed before and after estrogen treatment, are shown in Fig. 11. Estrogen treatment of patients increased both receptor levels, but this effect was less consistent in undifferentiated tumors than in more differentiated tumor forms. In contrast, after gestagen treatment of patients, the estradiol and progesterone receptor values decreased during the treatment period (Fig. 12).

The relationship between progesterone receptor concentration and clinical response of the carcinomas to treatment with medroxyprogesterone acetate (Upjohn) is shown in Table 2. A total of 22 endometrial carcinomas have been treated with medroxyprogesterone acetate, but we observed only nine responses. (The primary therapy consisted of irradiation and hysterectomy.) It is apparent that only the endometrial carcinoma with relatively high progesterone binding capacity showed a response to gestagen therapy.

DISCUSSION

The results presented in this investigation show the occurrence in normal human endometrial tissue as well as in endometrial carcinoma of high affinity, low capacity binding components in the cytoplasmic and nuclear fractions that reversibly bind estradiol and R5020. This result closely corresponds with other reports (3,5,6,11,12, 14,15,20,24,33,38).

When the characteristics of both sex hormone binding proteins from normal and neoplastic endometrium were compared, no differences could be found with regard to their affinity for estradiol or R5020, their sedimentation properties, or chromatographic patterns. These findings indicate that the neoplastic tissue may contain sex hormone receptors similar or identical to those from normal endometrial cytosol.

A notable observation of this investigation is that the number of cytoplasmic and nuclear binding sites for estradiol and progesterone has been found to change during the menstrual cycle. Variations in the levels of nuclear hormone binding proteins during the cycle are, however, of particular interest, as these receptor macromolecules have a direct effect in nuclear control. Similar results have been reported by other investigators (1).

In contrast, Robertson et al. (34) found the highest receptor concentration for estradiol during the luteal phase. Haukkamaa and Luukkainen (13) failed to detect any differences in the receptor levels in endometrial tissue samples collected during the proliferative and secretory phase of the menstrual cycle, although the highest binding activity was observed in hyperplastic endometria. The reason for these discrepancies is unknown at present.

Whether or not the total number of hormone receptors in the cells throughout the menstrual cycle is influenced by serum levels of steroid hormones remains to be clarified. As expected near the time of ovulation, at which the estradiol plasma level reaches its highest value (37), the total binding sites for both steroid hormones have their highest levels, indicating that the increase of estrogens during the proliferative phase leads to the synthesis of more receptor protein in the cytosol followed by the transfer of hormone receptor complexes into the nuclei. During the secretory phase when the hormone has completed its stimulation of endometrial secretion and when the blood level of progesterone is quite high, the number of binding sites for both hormones becomes low. The decrease of the total receptor content is explainable on the basis of the negative effect of gestagens on its own receptor and on the levels of estradiol binding sites.

Further, a correlation was noted between the number of nuclear and cytoplasmic binding sites of progesterone and the degree of differentiation of the endometrial carcinoma, which parallels the progestational sensitivity of these tumors. The concentration of progesterone binding sites in undifferentiated tumor was as low as in late secretory endometrium. In contrast, well-differentiated tumors contained a relatively high concentration of progesterone binding sites. This might explain why progestational agents play a definite role in the management of advanced adenocarcinoma of the endometrium and why response to progestational agents is more likely in those patients with well-differentiated tumors (25–32,37). No significant correlation was observed between the number of estradiol binding sites and the degree of differentiation of the tumor.

These data are in agreement with those of other investigators (33,42–45) indicating that the number of progesterone binding sites in human endometrial carcinomata is related to the degree of differentiation.

In addition, an increase in the endometrial estradiol and progesterone receptor levels occurred after treatment of patients with ethinylestradiol, whereas a drop in receptor levels for both steroid hormones could be observed when patients were treated with potent synthetic gestagens. These findings are in agreement with data obtained from animal experiments. Milgrom et al. (18,19) found that steroid hormone receptors in guinea pig uterus are under dual steroidal control: Estrogens induce the biosynthesis of new receptor protein, whereas progesterone displays a negative control over receptor levels.

Taken together, there seems to be support for the idea that an "estrogen priming" could be of value in progestogen treatment of endometrial cancer. It is well known that the likelihood of response to progestogen therapy is increased considerably when there is evidence of an adequate endogenous estrogen production (17). Estrogens have also been found to potentiate the effect of progesterone on endometrial cancer tissue in organ culture (22). It is thus tempting to speculate that a long-term progestagen treatment should be supplemented periodically by estrogen treatment.

REFERENCES

1. Bayard, F., Damilano, S., Robel, P., and Baulieu, E.-E. (1978): Cytoplasmic and nuclear estradiol and progesterone receptors in human endometrium. *J. Clin. Endocrinol. Metab.*, 46:635–648.
2. Brush, M. G., Taylor, R. W., and King, R. J. B. (1967): The uptake of [6,7-³H]-oestradiol by the normal human female reproductive tract. *J. Endocrinol.*, 39:599–607.
3. Brush, M. G., King, R. J. B., Taylor, R. W., eds. (1978): *Endometrial Cancer*. Bailliere Tindall, London.
4. Burton, K. (1968): Determination of DNA concentration with diphenylamine. In: *Methods of Enzymology*, edited by L. Grossmann and K. Moldave, pp. 163. Academic Press, New York.
5. Ehrlich, C. E., Yound, P. C. M., and Cleary, R. E. (1981): Cytoplasmic progesterone and estradiol receptors in normal, hyperplastic, and carcinomatous endometria: Therapeutic implications. *Am. J. Obstet. Gynecol.*, 141:539–546.
6. Evans, L. H., and Hähnel, R. (1971): Oestrogen receptors in human uterine tissue. *J. Endocrinol.*, 50:209–229.
7. Gurpide, E., Gusberg, S. B., and Tseng, L. (1976): Estradiol binding and metabolism in human endometrial hyperplasia and adenocarcinoma. *J. Steroid Biochem.*, 7:891–896.
8. Gurpide, E., and Tseng, L. (1976): Estrogens in normal human endometrium. In: *Receptors and Mechanism of Action of Steroid Hormones*, edited by J. R. Pasqualini, pp. 109–158. Marcel Dekker, New York and Basel.
9. Gurpide, E., Tseng, L., and Gusberg, S. B. (1977): Estrogen metabolism in normal and neoplastic endometrium. *Am. J. Obstet. Gynecol.*, 129:809–816.
10. Gurpide, E., and Tseng, L. (1978): Potentially useful tests for responsiveness of endometrial cancer to progesterone therapy. In: *Endometrial Cancer*, edited by M. G. Brush, R. J. B. King, and R. W. Taylor, pp. 252–257. Bailliere Tindall, London.
11. Gustafsson, J.-Ä., Einhorn, N. Elfström, G., Nordensköld, B., and Wrange, O. (1977): Progestin receptor in endometrial carcinoma. In: *Progesterone receptors in normal and neoplastic tissues*, edited by W. L. McGuire, J.-P. Raynaud, E.-E. Baulieu, pp. 299–312. Raven Press, New York.
12. Haukkamaa, M., Karjalainen, O., and Luukkainen, T. (1971): In vitro binding of progesterone by the human endometrium during the menstrual cycle and by hyperplastic, atrophic, and carcinomatous endometrium. *Am. J. Obstet. Gynecol.*, 111:205–210.
13. Haukkamaa, M., and Luukkainen, T. (1974): The cytoplasmic progesterone receptor of human endometrium during the menstrual cycle. *J. Steroid Biochem.*, 5:447–452.
14. Jänne, O., Kauppila, A., Kontula, K., Syrjälä, P., and Vihko, R. (1979): Female sex steroid receptors in normal hyperplastic and carcinomatous endometrium. The relationship to serum steroid hormones and gonadotropins and changes during medroxyprogesterone acetate administration. *Int. J. Cancer.*, 24:545–554.
15. Kontula, K., Jänne, O., Luukkainen, T., and Vihko, R. (1973): Progesterone-binding protein in human myometrium. Ligand specificity and some physicochemical characteristics. *Biochim. Biophys. Acta*, 328:145–153.
16. Lowry, O. H., Rosebrough, N. J., Farr, A. L., and Randall, R. J. (1951): Protein measurement with the Folin phenol reagent. *J. Biol. Chem.*, 193:265–275.
17. Lucas, W. E. (1974): Causal relationships between endocrine-metabolic variables in patients with endometrial carcinoma. *Obstet. Gynecol. Survey*, 29:507–512.
18. Milgrom, E., and Baulieu, E.-E. (1970): Progesterone in uterus and plasma. I. Binding in rat uterus; 05,000 g supernatant. *Endocrinology*, 87:276–287.
19. Milgrom, E., Atger, M., Perrot, M., and Baulieu, E.-E. (1972): Progesterone in uterus and

plasma. VI. Uterine progesterone receptors during the estrus cycle and implantation in the guinea pig. *Endocrinology*, 90:1071–1078.

20. Milton, P. J. D., Taylor, R. W., and Crocker, S. G. (1973): Oestradiol receptors in the cytoplasm of pre-cancerous and cancerous human endometrium. *Acta Endocrinol. (Suppl.)*, 177:245.
21. Morrow, C. P., DiSaia, P. J., and Townsend, D. E. (1973): Current management of endometrial carcinoma. *Obstet. Gynecol.*, 42:399–406.
22. Nordqvist, S. (1973): Aspects of the cellular action of progesterone with particular reference to endometrial carcinoma. In: *Symposium on endometrial carcinoma*, edited by M. G. Brush, R. W. Taylor, and D. C. Williams, pp. 34–48. Heinemann, London.
23. Noyes, R. W., Hertig, A. T., and Rock, J. (1950): Dating the endometrial biopsy. *Fertil. Steril.*, 1:3–25.
24. Philibert, D., and Raynaud, J. P. (1974): Binding of progesterone and R5020, a highly potent progestin, to human endometrium and myometrium. *Contraception*, 10:457–466.
25. Pollow, K., Lübbert, H., Boquoi, E., Kreuzer, G., and Pollow, B. (1975): Characterization and comparison of receptors for estradiol and progesterone in human proliferative endometrium and endometrial carcinoma. *Endocrinology*, 96:319–328.
26. Pollow, K., Boquoi, E., Lübbert, H., and Pollow, B. (1975): Effect of gestagen therapy upon 17β-hydroxysteroid dehydrogenase in human endometrial adenocarcinoma. *J. Endocrinol.*, 67:131–132.
27. Pollow, K., Lübbert, H., Boquoi, E., Kreuzer, G., Jeske, R., and Pollow, B. (1975): Studies on 17β-hydroxysteroid dehydrogenase in human endometrium and endometrial carcinoma. I. Subcellular distribution and variations of specific enzyme activity. *Acta Endocrinol.*, 79:134–145.
28. Pollow, K., Boquoi, E., Schmidt-Gollwitzer, M., and Pollow, B. (1976): The nuclear estradiol and progesterone receptors of human endometrium and endometrial carcinoma. *J. Mol. Med.*, 1:325–342.
29. Pollow, K., Lübbert, H., and Pollow, B. (1976): Partial purification and evidence for heterogeneity of the cytoplasmic 17β-hydroxysteroid dehydrogenase from normal human endometrium and endometrial carcinoma. *J. Steroid Biochem.*, 7:315–320.
30. Pollow, K., Schmidt-Gollwitzer, M., and Nevinny-Stickel, J. (1977): Progesterone receptors in normal human endometrium and endometrial carcinoma. In: *Progesterone Receptors in Normal and Neoplastic Tissues*, edited by W. L. McGuire, J.-P. Raynaud, and E.-E. Baulieu, pp. 313–338. Raven Press, New York.
31. Pollow, K., Schmidt-Gollwitzer, M., Boquoi, E., and Pollow, B. (1978): Influence of estrogens and gestagens on 17β-hydroxysteroid dehydrogenase in human endometrium and endometrial carcinoma. *J. Mol. Med.*, 3:81–89.
32. Pollow, K. (1981): Oestradiol and progesterone in normal and abnormal human uterine tissue. In: *Hormones in Normal and Abnormal Human Tissues*, edited by K. Fotherby, and S. B. Pal, pp. 373–408. Walter de Gruyter, Berlin, New York.
33. Richardson, G. S., and MacLaughlin, D. T., eds. (1978): *Hormonal Biology of Endometrial Cancer, Vol. 43*. UICC Technical Report Series.
34. Robertson, D. M., Mester, J., Beilby, J., Steele, S. J., and Kellie, A. E. (1971): The measurement of high-affinity oestradiol receptors in human uterine endometrium and myometrium. *Acta Endocrinol.*, 68:534–542.
35. Rozier, J. C., and Underwood, P. B. (1974): Use of progestational agents in endometrial adenocarcinoma. *Obstet. Gynecol.*, 44:60–64.
36. Scatchard, G. (1949): The attraction of proteins for small molecules and ions. *Ann. NY Acad. Sci.*, 51:660–672.
37. Schmidt-Gollwitzer, M., Genz, T., Schmidt-Gollwitzer, K., Pollow, B., and Pollow, K. (1978): Correlation between oestradiol and progesterone receptor levels, 17β-hydroxysteroid dehydrogenase activity and endometrial tissue levels of oestradiol, oestrone and progesterone in women. In: *Endometrial Cancer*, edited by M. G. Brush, R. J. B. King, and R. W. Taylor, pp. 227–241. Bailliere Tindall, London.
38. Terenius, L., Lindell, A., and Persson, B. H. (1971): Binding of estradiol to human cancer tissue of the female genital tract. *Cancer Res.*, 31:1895–1898.
39. Tseng, L., and Gurpide, E. (1972): Changes in the in vitro metabolism of estradiol by human endometrium during the menstrual cycle. *Am. J. Obstet. Gynecol.*, 114:1002–1008.
40. Tseng, L., and Gurpide, E. (1975): Induction of human endometrial estradiol dehydrogenase by progestin. *Endocrinology*, 97:825–833.

41. Tseng, L. (1978): Steroid specificity in the stimulation of human endometrial estradiol dehydrogenase. *Endocrinology*, 102:1398–1403.
42. Tseng, L., Gusberg, S. B., and Gurpide, E. (1977): Estradiol receptor and 17β-dehydrogenase in normal and abnormal human endometrium. *Ann. N.Y. Acad. Sci.*, 286:190–198.
43. Wrange, Ö., Nordenskjöld, B., and Gustafsson, J.-Ä. (1978): Cytosol estradiol receptor in human mammary carcinoma: An assay based on isoelectric focusing in polyacrylamide gel. *Anal. Biochem.*, 85:461–475.
44. Young, P. C. M., and Cleary, R. E. (1974): Characterization and properties of progesterone-binding components in human endometrium. *J. Clin. Endocrinol. Metab.*, 39:425–439.
45. Young, P. C. M., Ehrlich, C. E., and Cleary, R. E. (1976): Progesterone binding in human endometrial carcinomas. *Am. J. Obstet. Gynecol.*, 125:353–360.

Steroids and Endometrial Cancer,
edited by V. M. Jasonni, et al.
Raven Press, New York © 1983.

Estrogen and Progesterone Receptors in Postmenopausal Endometrial Carcinoma: The Potential of a Dynamic Test Using Tamoxifen

*Etienne-Emile Baulieu, *Paul Robel, **Rodrigue Mortel, and †Carlos Lévy

*INSERM U 33 and CNRS ER 125, Lab Hormones, 94270 Bicêtre, France;
**The Milton S. Hershey Medical Center, The Pennsylvania State University,
Hershey, Pennsylvania 17033; and †Institute of Oncology "Angel H. Roffo,"
Buenos Aires, Argentina

Endometrial carcinoma occurs most frequently in postmenopausal women, and epidemiological studies have shown an increased risk in women exposed to prolonged unopposed estrogenic stimulation (9,33,35). It is equally well accepted that progestational agents achieve objective remission in 30 to 35% of patients with advanced or metastatic endometrial cancer (16,32,33). However, based on clinical criteria, it is not possible to select those patients likely to benefit from hormonal therapy. Therefore, we have tried to set up an *in vivo* biochemical test to relate receptors and hormonal sensitivity in endometrial cancers.

Two tumor samples could be obtained, the first before and the second one after administration of tamoxifen. Tamoxifen binds to estradiol receptor (ER), and tamoxifen-receptor complexes accumulate into the nucleus. It was anticipated that the exposure of tumor cells to the drug would be indicated by the increase of nuclear estrogen receptor. The tumor response to tamoxifen, on the other hand, would be demonstrated by the increase of progesterone receptor (2,23,25).

MATERIALS AND METHODS

Forty-three patients with histologically proven adenocarcinoma of the endometrium were seen in consultation and treated by Dr. J. P. Wolff at the Institut Gustave Roussy, Villejuif. Their age ranged from 43 to 75 years with a mean of 62. All patients menopaused spontaneously for at least 3 years. A minimum of 200 mg of tumor tissue was obtained by uterine curettage, part of which was submitted to pathology for histologic confirmation. The degree of tumor differentiation was reported according to the FIGO classification; Grade 1, well-differentiated; Grade 2, moderately differentiated; and Grade 3, anaplastic tumors.

Two partial outpatient uterine curettages were performed on 25 patients; the first at the time of referral, the second during surgery or immediately before radiotherapy. After the first biopsy, 15 patients received 40 mg of tamoxifen orally each day for 5 to 7 days (Group 1); the second endometrial sampling was performed 12 to 18 hr after the last dose. Ten patients ingested 10 mg 8 hr and 4 hr before the second curettage (Group 2). Receptor concentrations were determined in all samples as reported in detail by Bayard et al. (2) and Lévy et al. (19,20). In addition, the activities of ornithinedecarboxylase (ODC) (15), estradiol 17β-hydroxysteroid dehydrogenase (EDH), (28,30) and serum hormones were evaluated before and after tamoxifen treatment.

RESULTS

Estradiol and Progesterone Receptors

No receptors in either cytosol or nuclei were detected in one tumor examined for estradiol receptor or in five tumors assayed for progesterone receptor (Table 1). When present, most estradiol and progesterone receptors were found in the cytosol. However, the totality or majority of receptors were located in the nuclei of 11 samples assayed for estradiol and in five tumors examined for progesterone. No attempt was made in this study to determine if nuclear receptors were occupied by endogenous hormones.

Although the difference was not statistically significant among the groups, there was a clear tendency for the well-differentiated Grade 1 tumors to contain higher levels of estradiol and progesterone receptors than the Grade 2 carcinomas. The small number of Grade 3 cases allowed no comparison.

Hormonal Correlations of Receptors

Estradiol values did not change with the degree of tumor differentiation, but a highly significant difference ($P < 0.01$) was observed in the mean estrone levels of patients from well to moderately differentiated cancers (Table 2). It may be related to a difference in body weight (63.6 ± 13.6 in Grade 1 versus 76.6 ± 16.0 kg in Grade 2 patients).

We found no significant correlation between estradiol and progesterone receptors and serum levels of estrone, estradiol, or progesterone even within the histologically defined groups.

Effects of Tamoxifen

Following tamoxifen administration, Group 1 and Group 2 patients did not demonstrate any significant increase in estrogen receptor concentration in their tumors. In Group 2, where tamoxifen administration immediately preceded the curettage, the ratio of cytoplasmic to nuclear receptors shifted in favor of nuclear receptors, as previously observed in animal model experiments (36).

TABLE 1. *Estradiol and progesterone receptors in postmenopausal endometrial carcinoma (pmoles/mg DNA)*

			Estradiol receptor		Progesterone receptor	
Grade	Id	Age	Total	C/N	Total	C/N
1	W4	49	1.63	1.94	1.33	2.02
(N = 22)	W16	76	1.57	>10	1.02	1.42
	W17	64	0.79	4.64	0.24	>10
	W23	53	0.64	>10	N.D.	N.D.
	W26	74	1.43	>10	0.70	>10
	W45	47	5.71	4.14	12.01	62.20
	W46	67	5.67	3.26	14.38	22.97
	W71	43	1.25	0.64	0.41	2.73
	W101	58	0.62	2.44	0.50	1.94
	W32	63	8.80	4.20	1.39	3.21
	W35	53	4.40	14.70	0.94	3.70
	W40	70	0.82	5.80	0.71	6.10
	W41	70	0.39	0	0.27	>10
	W51	65	2.54	>10	2.06	>10
	W53	60	0.92	>10	0.72	>10
	W55	67	0.99	0.50	0	—
	W59	68	0.92	2.83	1.79	16.90
	W65	57	0.34	0	0	0
	W67	76	7.34	3.80	1.61	>10
	W69	64	1.75	0	2.72	0
	W75	65	0.67	0.56	3.39	16.00
	W103	52	1.13	6.06	1.39	5.04
2	W18	71	0.72	4.53	0.11	>10
(N = 13)	W21	54	0.74	1.47	1.23	1.92
	W30	56	3.18	9.96	0.66	0.47
	W57	66	0.83	0.66	0.45	>10
	W81	65	0.36	1.57	0.65	>10
	W83	68	2.05	0	1.20	0.90
	W95	64	1.24	4.39	2.83	6.64
	W98	68	0.53	>10	0.80	>10
	W107	54	0.62	>10	1.51	>10
	W110	59	0	—	0	—
	W113	55	0.36	0.89	0	—
	W115	60	0.24	0	0.58	>10
	R1	65	0.57	0.78	0.16	0
3	W28	68	0.29	>10	0	—
(N = 4)	W34	75	3.25	10.6	0	—
	W61	69	4.03	3.48	3.11	>10
	W109	70	N.D.	N.D.	0.72	>10

Id = identification; C/N = cytosol to nuclear ratio; N.D. = not determined.

Progesterone receptor sites increased significantly in all but four samples in Group 1 patients (Table 3) and even appeared in three tumors (two Grade 1, one Grade 3) where the receptor was not measurable before tamoxifen. In Group 2 patients, no increase of the progesterone receptors was generally observed.

No statistical difference was observed in ODC and EDH activities or serum estrogens and progesterone for either group before and after tamoxifen treatment. We also found no correlation between tumor grading and ODC or EDH activity.

TABLE 2. *Serum levels of estrone, estradiol, and progesterone in patients with postmenopausal endometrial carcinoma[a]*

Endometrial carcinoma	Estrone	Estradiol	Progesterone
Whole series	33.8 ± 2.5 (43)	23.6 ± 1.5 (42)	435.6 ± 48.6 (42)
Grade 1	29.3 ± 2.9 (24)	22.0 ± 1.6 (23)	439.9 ± 55.9 (23)
Grade 2	43.0 ± 4 (15)[b]	25.6 ± 2.9 (15)	451.0 ± 102.0 (15)
Grade 3	57.2 ± 15.3 (4)	27.2 ± 7.7 (4)	361.0 ± 10.3 (4)

Number of cases in parentheses.
[a]pg/ml serum, mean ± standard error.
[b]$P < 0.01$ (nonparametric Wilcoxon rank order test).

DISCUSSION

Widespread concentrations of estradiol receptors were measured in 36 of 37 tumors examined. The mean values observed in this study support the findings of Tseng et al. (38) that in postmenopausal endometrial carcinoma the level of estradiol receptors is similar to that in the endometrium of normal women in the proliferative phase of the cycle. Crocker et al. (4) and Pollow et al. (30) found estradiol receptors in all endometrial cancer samples, but Grilli et al. (7) and Muechler et al. (26) reported estrogen receptors in 67 to 92% of the specimens assayed. Therefore, it appears that estradiol receptors are present in a large majority of endometrial adenocarcinomas.

Of 38 tumors assayed for progesterone receptors, 10 contained undetectable or insignificant amounts of receptors (<0.3 pmole/mg DNA). In 6 cases, the concentration was comparable to that of normal proliferative phase. In the majority of samples, as also reported by Pollow et al. (31), the range and mean values were similar to those observed in late secretory endometrium. Consequently, the estrogen/progesterone receptor ratio in these postmenopausal adenocarcinomas was generally greater than in normal premenopausal endometrium. Unexpectedly, the receptor concentration was much higher in the nuclear fractions from six specimens examined for estradiol and from two tumors tested for progesterone. In addition, all receptors were located in the nuclei of five samples assayed for estradiol and of two specimens examined for progesterone. Such findings are in keeping with the recent observations suggesting that unoccupied estrogen receptor sites are present in the nuclei of normal endometrium (6,18). Therefore, it appears that simultaneous measurement of both cytoplasmic and nuclear receptor sites is necessary to report accurately the total intracellular receptor concentration and before tumors could be classified as so-called "receptor negative."

The relationship between receptor levels and the degree of tumor differentiation has been the subject of conflicting reports. Our study provided no clear-cut answer to this question, as no statistical difference was found among the groups. However,

TABLE 3. *Estradiol and progesterone receptors (pmol/mgDNA)
in endometrial carcinoma before and after tamoxifen*

			Before					After			
			Estradiol receptors		Progesterone receptors		Tamoxifen	Estradiol receptors		Progesterone receptors	
Id #	Age	Grade	Total	C/N	Total	C/N		Total	C/N	Total	C/N
W30	56	2	3.18	9.96	0.66	0.46	Group 1 40 mg daily × 5–7 days	9.63	9.24	1.42	5.70
W31	63	1	8.80	4.20	1.29	3.21		6.16	8.33	8.96	37.95
W34	75	3	3.25	10.60	0	—		4.55	17.20	0.39	1.60
W35	53	1	4.40	14.71	0.94	3.70		6	21.22	1.24	5.52
W40	70	1	0.82	5.83	0.71	6.10		0.65	>10	1.50	>10
W41	70	1	0.39	0	0.27	>10		0.25	0	0.76	0
W51	65	1	2.54	>10	2.06	>10		2.15	3.30	5.88	>10
W53	60	1	0.92	>10	0.72	>10		2.60	1.54	6.78	>10
W55	67	1	0.99	0.50	0	—		0	—	0.30	>10
W57	66	2	0.83	0.66	0.45	>10		1.91	1.37	1.74	>10
W59	68	1	0.92	2.83	1.79	16.9		0	—	0.31	0
W65	57	1	0.34	0	0	—		0.84	0.29	0.58	3.46
W67	76	1	7.34	3.79	1.61	>10		7.28	0.39	6.35	13.43
W69	64	1	1.75	0	2.72	0		2.88	1.04	1.73	0.13
W115	60	2	0.24	0	0.58	>10		0	—	0.58	1.76
R1	65	2	0.57	0.78	0.16	0	Group 2 10 mg at – 8 and – 4 hr	0.65	0	0.39	0
W75	65	1	0.67	0.55	3.39	16		1.31	0.45	3.92	—
W81	65	2	0.36	1.57	0.64	>10		1.72	2.58	0.82	1.7
W83	68	2	2.05	0	1.20	0.9		>3	—	2.19	0
W95	64	2	1.24	4.39	2.83	6.6		0.63	1.1	1.21	>10
W98	68	2	0.53	>10	0.80	>10		0.97	4.7	3.11	27
W103	52	1	1.13	6.06	1.39	5		0.45	3.09	0.86	1.3
W107	54	2	0.62	>10	1.51	>10		0.74	5.72	1.19	>10
W109	70	3	N.D.	N.D.	0.72	>10		N.D.	N.D.	0.13	0
W110	59	2	0	—	0	—		0	—	0	—

C/N = cytosol to nuclear ratio.
N.D. = not determined.

as reported by other investigators (10,30,39), this study showed a clear tendency for well-differentiated tumors to contain higher levels of both estrogen and progesterone receptors.

The role played by estrogens in the etiology of endometrial cancer and the high estradiol receptor to progesterone receptor ratio found in carcinoma samples prompted us to investigate the biochemical changes following antiestrogen administration as a test of *in vivo* tumor sensitivity. Contrary to the test with medroxyprogesterone acetate, which acts via the progesterone receptor (8,29), tamoxifen is active via the estrogen receptor of the tumor. In the rodent uterus, it increases progesterone receptor concentrations (12,13). In addition, in human breast cancer cells in culture, tamoxifen stops estrogen promoted-growth but at some concentrations increases progesterone receptors (21). Moreover, tamoxifen has been used with good results in the treatment of advanced human breast cancer (17,22), particularly in postmenopausal women (24) and the increased sex hormone binding plasma protein observed in these patients was attributed to an estrogenic effect (34). In our study, when tamoxifen was given at a dose of 40 mg daily for 5 to 7 days, large increase of the progesterone receptor concentration was noted in about 60% of Group 1 estradiol and progesterone receptor positive tumors. Similar findings were observed in patients with metastatic breast cancers (27). Such effects were not apparent when the antiestrogen was administered in short term (8 hr and 4 hr before the second endometrial sampling) (5).

Ornithinedecarboxylase is an enzyme whose activity has been associated with a variety of cell proliferative responses (3,15,37). No changes in ODC activity were observed in our patients. These results are in keeping with observations that in the rat uterus and cultured mouse L cells tamoxifen does not accelerate cell division (13,14).

A serious difficulty related to receptor studies in malignant tumors is the heterogeneity of the sample. Such difficulty may have been increased by repeated curettage of the same tumors. In addition, complex hormonal changes may be elicited at the pituitary, adrenal, or ovarian level following administration of antiestrogen. However, such changes are unlikely to be very prominent in postmenopausal women, and no change of plasma sex steroid has been recorded.

Progestagens are of definite value in the treatment of patients with advanced or metastatic endometrial carcinoma (16,32,33). As demonstrated for breast cancers, responders are likely to have receptor-positive tumors (1). However, one drawback of progesterone therapy is the decrease of progesterone receptor concentration (11). Thus, any product which, like tamoxifen, could increase progesterone receptors without enhancing tumor growth would be helpful in increasing the magnitude and/ or duration of response in patients with endometrial cancer. However, further investigations are needed to establish the therapeutic merits of tamoxifen and the predictive value of the tamoxifen challenge test for the selection of patients with endometrial carcinoma likely to respond to hormone therapy.

ACKNOWLEDGMENTS

We are indebted to Bernard Eychenne and Monique Synguelakis for their expert technical assistance, to Jean Claude Nicolas for the assay of estradiol-dehydrogenase, and to Martine Rossillon for preparing the manuscript.

REFERENCES

1. Allegra, J. C., Lippman, M. E., Thompson, E., Simon, R., Barlock, A., Green, L., Huff, K. K., Hoan, M. Y. T., Do, Aitken, S. C., and Warren, R. (1979): Relationship between the progesterone, androgen and glucocorticoid receptor and response rate to endocrine therapy in metastatic breast cancer. *Cancer Res.*, 39:1973–1979.
2. Bayard, F., Damilano, S., Robel, P., and Baulieu, E. E. (1978): Cytoplasmic and nuclear estradiol and progesterone receptors in human endometrium. *J. Clin. Endocrinol. Metab.*, 46:635–648.
3. Bulger, W. H., and Dupfer, D. (1977): Inhibition of the 1-(*o*-chlorophenyl)-1-(-*p*-chlorophenyl) 2,4,2-trichloroethane (*O*,*p*'DDT) and estradiol mediated induction of rat uterine ornithine decarboxylase by prior treatment with *O*,*p*'DDT, estradiol and tamoxifen. *Arch. Biochem. Biophys.*, 182:138–146.
4. Crocker, S. G., Milton, P. J. D., and King, R. J. B. (1974): Uptake of 6,7 ^{3}H-estradiol 17β by normal and abnormal human endometrium. *J. Endocrinol.*, 62:145–152.
5. Davies, P., Syne, J. S., and Nicholson, R. I. (1979): Effects of estradiol and the antiestrogen tamoxifen on steroid hormone receptor concentration and nuclear ribonucleic acid polymerase activities in rat uterus. *Endocrinology*, 105:1336–1342.
6. Fleming, H., and Gurpide, E. (1980): Available estradiol receptors in nuclei from human endometrium. *J. Steroid Biochem.*, 13:3–11.
7. Grilli, S., Ferrari, A. M., Gola, G., Rochetta, R., Orlandi, C., and Prodi, G. (1977): Cytoplasmic receptors for 17β-estradiol, 5α-dihydro-testosterone and progesterone in normal and abnormal uterine tissue. *Cancer Lett.*, 2:247–258.
8. Gurpide, E., and Tseng, L. (1978): Potentially useful test for responsiveness of endometrial cancer to progestagen therapy. In: *Endometrial Cancer*, edited by M. G. Brush, R. J. B. King, and R. W. Taylor, pp. 252–257. Bailliere Tindall, London.
9. Gusberg, S. B. (1976): The individual at high risk for endometrial carcinoma. *Am. J. Obstet. Gynecol.*, 126:535–542.
10. Gustafsson, J. A., Einhorn, N., Elfstrom, G., Nordenskjold, B., and Wrange, O. (1977): Progestin receptor in endometrial carcinoma. In: *Progesterone Receptors in Normal and Neoplastic Tissues*, edited by W. L. McGuire, J. P. Raynaud, and E. E. Baulieu, pp. 299–312. Raven Press, New York.
11. Jänne, O., Kauppila, A., Kontula, K., Syrjälä, P., Vierikko, P., and Vihko, R. (1980): Female sex steroid receptors in human endometrial hyperplasia and carcinoma. In: *Steroid Receptors and Hormone Dependent Neoplasia*, edited by J. L. Wittliff, and I. Dapunt, pp. 37–44. Masson Publishing USA, Inc., New York.
12. Jordan, V. C., Dix, C. J., Rowsby, L., and Prestwich, G. (1977): Studies on the mechanism of action of the nonsteroidal antioestrogen tamoxifen (ICI 46,474) in the rat. *Mol. Cell. Endocrinol.*, 7:177–192.
13. Jordan, V. C., and Dix, C. J. (1979): Effect of estradiol benzoate, tamoxifen and monohydroxytamoxifen on immature rat uterine progesterone receptor synthesis and endometrial cell division. *J. Steroid Biochem.*, 11:285–291.
14. Jung-Testas, I., and Baulieu, E. E. (1979): Effects of sex steroids and antihormones on growth, adhesiveness and receptors of L-929 cells cultured in serum containing and serum free media. *Exp. Cell Res.*, 119:75–85.
15. Kaye, A. M., Icekson, I., and Lindner, H. R. (1971): Stimulation by estrogens of ornithine and *S*-adenosyl methionine decarboxylase in the immature rat uterus. *Biochim. Biophys. Acta*, 252:150–159.
16. Kohorn, E. I. (1976): Gestagens and endometrial carcinoma. *Gynecol. Oncol.*, 4:398–411.
17. Lerner, H. Jr., Band, P. R., Israel, L., and Leung, B. S. (1976): Phase II. Study of tamoxifen: Report of 74 patients with stage IV breast cancer. *Cancer Treat. Rep.*, 60:1431–1435.

18. Lévy, C., Mortel, R., Eychenne, B., Robel, P., and Baulieu, E. E. (1980): Unoccupied nuclear oestradiol-receptor sites in normal human endometrium. *Biochem. J.*, 185:733–738.
19. Lévy, C., Eychenne, B., and Robel, P. (1980): Assay of nuclear estradiol receptors by exchange on glass fiber filters. *Biochim. Biophys. Acta*, 630:301–305.
20. Lévy, C., Robel, P., Gautray, J. P., DeBrux, J., Verma, U., Descomps, B., and Baulieu, E. E. (1980): Estradiol and progesterone receptors in human endometrium: Normal and abnormal menstrual cycles and early pregnancy. *Am. J. Obstet. Gynecol.*, 136:646–651.
21. Lippman, M., Bolan, G., and Huff, K. (1976): The effects of oestrogens and antioestrogens on hormone responsive human breast cancer in long-term tissue culture. *Cancer Res.*, 36:4595–4601.
22. Manni, A., Trujillo, J. E., Marshall, J. S., Brodkey, S., and Pearson, O. (1979): Antihormone treatment of stage IV breast cancer. *Cancer*, 43:444–450.
23. Milgrom, E., Luu Thi, M., Atger, M., and Baulieu, E. E. (1973): Mechanisms regulating the concentration and the conformation of progesterone receptor(s) in the uterus. *J. Biol. Chem.*, 248:6366–6374.
24. Morgan, L. R., Schein, P. S., Wooley, P. V., Hoth, D., McDonald, J., Lippman, M., Posey, L. E., and Beasley, R. W. (1976): Therapeutic use of tamoxifen in advanced breast cancer. Correlation with biochemical parameters. *Cancer Treat. Rep.*, 60:1437–1443.
25. Mortel, R., Lévy, C., Wolff, J. P., Nicolas, J. C., Robel, P., and Baulieu, E. E. (1981): Female sex steroid receptors in postmenopausal endometrial carcinoma and biochemical response to an antiestrogen. *Cancer Res.*, 41:1140–1147.
26. Muechler, E. K., Flickinger, G. L., Mangan, C. E., and Mikhail, G. (1975): Estradiol binding by human endometrial tissue. *Gynecol. Oncol.*, 3:244–250.
27. Namer, M., Lalanne, C., and Baulieu, E. E. (1980): Increase of progesterone receptor by tamoxifen as a hormonal challenge test in breast cancer. *Cancer Res.*, 40:1750–1752.
28. Pollow, K., Lubbert, H., Jeske, R., and Pollow, B. (1975): Studies on 17β-hydroxysteroid dehydrogenase in human endometrium and endometrial carcinoma: Characterization of the soluble enzyme from secretory endometrium. *Acta Endocrinol.*, 79:146–156.
29. Pollow, K., Boquoi, E., Lubbert, H., and Pollow, B. (1975): Effect of gestagen therapy upon 17β-hydroxysteroid dehydrogenase in human endometrial adenocarcinoma. *J. Endocrinol.*, 67:131–132.
30. Pollow, K., Lubbert, H., Boquoi, E., Kreuzer, G., and Pollow, B. (1975): Characterization and comparison of receptors for 17β-estradiol and progesterone in human proliferative endometrium and endometrial carcinoma. *Endocrinology*, 96:319–328.
31. Pollow, K., Schmidt-Gollwitzer, M., and Nevinny Stickel, J. (1977): Progesterone receptors in normal human endometrium and endometrial carcinoma. In: *Progesterone Receptors in Normal and Neoplastic Tissues*, edited by W. L. McGuire, J. P. Raynaud, and E. E. Baulieu, pp. 313–338. Raven Press, New York.
32. Reifenstein, E. C. (1974): The treatment of advanced endometrial cancer with hydroxy-progesterone caproate. *Gynecol. Oncol.*, 2:377–389.
33. Richardson, G. S., and McLaughlin, D. H. (1978): The hypothesis of unopposed estrogen. *Hormonal Biology of Endometrial Cancer, UICC Technical Report Series*, (8), 42:13–14.
34. Sakai, F., Cheix, F., Clavel, M., Colon, J., Mayer, M., Pommatau, E., and Saez, S. (1978): Increases in steroid binding globulins induced by tamoxifen in patients with carcinoma of the breast. *J. Endocrinol.*, 76:219–226.
35. Smith, D. C., Prentice, R., Thomson, D. J., and Hermann, W. L. (1975): Association of exogenous estrogen and endometrial carcinoma. *N. Engl. J. Med.*, 293:1164–1167.
36. Sutherland, R. L., Mester, J., and Baulieu, E. E. (1977): Hormonal regulation of sex steroid hormone receptor concentration and subcellular distribution in chick oviduct. In: *Hormones and Cell Regulation*, edited by J. Dumont, and J. Nunez, pp. 31–48. North Holland Publishing Co., Amsterdam.
37. Tabor, C. W., and Tabor, H. (1976): 1,4-Diaminobutane (putrescine) spermidine and spermine. *Annu. Rev. Biochem.*, 45:285–306.
38. Tseng, L., Gusberg, S., and Gurpide, E. (1977): Estradiol receptor and 17β-dehydrogenase in normal and abnormal human endometrium. *Ann. NY Acad. Sci.*, 286:190–198.
39. Young, P. C. M., Ehrlich, C. E., and Cleary, R. E. (1976): Progesterone binding in human endometrial carcinomas. *Am. J. Obstet. Gynecol.*, 125:353–360.

Steroids and Endometrial Cancer,
edited by V. M. Jasonni, et al.
Raven Press, New York © 1983.

Estrogen Induced Proteins in Human Endometrial Cells

*S. Iacobelli, *P. Marchetti, *V. Natoli, *G. Scambia,
**N. A. Reiss, and **A. M. Kaye

*Laboratory of Molecular Endocrinology, Catholic University of San Cuore,
00168 Rome, Italy; and **Department of Hormone Research,
The Weizmann Institute of Science, Rehovot, 76100 Israel*

Studies on the regulation of macromolecular synthesis by steroid hormones offer further insight into the means by which these hormones affect both normal cells and those cells that ultimately develop into cancer in responsive organs such as the uterus. These studies also supply useful information on the possible dangers of contraceptive and therapeutic uses of steroids.

Classically, once inside the cell, apparently by passive diffusion, the steroid molecule interacts with the receptor protein to form a receptor-hormone complex. The receptor-hormone complex undergoes a conformational change, i.e., activation, which makes it able to interact with the genetic material of the cell to cause an increase in messenger RNA (mRNA) synthesis for specific proteins (1,4).

Although the various phases of the receptor mechanism are generally well understood, relatively little is known about the sequence of events that follow the binding of the steroid-receptor complex to chromatin, especially those events that occur during the processing period, which has been defined as the time between the initial appearance of the steroid-receptor complex in the nucleus and its final disappearance (5). Pioneer studies by Gorski et al. (11) have demonstrated that one of the earliest events following the interaction of the steroid-receptor complex with chromatin is the induction of a specific uterine protein in the rat known as the "induced protein" (IP). The time-dependent relationship between IP synthesis and other estrogen-dependent events is schematically shown in Table 1. An increase in total protein synthesis does not occur until at least 6 hr after estrogen stimulation, whereas an increase in IP synthesis is seen after only 30 to 60 min. This rapidity of IP induction in uterine tissue both *in vitro* and *in vivo* (8), and the dependence of induction on an actinomycin D-sensitive step (3) make IP a valuable tool for studying the mechanism of action of the estrogen-receptor complex.

METHODOLOGICAL ASPECTS

Two different methods can be used to analyze IP synthesis. The first consists of incubating uteri from control animals in medium containing leucine or other amino

TABLE 1. *Estradiol-induced events in the rat uterus*

Event	Time (hr)
Estrogen binding in cytoplasm Estrogen binding in nucleus	0.01
IP–RNA synthesis (other RNAs?) Nucleoplasmic RNA polymerase II	0.2
IP synthesis Nucleolar RNA polymerase I; phospholipid synthesis; glucose metabolism	1
Protein synthesis Water imbibition	3
Net RNA	7
Net protein Histone synthesis; DNA synthesis Cell division	20

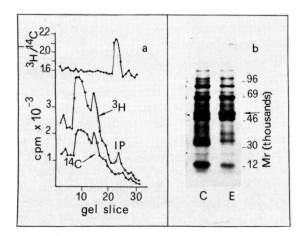

FIG. 1. a: Detection of IP using leucine labeled with ^{3}H and ^{14}C. **b:** Fluorography of newly synthesized proteins of rat uterus. C, control; E, 17-β-estradiol (5 each animal i.p. for 1 hr).

acids labeled with one isotope, such as ^{3}H, and uteri from animals treated with estrogens in medium containing the same labeled amino acids with a different isotope, such as ^{14}C. The uteri are then homogenized and the soluble proteins analyzed by polyacrylamide gel electrophoresis under nondenaturing conditions. The gel is sliced and the radioactivity of the two isotopes determined for each slice (7). Under these conditions (Fig. 1a), there is a single peak of estrogen-stimulated leucine incorporation visible on the gel.

The second method consists of labeling the uterine proteins of both control and estrogen-treated animals with the same isotope, such as [^{35}S]methionine, and then analyzing the proteins by polyacrylamide gel electrophoresis under denaturing conditions followed by fluorography (Fig. 1b) (17).

IP in Dimethylbenzanthracene-Induced Tumors

Using a specific radioimmunoassay, we were recently able to demonstrate the presence of IP in dimethylbenzanthracine (DMBA)-induced rat mammary tumors (9). In all tumors examined IP was detected. In six of ten tumors, the levels were increased after estradiol treatment.

IP in the Thymus

The recent detection of estrogen receptor (ER) in the thymus (13) prompted us to test for the induction of IP in this organ. For these experiments, the animals were treated with hydrocortisone (two intraperitoneal injections 24 hr apart) to eliminate the lymphocyte component of the thymus. The rest of the experiment was the same as that already used to demonstrate the induction of IP in rat uterus.

The fluorograph in Fig. 2 shows that also in the thymus, after 60 min of 17-β-estradiol treatment, the induction of a protein with electrophoretic migration identical to that of uterine IP is detectable.

This result is particularly interesting if we consider the fact that estrogen exerts a trophic effect on the uterus but causes atrophy of the thymus (16). This would suggest that the induction of IP in the two organs has opposite final effects.

IP in Human Endometrium

On the basis of the evidence that estrogen induces the rapid synthesis of specific proteins in the animal uterus, we have extended these studies to include human endometrium (6), with the dual purpose of first seeing whether IP synthesis is a more general event of estrogen action independent of the species to which the

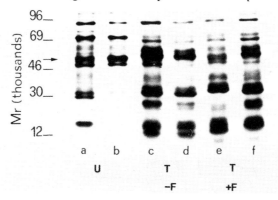

FIG. 2. Fluorography (F) of newly synthesized proteins of rat thymus. *a*, control and *b*, 17 β estradiol-treated, uterus (U); *c*, control and *d*, 17 β estradiol-treated, thymus (T); *e*, control and *f*, 17 β estradiol-treated, thymus (T) after hydrocortisone treatment.

responsive cell belongs (given that the mechanism of receptor action seems to be the same in different species) and, secondly, exploring the use of these proteins as end-products of estrogen action, as markers of estrogen-stimulated cell growth and proliferation in potential hormone-responsive tumors in conjunction with other already existing indicators such as steroid receptors. Human endometrium obtained by biopsy from women with normal menstrual cycles in the absence of endometrial pathology was used for these studies. Immediately after biopsy, the tissue was washed and incubated in medium containing [^{35}S]methionine in the absence and the presence of physiological concentrations of estradiol. The soluble proteins were then analyzed by polyacrylamide gel electrophoresis under denaturing conditions. In some cases, estrogens were administered *in vivo* by injecting 20 mg of conjugated equine estrogens immediately after anesthetization.

With the above procedures the endometrial proteins were separated into numerous sharp bands, as illustrated in Fig. 3, which reports the densitometric profiles of polyacrylamide gels. In this figure, single bands or groups of minor components have been arbitrarily divided into 12 groups.

We first attempted to determine whether endometrial proteins undergo qualitative or quantitative alterations during the menstrual cycle as a result of variations in endogenous steroid levels. If the proteins are divided according to molecular weight, there is a group corresponding to a protein with a molecular weight of 41,000 to 65,000 daltons, whose synthesis is significantly more marked in the endometrium secretory phase than in the proliferative phase (Fig. 4). It is interesting to note that this same group of proteins includes IP, which has a molecular weight of approximately 46,000 daltons (7).

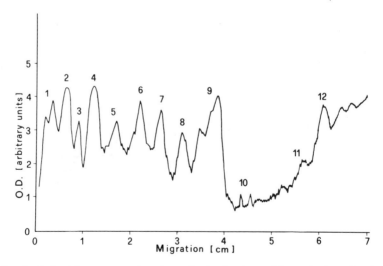

FIG. 3. Analysis of fluorograms of newly synthesized endometrial proteins by a densitometer equipped with a linear/log integrator.

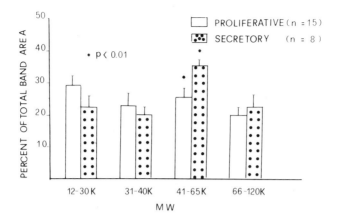

FIG. 4. Changes in endometrial protein synthesis throughout the menstrual cycle. The values shown are the means ± S.D. of three determinations.

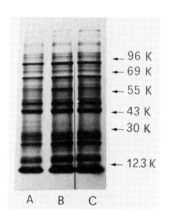

FIG. 5. SDS-polyacrylamide gel of soluble proteins in the secretory endometrium (day 23 of cycle **(A)** control; **(B)** estrogen-treated; **(C)** 17-β-estradiol-treated.

Having observed these alterations in the pattern of endometrial protein synthesis as a probable result of parallel variations in the endogenous steroid concentrations, we subsequently studied the effects of exogenous stimulation with estrogens. The addition of estradiol to endometrial tissue fragments taken during the secretory phase induces a slight increase in the rate of [^{35}S]methionine incorporation in at least one protein band with a molecular weight of about 55,000 daltons (Fig. 5). In this particular experiment, the time of exposure to estrogens was 60 min. The increase in the rate of synthesis of this protein was specifically induced by steroids with estrogenic activity, inasmuch as neither dexamethasone nor progesterone was capable of reproducing the effect (data not shown).

To characterize these estrogen-induced proteins further, two-dimensional electrophoresis was done as illustrated in Fig. 6. By means of this very sensitive

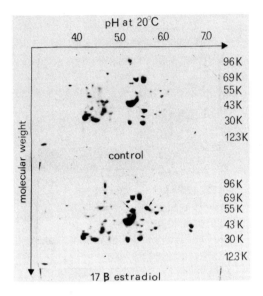

FIG. 6. Fluorography of two-dimensional gels of soluble proteins synthesized in secretory (day 23 of cycle) endometrium.

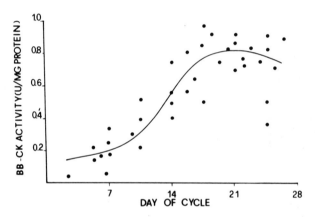

FIG. 7. Levels of BB-CK activity in human endometrium during menstrual cycle.

technique, the protein was resolved into two spots of almost identical molecular weight having different isoelectric points (pI).

As previously shown, the stimulation of estrogen-induced protein synthesis was observed only in secretory endometrium. It is interesting to note the different possible reasons for the variations in response to estrogens during the two phases of the menstrual cycle. One is that there is a difference in the proportions of estrogen-responsive and estrogen-unresponsive cells throughout the menstrual cycle (12). Another is that since the studies are based on the addition of exogenous steroids, there may be no visible response to this addition in the presence of already optimal concentrations of circulating or endometrial estrogens (15) if there is not simultaneous counteraction by a high concentration of progesterone (2). On the other hand, the maximum rate of synthesis of some proteins may depend on the synergistic effect of estrogens in combination with progesterone, which exists only during the secretory stage of the menstrual cycle (see following section).

IDENTIFICATION OF IP AS THE BB ISOZYME OF CREATINE KINASE: IMPLICATION FOR NORMAL AND TUMOR CELLS

The endometrium of various animal species, including rats and humans, responds to estrogen stimulation by increased synthesis of specific proteins, presumably expressing the increase by way of early genetic activation that follows interaction of the estrogen-receptor complex with nuclear chromatin. It is not yet known which of these proteins is involved in estrogen-stimulated cell proliferation, but some of them may prove to have interesting implications in estrogen-related tumors.

Although the exact biological function of IP is not yet known, our recent studies at the Weizmann Institute have demonstrated that the major constituent of rat uterine IP is the BB isozyme of creatine kinase (CK-BB) (14) and that its rapid induction by estrogen is indeed a consequence of an increased concentration of mRNA for IP (18). When CK activity of human endometrium is assayed (10) throughout the menstrual cycle, an increase is seen during the late secretory stage (Fig. 7) in accord with the stimulation of IP synthesis described above.

The function of CK is to act as part of an energy buffer system to maintain the physiological concentration of ATP. Thus, CK could play a role in energy mobilization for estrogen-stimulated growth and cell division. In addition, the finding of an easily measurable enzymic activity for IP makes it an extremely more convenient marker protein for exploring the estrogen dependence of normal and tumor cells (10). Indeed, both in the animal model, the GR mouse mammary tumor, and in human breast carcinoma, the steroid-dependent state may be characterized by a preponderance of the estrogen-dependent BB isozyme of CK, whereas steroid-independent tumors rely on the MM (muscle type) isozyme of creatine kinase.

ACKNOWLEDGMENTS

This work was supported by the National Research Council Project "Biologia della Riproduzione."

REFERENCES

1. Baulieu, E. E. (1975): Steroid receptor and hormone receptivity: New approaches in pharmacology and therapeutics. *Biochem. Pharmacol.*, 24:1743–1748.
2. Clark, J. H. (1979): *Female Sex Steroids: Receptor and Function.* Springer-Verlag, New York.
3. De Angelo, A. B., and Gorski, J. (1970): Role of RNA synthesis in the estrogen induction of a specific uterine protein. *Proc. Natl. Acad. Sci. USA.*, 66:693–700.
4. Higgins, S. J., and Gehring, V. (1978): Molecular mechanisms of steroid hormone action. *Adv. Cancer Res.*, 28:313–317.
5. Horwitz, K. B., and McGuire, W. L. (1980): Studies on mechanisms of estrogen and antiestrogen action in human breast cancer. In: *Endocrine Treatment of Breast Cancer, A New Approach,* edited by B. Henningsen, F. Linder, and C. Steichele, pp. 45–58. Springer-Verlag, Berlin.

6. Iacobelli, S., Marchetti, P., Bartoccioni, E., Natoli, V., Scambia, G., and Kaye, A. M. (1981): Steroid-induced proteins in human endometrium. *Mol. Cell. Endocrinol.*, 23:321–331.
7. Iacobelli, S., Paparatti, L., and Bompiani, A. (1973): Oestrogen-induced protein (IP) of rat uterus. Isolation and preliminary characterization. *FEBS Lett.*, 32:199–203.
8. Katzenellenbogen, B. A., and Gorski, J. (1972): Estrogen action *in vitro*: Induction of the synthesis of a specific uterine protein. *J. Biol. Chem.*, 247:1299–1305.
9. Kaye, A. M., Reiss, N., Iacobelli, S., Bartoccioni, E., and Marchetti, P. (1980): The "Estrogen-induced Protein" in normal and neoplastic cells. In: *Hormones and Cancer*, edited by S. Iacobelli, R. J. B. King, H. R. Lindner, and M. E. Lippman, pp. 41–52. Raven Press, New York.
10. Kaye, A. M., Reiss, N., Shaer, A., Sluyser, M., Iacobelli, S., Amroch, D., and Soffer, Y. (1981): Estrogen responsive creatine kinase in normal and neoplastic cells. *J. Steroid Biochem.*, 15:69–75.
11. Notides, A., and Gorski, J. (1966): Estrogen induced synthesis of a specific uterine protein. *Proc. Natl. Acad. Sci. USA*, 56:230–235.
12. Prianishnikov, V. A. (1978): A functional model of the structure of the epithelium of normal, hyperplastic and malignant human endometrium: a review. *Gynecol. Oncol.*, 6:420–428.
13. Reichman, M. E., and Villee, C. A. (1978): Estradiol binding by rat thymus cytosol. *J. Steroid Biochem.*, 9:637–641.
14. Reiss, N., and Kaye, A. M. (1981): Identification of the major component of the estrogen induced protein of the rat uterus as the BB isozyme of creatine kinase. *J. Biol. Chem.*, 256:5741–5749.
15. Schmidt-Gollwitzer, M., Genz, T., Schmidt-Gollwitzer, K., Pollow, B., and Pollow, K. (1978): Correlation between oestradiol and progesterone receptor levels, 17βhydroxysteroid dehydrogenase activity and endometrial tissue levels of oestradiol, oestrone and progesterone in women. In: *Endometrial Cancer*, edited by M. G. Brush, R. W. Taylor, and R. J. B. King, pp. 227–241. Bailiere Tindall, London.
16. Sobhon, P., and Jirasattham, C. (1974): Effect of sex hormones on the thymus and lymphoid tissue of ovariectomized rats. *Acta Anat. (Basel)*, 89:211–225.
17. Walker, M. D., Gozes, I., Kaye, A. M., Reiss, N., and Littauer, U. Z. (1976): The "estrogen-induced protein": Quantitation by autoradiography of polyacrylamide gels. *J. Steroid Biochem.*, 7:1083–1085.
18. Walker, M. D., and Kaye, A. M. (1981): mRNA for the rat uterine estrogen induced protein: Translation *in vitro* and regulation by estrogen. *J. Biol. Chem.*, 256:23–26.

Steroids and Endometrial Cancer,
edited by V. M. Jasonni, et al.
Raven Press, New York © 1983.

Specificity of an Estrogen Binding Protein in the Human Vagina Compared with that of Estrogen Receptors in Different Tissues from Different Species

*E. W. Bergink, *H. J. Kloosterboer, **W. H. M. van der Velden, *J. van der Vies, and *M. S. de Winter

*Scientific Development Group, Organon International B.V., Oss, The Netherlands; and **St. Josephziekenhuis, Eindhoven, The Netherlands

Several studies have indicated that estrogen receptors found in different tissues have similar specificities (1,8–10,12,16,17,19–21). However, clinical studies with estriol or estriol succinate have indicated that the effect of estrogenic compounds on the human vagina may be different from that on the endometrium. The dose-dependent stimulatory effect of estriol on the endometrium and on liver protein synthesis is low compared with its effect on vaginal atrophy and urinary incontinence (3,11,15). Estriol has been defined as a short-acting estrogen because of its weak estrogenic effect on long-term estrogenic events, such as endometrial proliferation and its strong effect on short-term estrogenic events (5,6,18). However, there is no explanation for the full estrogenic effect of estriol on the stimulation of the human vagina; in the present study, we investigated the specificity of the estrogen binding protein in the human vagina. A comparison was made between the specificities of the human vaginal estrogen binding protein and the specificities of estrogen receptors in different rabbit, rat, and human tissues. The interaction between estriol and the estrogen binding protein in the human vagina was further investigated in an attempt to explain the specific vaginographic effects of estriol.

MATERIAL AND METHODS

The details of the procedure for receptor binding studies (saturation analysis and competitive binding studies) have been previously described (1,2). In brief, frozen tissues or freeze dried powder was homogenized in TE buffer (10 mM Tris-HCl, 1 mM ethylenediaminetetracetate [EDTA], 0.5 mM dithioerythritol, 0.002% NaN$_3$, pH 7.4). Cytosol fractions were collected following centrifugation (30 min, 100,000 g), and aliquots of the cytosol fractions were incubated with tritiated ligand (either [^{3}H]17β-estradiol or [^{3}H]estriol; specific activity 90 Ci/mmole), either alone or in the presence of increasing concentrations of competitor as described previously (2). Unbound ligand was removed by incubating the mixture with the same volume of a charcoal suspension (0.25% charcoal, 0.025 dextran T70 in TE buffer). All procedures were performed at 4°C. Human myometrial and vaginal tissues were obtained from postmenopausal patients (age 60–82 years) who underwent surgery for nononcological disorders (vaginal repair with hysterectomy) and who were treated with estriol succinate (2 mg daily for at least 3 months; last administration 24 hr before surgery). Human breast tumor tissue (obtained from a number of patients) was stored at 0°C as a freeze-dried powder. The MCF-7 human breast tumor cell line was generously provided by Dr. McGrath (Michigan Cancer Foundation).

RESULTS AND DISCUSSION

Specificity of the Estrogen Receptor in a Cytosol Fraction Obtained from Rabbit Myometrium

Several studies have indicated that the interaction between estrogens and estrogen receptors is determined by several factors and, in particular, the following elements appear to be important (4,7,13,14,17,24): (a) functional hydroxyl groups at positions 3 and 17 of the steroid molecule, (b) hydrophobic bonding, and (c) complex formation by the aromatic ring A. However, these studies comparing steroid structure and receptor affinity are incomplete because not all steroids belonging to a particular structural series have been available to the investigators. Figure 1 shows the influence of various substituents at position C-3 of 17β-estradiol or ethinylestradiol and at position C-17β of 17β-estradiol on receptor binding. Removal of the hydroxyl group at the C-3 or C-17β site of 17β-estradiol decreases its affinity 30-fold, which corresponds to a loss of a hydrogen bond (24). The nature of the hydrogen bond

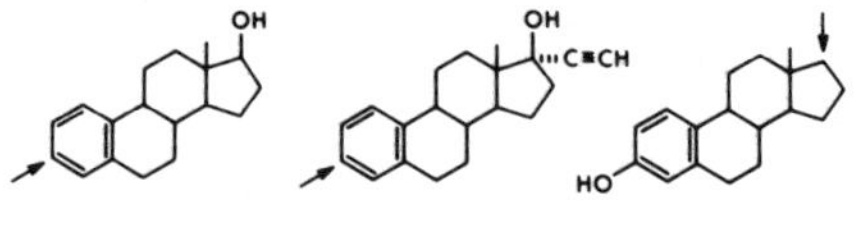

Substitution	Relative affinity (17 β -oestradiol = 100%)		
- OH	100	75	100
- H	3	4	3
- CH$_3$	3		2
- CH$_2$OH	4		41
- OCH$_3$	4	3	19
- OCH$_2$OCH$_3$			8

FIG. 1. Effect of substitution at positions C-3 and C-17β on the relative affinity for the estrogen receptor in the cytosol fraction from rabbit myometrium.

at site C-3 is different from that at position C-17β. The only substituent allowed at position C-3 in estradiol 17β is the hydroxyl group. The earlier reported high affinities of ester derivatives of 17β-estradiol are probably due to hydrolysis of the esters during incubation (17). Replacement of the hydroxyl at position C-17β with either a methoxy or a methoxymethylether reduced the affinity only 5 or 10 times, respectively, whereas a 30-fold reduction in affinity was found after replacement with a methoxy-group at position C-3.

We further investigated the effect of substitution at positions C-3α and β of 7α-methyllynestrenol (Fig. 2). Recent studies (1,2,22) indicate that 19-norsteroids with a double bond at position C4-5 may bind relatively strongly to the estrogen receptor, depending on the substituent at site C-3. We confirmed these observations and found the following rank in affinities for the 7α-methyllynestrenol derivatives: 3β-OH > 3α-OH >> 3-deoxy > 3-keto. The keto group at site C-3 is inhibitory. This is not the case at site C-17, as estrone binds relatively strongly to the estrogen receptor. We concluded that the hydroxyl group at site C-3 of 17β-estradiol maintains a hydrogen bond with a hydrogen acceptor site in the binding groove of the receptor. The hydroxyl group at site C-17 may interact with a hydrogen donor or acceptor site.

We analyzed the influence of hydrophobic binding on the stability of the receptor complex and estimated the effects of substitution with a hydroxyl or a methyl group at various sites of 17β-estradiol on receptor binding (Fig. 3). An extra hydroxyl group in 17β-estradiol, especially in rings B or C, decreased the affinity for the receptor. The introduction of a methyl group into 17β-estradiol at the sites C-11β or C-7α did not influence binding; the expected effect of increased hydrophobic binding was counteracted, presumably by steric hindrance (24). These data suggest the following characteristics for the steroid binding site in the estrogen receptor:

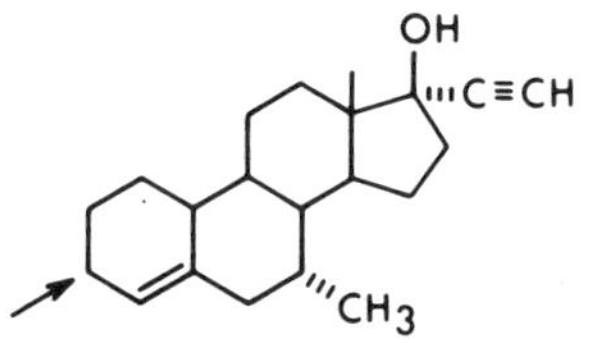

Substitution	Relative affinity (17 β-oestradiol = 100%)
- OH	26
''' OH	10
= O	1
- H	4

FIG. 2. Effect of substitution at position C-3 of 7α-methyllynestrenol on the relative affinity for the estrogen receptor in the cytosol fraction from rabbit myometrium.

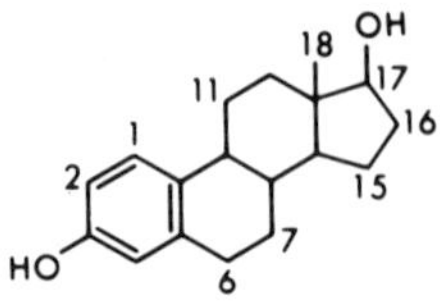

Position of "OH"	Relative affinity (17 β -oestradiol = 100%)	Position of "CH₃"	Relative affinity (17 β -oestradiol = 100%)
2	3	1	15
6 α	1	2	36
7α	1	6 β	31
11α	1	7α	104
11 β	7	9 α	40
15 α	1	11 β	83
16 α	17	17 α	83
		18	44

FIG. 3. Effect of hydroxyl and methyl groups at different positions in 17β-estradiol on the relative affinity for the estrogen receptor in the cytosol fraction from rabbit myometrium.

(a) A hydrogen acceptor at the inside of the binding groove forms a hydrogen bond with the 3-OH group of 17β-estradiol.

(b) A hydrogen acceptor/donor probably at the entrance of the groove may form a hydrogen bond with the 17β-OH group of 17β-estradiol or with the 17-keto group of estrone.

(c) The sites in the binding groove, lining rings B and C, are strictly hydrophobic in nature; the hydrophobic binding can be disturbed by steric hindrance.

Comparison of the Specificity of Estrogen Binding Proteins in Different Target Tissues

The information obtained in our studies on the specificity of the rabbit myometrial estrogen receptor was used to select a list of reference compounds for specificity studies with estrogen binding proteins in different tissues from rabbit, rat, and human. Compounds were selected with different structural features representing the various elements and factors considered to be of importance for binding. The results of these competitive binding studies are presented in Tables 1, 2, and 3. The relative affinities of most of the individual test compounds were similar in the various tissues from rabbit (Table 1), rat (Table 2), and in human sources (Table 3). This suggests that the specificities of these estrogen binding proteins are similar. These proteins appear to have the characteristics of estrogen receptors. These results confirmed the result of Payne and Katzenellenbogen (21), who reported that the specificity of estrogen receptors in rabbit uterus and vagina is similar.

TABLE 1. *Relative affinities of test compounds for various estrogen receptors in rabbit[a] tissues*

	Relative affinity (%, 17β-estradiol = 100%)			
Compound	Myometrium	Pituitary	Thymus	Vagina
1. Ethinylestradiol (EE)	100	101	56	68
2. 11β-Methyl-EE	90	87	150	84
3. 7α-Methyl-E$_2$	104	98	123	80
4. 7α, 18-Dimethyl-EE	62	41	68	33
5. 7α-Hydroxymethyl-EE	0.2	0.2		0.1
6. 11β-Methoxymethyl-EE	34	31	20	45
7. 7α-Methoxymethyl-EE	37	37	38	36
8. 11β-Methoxymethylestriol	7		3	8
9. 3-Desoxy-EE	3.6	2.6	0.5	3.1
10. 17α-Estradiol	28	23	13	22
11. Estriol	17	13	6	28
12. Diethylstilbestrol	29	14	19	51
13. 11β-Methoxy-EE	18			18
14. 3β-OH,7α-Methyllynestrenol	26		23	22
15. 3β-OH-Lynestrenol	6	12	6	13
16. Lynestrenol	0.6	1.2	0.5	1
17. 17β-Ethyl,17-desoxy-E$_2$	0.9	0.6	0.5	0.9
18. 7α,18-Dimethyl-E$_2$	89			90
19. 18-Methyl-E$_2$	44			73

[a]Rabbits were castrated and after 7 days treated daily for 7 days with a subcutaneous dose of 10 μg 17β-estradiol (100 ng/ml arachis oil). Tissues were collected 24 hr after the last injection.

However, our studies show that the specificity of an estrogen binding protein in the human vagina differs from that of the estrogen receptor in human myometrium and human breast tumor tissue (Table 3).

When measured against [^{3}H]17β-estradiol, the human vaginal binding protein was competed for strongly by estriol and 17α-estradiol and weakly by diethylstilbestrol, whereas binding sites in human myometrium breast tumor tissue and MCF-7 cells interacted more strongly with diethylstilbestrol than with estriol and 17α-estradiol. When measured against [^{3}H]estriol (Table 3), the human vaginal binding protein was also competed for strongly by 17α/β-estradiol and weakly by diethylstilbestrol, suggesting characteristics different from that of estrogen receptors present in myometrium and breast tumor tissue.

Cytoplasmic binding of [^{3}H]17β-estradiol-17β and [^{3}H]estriol in cytosol from human myometrium was studied. At 4°C 17β-oestradiol (equilibrium dissociation constant = 1.0 × 10^{-10}M) binds more strongly than estriol (equilibrium dissociation constant = 9 × 10^{-10}M) to the estrogen receptor in human myometrium.

The human vaginal estrogen binding protein was also characterized in saturation studies with radioactive ligands. We demonstrated a high-affinity binding site for [^{3}H]estriol (equilibrium dissociation constant 4.3 × 10^{-10}M) and [^{3}H]17β-estradiol (equilibrium dissociation constant 4.0 × 10^{-10}M). This is in agreement with our competitive binding studies (Table 3), which show that estriol and 17β-estradiol

TABLE 2. *Relative affinities of test compounds for various estrogen receptors in rat[a] tissues*

	Relative affinity (%, 17β-estradiol = 100%)		
Compound	Myometrium	Endometrium	Vagina
1. Ethinylestradiol (EE)	126	88	116
2. 11β-Methyl-EE	84	107	95
3. 7α-Methyl-E$_2$	123	115	110
4. 7α,18-Dimethyl-EE	33	30	46
5. 7α-Hydroxymethyl-EE		0.1	0.3
6. 11β-Methoxymethyl-EE	26	50	45
7. 7α-Methoxymethyl-EE	26	39	22
8. 11β-Methoxymethylestriol	3	4	7
9. 3-Desoxy-EE	0.5	0.4	1.0
10. 17α-Estradiol	3	2	9
11. Estriol	7	4	17
12. Diethylstilbestrol		36	34
13. 11β-Methoxy-EE	10		
14. 3β-OH,7α-Methyllynestrenol	10	12	14
15. 3β-OH-Lynestrenol	10		
18. 7α, 18-Dimethyl-E$_2$	66	65	65

[a]Rats were castrated and after 14 days treated with 2 × 15 mg estriol daily, orally for 4 days. Tissues were collected 24 hr after the administration of the last tablet.

compete equally strongly for binding to the estrogen binding protein in human vagina. The concentration of the estrogen binding protein in the vaginal tissue from postmenopausal women who all received estrogen medication (estriol succinate 2 mg daily) varied between 30 and 170 femtomoles/mg protein, with the exception of the tissue from a 82 year-old patient with undetectably low levels.

Wiegerinck et al. (23) found values between 4 and 119 femtomoles/mg protein in vaginal tissues from untreated postmenopausal patients. It may be concluded that the human vagina contains an estrogen-binding protein with characteristics different from those of estrogen receptors present in myometrium and breast tumor tissue. The presence of this binding protein could explain the preferential vaginotrophic effects of estriol.

SUMMARY

In the present study, we investigated the specificity of the estrogen binding proteins in various target tissues from different species. The structural requirements of different estrogenic compounds for the formation of complexes with the estrogen receptor in rabbit myometrium were determined. Compounds with hydroxyl groups in rings B or C of the steroid skeleton displayed weak binding for the estrogen receptor in rabbit myometrium, whereas hydroxyl groups at positions C-3 and C-17 of the steroid molecule were needed for the formation of hydrogen bonds with the receptor. The hydroxyl group at position C-3 interacts with a hydrogen acceptor on the receptor, whereas the hydroxyl group at position C-17 may react with a

TABLE 3. Affinities of test compounds relative to that of ^3H-17β-estradiol and ^3H-estriol for estrogen binding proteins in human tissues

| | | 17β Estradiol = 100% | | | Estriol = 100% | |
| | | Breast tumor | | | | |
Compound	Myometrium	Solid	MCF-7 cells	Vagina	MCF-7 cells	Vagina
1. Ethinylestradiol (EE)	103	98	102	58	>500	130
2. 11β-Methyl-EE	100	105	184	80	>500	114
3. 7α-Methyl-E$_2$	85	125	160	42	>500	66
4. 7α,18-Dimethyl-EE	50	41	96	68	>500	108
5. 7α-Hydroxymethyl-EE	0.2		0.2	10	0.9	9
6. 11β-Methoxymethyl-EE	44	37	47	39	250	69
7. 7α-Methoxymethyl-EE	41	35	28	190		
8. 11β-Methoxymethylestriol	5		4	68	6	47
9. 3-Desoxy-EE	0.5	0.5	3	0.5	40	5
10. 17α-Estradiol	14	4	6	140	21	80
11. Estriol	18	7	7	100	100	100
12. Diethylstilbestrol	32	42	82	4	>500	10
13. 11β-Methoxy-EE	20	7	9	18	180	31
14. 3β-OH, 7α-Methyllynestrenol	19	12	31	4		26
15. 3β-OH-Lynestrenol	15		10	2		7
16. Lynestrenol	0.6	0.2	0.5	0.3	4	2
17. 17β-Ethyl,17-desoxy-E$_2$	0.3	0.8	1.1	0.3	7	0.6
18. 7α-18-Dimethyl-E$_2$			157	41	>500	113
19. 18-Methyl-E$_2$			87	112	>500	197
20. Tamoxifen	0.2		0.2	0.2		
21. 2-OH-E$_2$	12			12		

hydrogen donor or acceptor site on the receptor. Estrogen binding proteins with similar specificities were found in the following tissues: myometrium, pituitary, thymus, and vagina of the rabbit; myometrium, endometrium, and vagina of the rat; and myometrium, breast tumour tissue, and MCF-7 cells of the human. These estrogen binding proteins displayed the characteristics of an estrogen receptor. However, the specificity of an estrogen binding protein in the human vagina was different from that of the human estrogen receptor; the estrogen binding protein displayed similar high affinities for 17β-estradiol, 17α-estradiol, and estriol and a relatively low affinity for diethylstilbestrol.

ACKNOWLEDGMENTS

The authors wish to thank Mr. E. W. Turpijn and Mr. J. L. Wagenaars for the technical assistance and Dr. H. D. Berkeley for his critical comments.

REFERENCES

1. Bergink, E. W. (1980): Oestriol receptor interactions: Their biological importance and therapeutic implications. Acta Endocrinol. [Suppl.] (Copenh.), 233:9–16.
2. Bergink, E. W., Hamburger, A. D., de Jager, E., and van der Vies, J. (1981): Binding of a

contraceptive progestogen Org 2969 and its metabolites to receptor proteins and human sex hormone binding globulin. *J. Steroid Biochem.*, 14:175–183.

3. Bergink, E. W., Crona, N., Dahlgren, E., and Samsioe, G. (1981): Effect of oestriol, oestradiol valerate and ethinyloestradiol on serum proteins in oestrogen-deficient women. *Maturitas*, 3:241–247.

4. Chernyaev, G. A., Barkova, T. I., Egorova, V. V., Sorokina, I. B., Ananchenko, S. N., Matarodze, G. D., Sokolova, N. A., and Rozen, V. B. (1975): A series of optical, structural and isomeric anologs of estradiol: A comparative study of the biological activity and affinity to cytosol receptor of rabbit uterus. *J. Steroid Biochem.*, 6:1483–1488.

5. Clark, J. H., Paszko, Z., and Peck, E. J. (1977): Nuclear binding and retention of the estrogen complex. Relation to the agonistic and antagonistic properties of oestriol. *Endocrinology*, 100:91–96.

6. Clark, J. H., Peck, E. J., and Anderson, J. N. (1976): Estrogen receptor binding: Relationship to estrogen-induced response. *J. Toxicol. Environ. Health*, 1:561–586.

7. Duax, W. L., Smith, G. D., Swenson, D. C., Strong, P. D., Weeks, C. M., Anachenko, S. N., and Egorova, V. V. (1981): Steroid structure and function-IX. Molecular conformation and receptor binding of isomeric analogs of d-homo-estradiol. *J. Steroid Biochem.*, 14:1–7.

8. Ginsburg, M., MacLusky, N. J., Morris, I. D., and Thomas, P. J. (1977): The specificity of oestrogen receptor in brain, pituitary and uterus. *Br. J. Pharmac.*, 59:397–402.

9. Hähnel, R., Twaddle, E., and Ratajzak, T. (1973): The specificity of the estrogen receptor of human uterus. *J. Steroid Biochem.*, 4:21–31.

10. Hähnel, R., and Twaddle, E. (1974): The steroid specificity of the estrogen receptor of human breast carcinoma. *J. Steroid Biochem.*, 5:119–122.

11. Henser, H. P., and Staemmler, H. J. (1973): Histological investigation into the effect of oestriol succinate on the corpus uteri in postmenopausal women. *Arzneim. Forsch.*, 23:558–562.

12. Jänne, O., Kontula, K., and Vihko, R. (1975): Steroid binding properties of oestrogen receptors in human breast cancer. *Med. Biol.*, 53:214–223.

13. Katzenellenbogen, J. A., Johnson, H. J., and Myers, H. N. (1973): Photoaffinity labels for estrogen binding proteins of rat uterus. *Biochemistry*, 12:4085–4092.

14. Katzenellenbogen, J. A. (1978): Comparative binding affinity of estrogen derivatives. *Cancer Treat. Rep.*, 62:1243–1249.

15. Kicovic, P. M., Cortes-Prieto, J., Milojevic, S., Haspels, A. A., and Aljinovic, A. (1980): The treatment of postmenopausal vaginal atrophy with ovestin vaginal cream or suppositories: Clinical, endocrinological and safety aspects. *Maturitas*, 2:275–282.

16. King, R. J. B., and Mainwaring, W. I. P. (1974): *Steroid-Cell Interactions.* Butterworths, London.

17. Korenman, S. G. (1969): Comparative binding affinity of estrogens and its relation to estrogenic potency. *Steroids*, 13:163–177.

18. Lan, N. C., and Katzenellenbogen, B. S. (1976): Temporal relationship between hormone receptor and biological responses in the uterus: Studies with short- and long-acting derivatives of estriol. *Endocrinology*, 98:220–227.

19. Malacarne, P., Piffanelli, A., Indelli, J., Fumero, S., Mondino, A., Gionchiglia, E., and Silvestri, S. (1980): Estradiol binding in rat thymus cells. *Horm. Res.*, 12:224–232.

20. Ojasoo, T., and Raynaud, J. P. (1978): Unique steroid congeners for receptor studies. *Cancer Res.*, 38:4186–4198.

21. Payne, D. W., and Katzenellenbogen, J. A. (1980): Differential effects of estrogens in tissues: A comparison of estrogen receptor in rabbit uterus and vagina. *Endocrinology*, 106:1345–1352.

22. Tamaya, T., Nioka, S., Furuta, N., Shimura, T., Takano, N., and Okada, H. (1977): Contribution of functional groups of 19-nor-progestogens to binding to progesterone and estradiol-17β receptors in rabbit uterus. *Endocrinology*, 100:1579–1584.

23. Wiegerinck, M. A. H. M., Poortman, J., Agema, A. R., and Thijssen, J. H. H. (1980): Estrogen receptors in human vaginal tissue. *Maturitas*, 2:59–67.

24. Zeelen, F. J., and Bergink, E. W. (1980): Structure-activity relationships of steroid estrogens. In: *Cytotoxic Estrogens in Hormone Receptive Tumours*, edited by J. Raus, H. Martens, and G. Leclerq, pp. 39–48. Academic Press, London.

Steroids and Endometrial Cancer,
edited by V. M. Jasonni, et al.
Raven Press, New York © 1983.

Effects of Progestins on the Binding of Estradiol with Rat Uterine Estrogen Receptors

Francesco Di Carlo, Elena Gallo, Silvia Racca, Camilla Reboani, and Giuseppe Conti

Institute of Pharmacology, Faculty of Medicine, University of Turin, 10125 Turin, Italy

Many drugs and hormones have been shown to have the capacity, when used at suitable doses or concentrations, to interfere with the binding of estradiol-17β with its specific cytoplasmic receptors (1,3,6,8,9,12,13).

Hsueh et al. (5) first demonstrated that progesterone, given in physiological doses, reduces the number of receptors available for binding estradiol-17β in the rąt uterus. It is generally thought that in this way progesterone can limit the biological effects of estradiol in the uterus and perhaps in other estrogen target tissues (1,2,5).

Recently, Di Carlo et al. (2,4) have demonstrated that, other than the natural hormone, some synthetic progestins (i.e., clogestone, medrogestone, and medroxy-progesterone acetate, all pregnane derivatives) can induce a marked decrease in the binding capacity of estradiol-17β to specific uterine receptors, both *in vivo* and *in vitro*.

In the studies described in the present chapter, we compared the effects of two pregnane derivatives (medroxyprogesterone acetate and chlormadinone) and two 19-nortestosterone derivatives (norgestrel and norethisterone) on the concentration of cytoplasmic estrogen receptors in the rat uterus.

This investigation was carried out to ascertain whether the influence on estrogen receptor levels, observed with some pregnane derivatives, is due to structural features particular to this group of progestins, or it is a property also common to 19-nortestosterone derivatives, i.e., to all steroids with progestational activity. It is known that pregnane derivatives are considered to be almost pure progestational agents, whereas 19-nortestosterone derivatives have, in addition, clear androgenic, estrogenic, and anabolic properties, that could modify the effects on estrogen receptor levels (10).

MATERIALS AND METHODS

Drugs and Buffer

[6,7-³H]Estradiol-17β (40 Ci/mmole) was obtained from the Radiochemical Centre, Amersham (England). Unlabeled estradiol-17β was purchased from Merck AG

Darmstadt (Germany), and chlormadinone from Prodotti Gianni S.R.L., Milan (Italy).

Medroxyprogesterone acetate (MPA) was obtained from Upjohn Italiana S.p.A, Milan, and norgestrel and norethisterone were a gift of Schering S.p.A., Milan.

The buffer solution (TED) contained 1 mM EDTA, 10 mM Tris-HCl, and 0.5 mM dithiothreitol, pH 7.4, at 4°C. The dextrancharcoal suspension contained 0.005% dextran and 0.5% activated charcoal in buffer solution.

Animals and Tissue Preparation

Two series of experiments were performed *in vivo* and *in vitro*. Intact female rats (160–180 g) in diestrus were used throughout this study to ensure low levels of estrogens in the circulation.

In a first series of experiments *in vivo*, the rats were given a single oral dose of the four tested progestins and killed after 1, 6, 24, or 48 hr.

In a second series of experiments *in vivo*, all animals received a single i.p. injection of 10 ng estradiol-17β and were then divided into five groups. One group received no further treatment and served as controls; the remaining four groups received either MPA or chlormadinone or norgestrel or norethisterone orally 5 min after the estradiol and were killed 1, 6, 15, 30, or 48 hr later.

For experiments *in vivo* and for those *in vitro*, uteri were removed immediately after sacrifice, homogenized in TED buffer (1:4, wt/vol), and the homogenates were then centrifuged at 105,000 g for 1 hr at 4°C to obtain the supernatant fraction (cytosol).

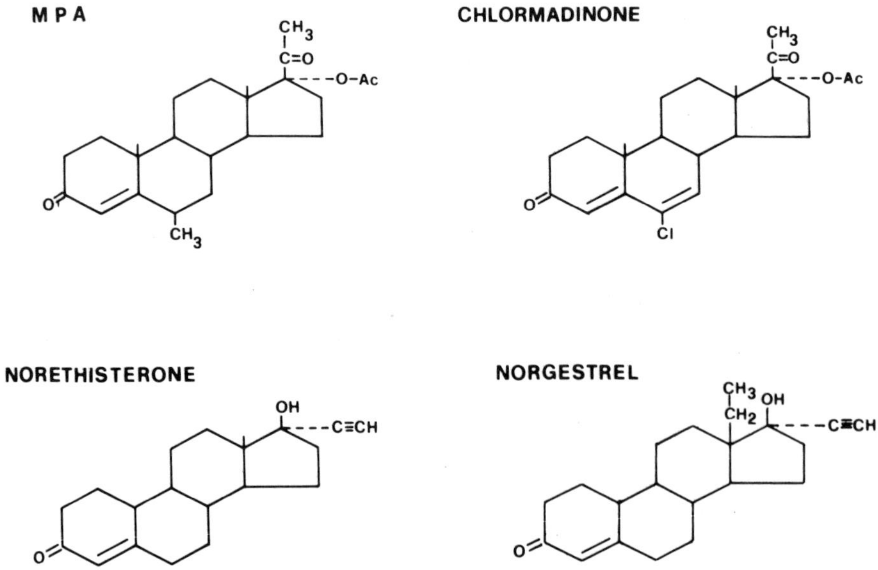

FIG. 1. Structural formulas of medroxyprogesterone acetate (MPA), chlormadinone, norethisterone, and norgestrel.

The concentration of protein in each cytosol sample was determined according to the method of Lowry et al. (10).

Preparation of Progestin Solutions

For the experiments performed *in vitro*, the progestins tested were carefully dissolved in ethanol and then diluted in TED buffer to give a stock solution containing 40 nmoles drug/ml. Thereafter, serial dilutions were made with buffer in order to obtain four solutions containing 0.8, 4, 20, or 40 nmoles/ml.

In the experiments performed *in vivo*, the progestins were suspended in 0.5% carboxymethyl cellulose to give an oral dose of 15 mg/kg body weight in a volume of 10 ml.

Binding Assay by Charcoal Adsorption

The specific binding of estradiol to its receptors and values for dissociation constants were obtained as described previously (2).

Duplicate samples of 150 μl cytosol (obtained from the uteri of untreated or treated rats), 50 μl buffer, and 50 μl [^{3}H]estradiol-17β (seven concentrations between 0.015 and 0.2 pmoles) were incubated overnight at 4°C.

In the experiments *in vitro* the interference of the progestins with the specific binding of estradiol-17β to its receptors was determined by preincubating each sample of cytosol (150 μl) with 50 μl buffer containing the progestins tested (instead of buffer alone) before adding [^{3}H]estradiol-17β.

Nonspecific binding was obtained by heating cytosol samples for 60 min at 45°C according to the method of Wagner (14).

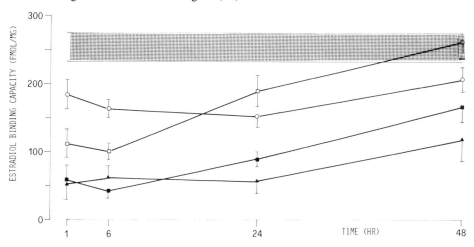

FIG. 2. Changes in the effect of chlormadinone *(open circles)*, medroxyprogesterone acetate (MPA) *(triangles)*, norethisterone *(open squares)*, or norgestrel *(solid squares)* (20 mg/kg orally) on the estradiol binding capacity in relation to time. Results are means ± SEM of four determinations with 16 rats in each group.

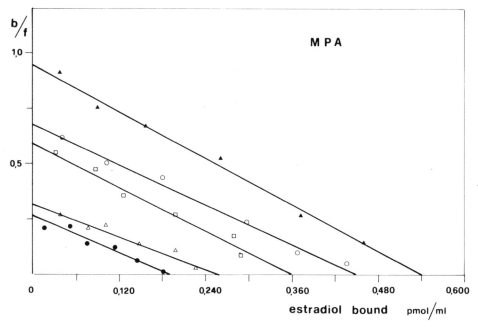

FIG. 3. Scatchard analysis of the binding of [³H]estradiol-17β *in vitro* in the absence of medroxyprogesterone acetate (MPA) (solid triangles) and in the presence of 0.8 *(open circles)*, 4 *(squares)*, 20 *(open triangles)* or 40 *(solid circles)* nmoles MAP/ml.

Specific binding was calculated by subtracting the nonspecific binding from the total binding. After incubation, 250 μl dextran-coated charcoal suspension were added (for 30 min at 4°C) to remove unbound radioactive estradiol.

The mixture was then centrifuged for 30 min at 2,000 *g* and the supernatant fraction (containing bound radioactive estradiol-17β) was transferred to scintillation vials. After addition of scintillation fluid (Instagel, Packard) the radioactivity was determined in a liquid scintillation counter (Wallac, LKB).

The results, obtained by Scatchard analysis, are expressed as fmoles [³H]estradiol-17β specifically bound/mg cytosol protein.

RESULTS

The structural formulas of the four progestins used in our experiments are reported in Fig. 1.

It clearly appears that chlormadinone differs from MAP only in having a double bond in ring B and a Cl atom in position 6 instead of a methyl group.

Norgestrel is the 13-ethyl analog of norethisterone; it is 100 times as progestational as norethisterone in the Clauberg test.

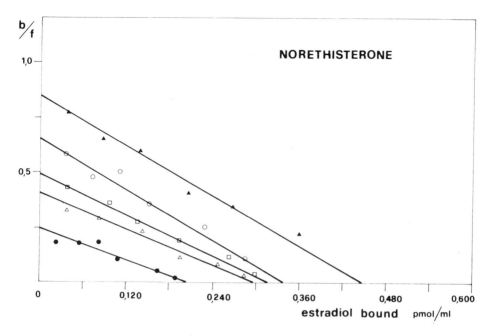

FIG. 4. Scatchard analysis of the binding of [³H]estradiol-17β *in vitro* in the absence of nor-ethisterone *(solid triangles)* and in the presence of 0.8 *(open circles)*, 4 *(squares)*, 20 *(open triangles)* or 40 *(solid circles)* nmoles norethisterone/ml.

In Vivo and *In Vitro* Effects on the Binding
of Estradiol to its Receptors

Figure 2 shows the effects of administration of a single dose of progestins on the estradiol binding capacity and the modification of this effect in relation to time.

MAP, norgestrel, and norethisterone induce a prompt and remarkable decrease in uterine estrogen receptor levels 1 hr after treatment. This reduction remains almost unchanged for 24 hr in rats treated with MAP or norgestrel, whereas it is much lower in the animals given norethisterone.

During the following hours the effect of MAP and norgestrel begins to decrease but is still noticeable after 48 hr when, on the contrary, the effect of norethisterone has completely disappeared.

It is clear that the effect of chlormadinone is completely different from that induced by MAP and norgestrel. In fact, the reduction of estradiol binding capacity obtained with this compound is much lower at all hours considered.

The results of these experiments performed *in vivo* show that all progestins tested can influence the levels of estrogen receptors, although both the intensity and the persistence of this effect are different from one compound to another.

In the experiments *in vitro*, these progestins confirmed their different ability to interfere with the binding capacity of estradiol to its receptors.

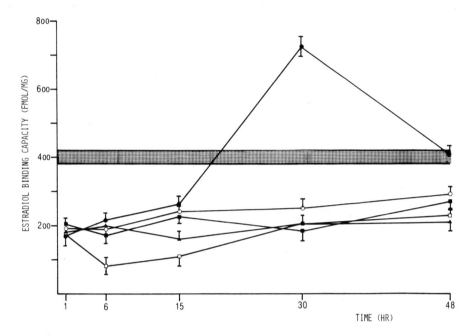

FIG. 5.   Effect of administration of 10 ng i.p. estradiol-17β alone *(solid circles)* or with chlor-madinone *(open circles)*, MAP *(triangles)*, norethisterone *(open squares)* or norgestrel *(solid squares)* (20 mg/kg orally), given 5 min later on the binding of [³H]estradiol-17β to its specific uterine cytosolic receptors in the rat. Results are means ± S.E.M. of four determinations with 20 rats in each group.

The results reported in Table 1 show that among the progestins used, MPA induces the highest inhibition of estradiol-receptor interaction. The progestin-induced interference, evaluated on the basis of Scatchard analysis, seems to be due to a noncompetitive inhibition.

Scatchard plots concerning the changes in the binding of estradiol in the presence of MPA or norethisterone are reported, as example of the results obtained, in Figs. 3 and 4, respectively.

In Vivo Effects on Cytoplasmic Levels of Estrogen Receptors

It is well known that the administration of estradiol induces a dose-dependent depletion in the number of its receptors in the cytoplasm, as the estrogen-receptor complexes translocate from the cytoplasmic into the nuclear compartment.

During the following hours, because of the resynthesis of estrogen receptors, their levels in the cytoplasm are gradually restored (replenishment phase).

Subsequently, the concentration of cytoplasmic receptors increases beyond the normal values (overshoot phase), and this effect lasts several hours.

Figure 5 shows the effects of MPA, chlormadinone, norgestrel, and norethisterone on cytoplasmic levels of estrogen receptors, administered orally after a single injection of estradiol (10 ng i.p., a dose that induces a 50% depletion in the number of estrogen receptors) (3).

TABLE 1. *Binding of [³H]estradiol-17β to its specific uterine receptors* in vitro[a]

Unlabeled steroid	Concentration (nmoles/ml)	Estradiol binding capacity (fmoles/ml cytosol protein)[b]	Dissociation constant (moles/liter)
Chlormadinone	0	369	$(1.4–1.8) \times 10^{-10}$
	0.8	345	
	4	322	
	20	307	
	40	275	
Medroxyprogesterone acetate	0	352	$(1.6–2.0) \times 10^{-10}$
	0.8	293	
	4	235	
	20	168	
	40	118	
Norethisterone	0	360	$(0.8–1.0) \times 10^{-10}$
	0.8	272	
	4	256	
	20	233	
	40	160	
Norgestrel	0	344	$(1.0–1.5) \times 10^{-10}$
	0.8	284	
	4	253	
	20	215	
	40	178	

[a]Estradiol-17β (0.06–0.8 pmole/ml); data obtained by Scatchard analysis.
[b]Results are means of two determinations.

It is clear that all progestins are devoid of activity on depletion phase, whereas they cause a significant inhibition both of replenishment and overshoot phases. No significant difference exists in this test among the four progestins used, although norethisterone seems to be the most effective in reducing the first part of replenishment.

DISCUSSION

The results reported in this chapter indicate that all of the synthetic progestins used are able to reduce the levels of estrogen receptors in the uterine cytoplasm. However, clear differences in intensity and duration of this effect exists from one progestin to another.

That progesterone and some pregnane derivatives can influence the estradiol–receptor interaction has been well known for some years (4,5). On the contrary, no data is available to date on the effect of 19-nortestosterone derivatives.

The results of our experiments show that both norgestrel and norethisterone interfere with the binding of estradiol both *in vivo* and *in vitro*. Therefore, we may conclude that all steroids with progestational activity have an inhibitory effect on the binding of estradiol to its specific uterine receptors.

The main mechanism by which progestins decrease *in vivo* the number of cytoplasmic estrogen receptors available for estradiol is probably related to a reduction in the synthesis of new receptors.

However, we have shown that progestins, at suitable concentrations, also reduce *in vitro* the binding of estradiol to its receptors. In addition, this *in vitro* effect has been observed by others (7) also in the hypothalamus, when using a high concentration (1×10^{-5}M) of progesterone.

Obviously, in these experiments performed *in vitro* we cannot presume that progesterone or progestins act by reducing the resynthesis of estrogen receptors.

Our results suggest that when high doses of progestins are used, as occurs in the therapy of hormone-dependent breast tumors, these drugs can decrease the number of estrogen receptors not only indirectly, by reducing their resynthesis, but also directly, by inhibiting the binding of estradiol to its cytosolic receptors.

This could explain, at least in part, the better results obtained in breast cancer therapy by using high doses (>500 mg/day) of MPA rather than low doses (11).

REFERENCES

1. Di Carlo, F., Conti, G., and Reboani, C. (1978): Interference of gestagens and androgens with rat uterine oestrogen receptors. *J. Endocrinol.*, 77:49–55.
2. Di Carlo, F., Pacilio, G., and Conti, G. (1975): Sul meccanismo d'azione dei progestinici nella terapia dei tumori mammari ormono-dipendenti. *Tumori*, 61:501–508.
3. Di Carlo, F., Reboani, C., Conti, G., and Genazzani, E. (1978): Changes in the concentration of uterine cytoplasmic oestrogen receptors induced by doxorubicin and methotrexate. *J. Endocrinol.*, 79:201–208.
4. Di Carlo, F., Reboani, C., Conti, G., Portaleone, P., Viano, I., and Genazzani, E. (1980): Changes in estrogen receptor levels induced by pharmacological agents. In: *Pharmacological Modulation of Steroid Action*, edited by E. Genazzani, F. Di Carlo, and W. I. P. Mainwaring, pp. 61–74. Raven Press, New York.
5. Hsueh, A. J. W., Peck, E. J., and Clark, J. H. (1976): Control of uterine estrogen receptor levels by progesterone. *Endocrinology*, 98:438–444.
6. Jordan, V. C., Prestwich, G., Dix, C. J., and Clark, E. R. (1980): Binding of antiestrogens to the estrogen receptor, the first step in antiestrogen action. In: *Pharmacological Modulation of Steroid Action*, edited by E. Genazzani, F. Di Carlo, and W. I. P. Mainwaring, pp. 81–98. Raven Press, New York.
7. Kato, J., Atsumi, Y., and Inaba, M. (1974): Estradiol receptors in female rat hypothalamus in the development stage and during pubescence. *Endocrinology*, 94:309–317.
8. Katzenellenbogen, B. S., Katzenellenbogen, J. A., Ferguson, E. R., and Krauthammer, N. (1978): Antioestrogen interaction with uterine oestrogen receptors. *J. Biol. Chem.*, 253:697–707.
9. Levy, J., Burshell, A., Marbach, M., Afflalo, L., and Glick, S. M. (1980): Estrogen activity of drugs known to cause gynecomastia. In: *Pharmacological Modulation of Steroid Action*, edited by E. Genazzani, F. Di Carlo and W. I. P. Mainwaring, pp. 111–122. Raven Press, New York.
10. Lowry, O. H., Rosebrough, N. J., Farr, A. L., and Randall, K. J. (1951): Protein measurement with the Folin phenol reagent. *J. Biol. Chem.*, 193:265–275.
11. Pannuti, F., Martoni, A., Lenaz, G. R., Piana, E., and Nanni, P. (1978): A possible new approach to the treatment of metastatic breast cancer: Massive doses of medroxyprogesterone acetate. *Cancer Treat. Rep.*, 62:499–504.
12. Rochefort, H. (1976): Régulation physiologique et pharmacologique des récepteurs des oestrogéns. In: *Hormones and Breast Cancer*, pp. 83–96. INSERM, Paris.
13. Rochefort, H., and Garcia, M. (1980): Interactions and actions of androgens on the estrogen receptor. In: *Pharmacological Modulation of Steroid Action*, edited by E. Genazzani, F. Di Carlo and W. I. P. Mainwaring, pp. 78–80. Raven Press, New York.
14. Wagner, R. K. (1972): Characterization and assay of steroid hormone receptors and steroid binding serum proteins by agar-gel electrophoresis at low temperature. *Hoppe Seylers Z. Physiol. Chem.*, 353:1235–1245.

Steroids and Endometrial Cancer,
edited by V. M. Jasonni, et al.
Raven Press, New York © 1983.

Analysis of Human Endometrial Protein Secretions *In Vivo* and *In Vitro*: Effects of Estrogens and Progesterone

*†David T. MacLaughlin, **†George S. Richardson,
and †Paul E. Sylvan

*Department of Obstetrics and Gynecology; **Department of Surgery, Harvard Medical
School, Boston, Massachusetts 02114; and †Vincent Research Laboratory, Department of
Gynecology, Massachusetts General Hospital, Boston, Massachusetts 02114*

The human endometrium is known to respond to the sequential action of estrogens and progestins. The morphological changes induced by these hormones are well established. Relatively little is known, however, concerning the biochemical changes that these steroids regulate. Most of the advances in these areas involve cytoplasmic events, such as the regulation of steroid receptors (5,14) and the induction of a variety of enzymes, including that of steroid oxidoreductase by progesterone (15) and malate dehydrogenase (17), a variety of glycolytic enzymes (12), and ornithine decarboxylase by estradiol. An overview of these findings is given in a recent review (8).

Endometrial secretions are believed to contain a transudate of human serum proteins, although a number of groups have reported quantitative differences in electrophoretic patterns of uterine luminal fluids and of radiolabeled proteins recovered from the media of cultured tissue (8). More studies are required before the exact nature of human uterine secretions and the effect of hormones on them can be established.

The importance of a biochemical description of the effects of steroid hormones on human endometrium is obvious in providing the basis of wide ranging basic and clinical studies.

MATERIALS AND METHODS

Chemicals

All reagents in this study were purchased in the highest grade available. Radiolabeled leucine (110 Ci/mmole) was purchased from New England Nuclear Corp., Boston, MA. The tissue culture media, fetal calf serum and balanced salt solutions were obtained from Grand Island Biological Company (GIBCO).

Human Subjects

This study was approved by the Internal Review Board (Human Studies Committee) of the Massachusetts General Hospital. Informed consent for the Gravlee procedure was obtained concurrently with the patient's consent for surgery.

Endometrium and Uterine Washings

Endometrium used in this study was obtained in the operating room as part of appropriate gynecological treatment for benign disease (dilatation and curettage [D & C], or hysterectomy). In all cases, the tissue delivered to the laboratory was that which remained after the staff pathologist had taken sufficient material for histological examination. In addition, endometrial washings obtained by the Gravlee method were retained for the present study only when the accompanying endometrium was found to be histologically normal. Endometrial dating established by the convention of Noyes et al. (9) was rechecked by Dr. R. E. Scully or Dr. S. J. Robboy of the Pathology Department of the Massachusetts General Hospital.

Collection of Human Uterine Luminal Fluid

Human uterine luminal fluid was collected by the Gravlee jet washer, a sterile disposable unit manufactured by the Upjohn Co. (Kalamazoo, MI) (4). The uterine lumen was rinsed with 10 to 15 ml of isotonic glycine buffer (0.15 M at neutral pH). The fluid was then chilled immediately to 4°C and centrifuged at 100,000 × g for 45 to 60 min. The supernatant was stored frozen at −80°C for further analysis.

Measurement of Soluble Protein

Proteins in solution were measured either by the technique of Lowry et al. (7), by the nondestructive optical method described by Waddell (16), or by the optical density observed at 280 nm.

Desalting of Sera, Media, and Uterine Washes

Proteins from uterine luminal fluids, sera, or media from tissue culture experiments were desalted by Sephadex G25 chromatography over a 1 × 30 cm column equilibrated and eluted with double-distilled water at 4°C, or by dialysis against distilled water or the appropriate buffer using Spectra Por-6 tubing with a 1,000 molecular weight cutoff.

Ion Exchange Chromatography

Cation exchange using CM Sephadex. Test material (luminal fluid proteins, culture media, sera) was equilibrated with 0.01 M citrate pH 7.5 by dialysis and loaded onto a 6.0-ml resin bed of the cation exchanger (CM Sephadex) equilibrated in the same buffer. Fractions of 1 ml were collected and the elution was carried out by a stepwise addition of the NaCl containing citrate buffer. Eluates were analyzed for protein by one of the optical methods discussed above and radioactivity was followed by liquid scintillation counting (see below).

Anion exchange using Sephadex DEAE-A-50. In a fashion analogous to the cation-exchange chromatography, test material (proteins not retained by the cation-exchanged column) was equilibrated with Tris 0.01 M, pH 8.0, buffer by dialysis and placed on a 6.0-ml bed of ion-exchange resin swollen in the same buffer. The sample was washed into the 6.0-ml column with 15 to 20 ml of Tris. 0.01 M buffer, and adhering proteins were eluted by adding 20-ml increments of Tris buffer containing successively higher concentrations of NaCl (0.05, 0.2, and 0.3 M). Fractions of 1 ml were collected and analyzed for protein by the Waddell technique or by monitoring the absorbance of material at 280 nm. Radioactivity was followed by liquid scintillation counting (see below).

Isoelectric Focusing

Isoelectric focusing of proteins in polyacrylamide tube gels was carried out exactly according to the method of O'Farrell (10).

Slab Gel Electrophoresis

The system described by O'Farrell (10) was used in all cases. Homogenous 7 or 10% acrylamide gels were used in these experiments. At the conclusion of these runs, the gels were either stained for protein using Coomassie brilliant blue or prepared for fluorography (see below).

Fluorography of Polyacrylamide Gels

Fluorographic analysis of labeled proteins in the second dimension gels was performed using the technique of Bonner and Laskey (1).

Immunological Screening of Endometrial Cell Culture-Secreted Proteins

Radiolabeled proteins secreted into the media of endometrial cell cultures (see below) were analyzed for crossreactivity to rabbit antisera directed against human serum preparations (GIBCO). Normal rabbit serum was used as a control. Media from the cultures were dialyzed extensively to remove free radiolabeled amino acids. The dialyzed proteins were then screened initially using the antisera mentioned above as follows: a constant level of antigen was incubated for 48 hr at 4°C with serially diluted antisera or normal rabbit serum. Following this period, goat anti-rabbit gamma globulin antiserum was added and the incubation continued for another 24 hr at 4°C. The incubate was then centrifuged at 3,000 × g for 20 min at 4°C and the pellet counted for radioactivity. I^{125}-labeled human serum protein was used as a control for the quality of the rabbit antihuman serum.

Cell Culture

Routine methods were used (11) as previously reported by this laboratory (6) with slight modification in establishing the monolayer cell cultures (2). The tissue was diced with a McIlwain slicer, incubated for 25 min at 32°C in 0.25% trypsin and 0.001% DNase in HEPES buffer with shaking, centrifuged for 10 min at 550 rpm, resuspended in 10 ml of HEPES buffer containing collagenase, 2500 U, incubated for 25 min for 32°C, and then centrifuged as before. The precipitate was resuspended in culture medium with antibiotics added (penicillin and streptomycin (No. 514, GIBCO) 2,000 U in 0.2 ml) and amphotericin B (No. 529, (GIBCO) 50 mcg in 0.2 ml added per 100 ml of medium). The cells plated out in a few hours and survived in high yield. Flasks were washed with Hanks buffered saline solution after 24 hr to remove red blood cells and debris, and new medium was added. When the cells reached confluency, the culture was considered ready for transfer. The culture medium consisted of equal parts of Ham F12 and Dulbecco's modified Eagle's (GIBCO) and 15% whole (3) or stripped fetal bovine serum (No. 614, GIBCO). The stripped sera were prepared by equilibration with 0.25% charcoal (w/v) for 16 hr shaking at 25°C followed by sterilization by passage through a Millex 0.22-μm filter. [³H]Progesterone (New England Nuclear, 1 μCi, specific activity 105 Ci/mmole), equilibrated with fetal bovine serum has been found to be completely removed by this procedure. The tightly closed flasks were incubated at 37°C. Under phase microscopy, most of the cells were seen to be attached to the flask wall at 24 hr. These cultures of mixed cell types usually became confluent within 2 weeks. When subculture was required, the medium was decanted and the monolayer cells were rinsed with calcium- and magnesium-free Hanks solution and incubated for 15 min at 37°C with 1.5 ml of the trypsin-EDTA solution. The detached cells were diluted to a final volume of 30 ml with nutrient mixture, and approximately half of the suspension was transferred to the new flask.

Preparation of Cultures for Experimentation

Flasks containing fresh cultures or cultures that had not been subcultured for more than three passages were detached as for subculture and pooled in a common suspension that was aliquoted to the experimental flasks. These flasks were maintained for 3 days in medium containing stripped fetal calf serum with daily additions of either vehicle alone, 10^{-8} M diethylstilbestrol (DES) or a combination of 10^{-8} M DES and 10^{-8} M progesterone. On the fourth day, the medium was changed to one containing the hormonal additions and 3, 4, 5 [³H]leucine (110 Ci/mmole, New England Nuclear) but without fetal calf serum. At the conclusion of the incubation,

TABLE 1. *Luminal fluid proteins*

Proliferative phase	(*N* = 11)	1.436 mg protein/ml wash
Secretory phase	(*N* = 10)	0.436 mg protein/ml wash

the flasks were chilled to 4°C, and the medium was centrifuged at 100,000 × *g* for 45 min. The incorporation of [³H]leucine into proteins recovered from the supernate was determined and the proteins were analyzed as described above.

Measurement of Radioactive Compounds

Radiolabeled substances were measured by counting in 2 ml Aquasol II (New England Nuclear) in disposable glass minivials (Rochester Scientific) in a Nuclear Chicago (Searle) Mark III or an Isocap 300 Liquid Scintillation spectrophotometer, accumulating 5000 or more counts per observation and using the automatic external standard. ¹²⁵Iodine-labeled serum proteins were counted in a Nuclear Chicago 1185 gamma counter.

RESULTS

Protein Content of Luminal Washes

The protein content of human uterine luminal washings varied with the stage of the menstrual cycle in which the samples were collected. The mean levels of protein were higher in the proliferative phase than in the secretory phase (Table 1). This difference approaches statistical significance.

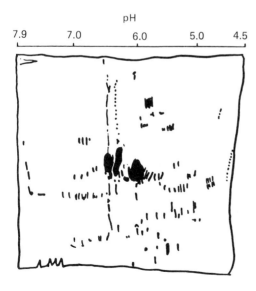

FIG. 1. Two-dimensional electrophoresis (25 mA, 2.5 hr) of human serum proteins (200 μg) stained for 48 hr in 50% ethanol, 7% acetic acid, 0.005% Coomassie blue followed by rehydration in 7% acetic acid. The isoelectric focusing gradient of the first dimension is given on the top of the figure. The second dimension was a homogenous 7% acrylamide gel in SDS. Migration was from top to bottom. This figure is a photograph of a tracing of the stained slab gel.

Polyacrylamide Gel Electrophoresis of Uterine Fluid and Serum

Standard 7% polyacrylamide tube gel electrophoresis followed by Coomassie blue staining showed marked qualitative similarities between serum and uterine luminal proteins (13). Two-dimensional electrophoretic analysis, however, revealed qualitative as well as quantitative differences between these samples. Figure 1 is a representative two-dimensional gel electrophoretic pattern of Coomassie blue stained serum proteins. No difference was noted between proliferative and secretory serum samples. A similar quantity of protein from a proliferative phase luminal wash sample reveals fewer stained spots than does serum (Fig. 2). In addition, three spots (arrow in the figure) were observed that appear to be unique to the wash proteins. Uterine luminal wash material from the secretory phase of the menstrual cycle contains even fewer spots, all of which co-migrate with serum proteins (Fig. 3).

Analysis of Proteins Secreted from Human Endometrial Cell Cultures

Monolayer cell cultures of human endometrium were prepared in sufficient quantity to perform *in vitro* experiments to assess the effects of added hormones on proteins appearing in the overlaying culture media. For these experiments [³H]leucine incorporation into media proteins was assessed as a function of time and hormone addition.

The rate of incorporation of [³H]leucine into proteins recovered from the media was maximal at about 3 hr of culture and decreased thereafter, independent of the hormonal additions. As expected, none of the protein recovered in the media cross-reacted with antihuman serum antibody. The media proteins collected from these cultures after control or hormonal stimulation were subjected to cation exchange

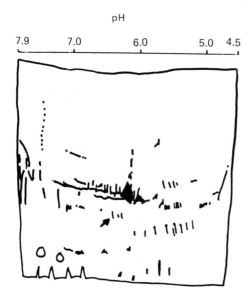

pH

| 7.9 | 7.0 | 6.0 | 5.0 | 4.5 |

FIG. 2. Details as in Fig. 1 except the sample was luminal fluid protein (400 μg) from the proliferative phase of the cycle. *Arrow* indicates protein spots not seen in serum.

pH

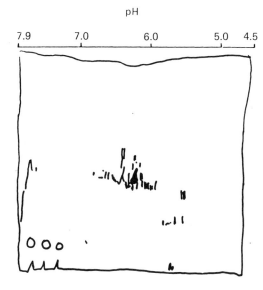

FIG. 3. Conditions as in Fig. 1 except the sample was luminal fluid protein (410 μg) from the secretory phase (day 25) of the menstrual cycle.

chromatography to separate acidic (flow-through) from basic (retained) proteins. Following this step, the acidic proteins were divided further into two pools of nearly equal size by anion exchange chromatography. In all cases, serum and luminal fluid proteins from the proliferative and secretory phase of the menstrual cycle were also run for comparison. A small proportion (5%) of the human serum was basic and was therefore retained by the cation exchange column (data not shown).

When media proteins were analyzed in a similar fashion, control cultures and those treated with estrogen also showed a very small content of basic protein. Addition of estrogen and progesterone to the cultures, however, increase the relative percentage of basic protein.

Anion-exchange chromatography of the acidic proteins in the estrogen treated cultures showed a nearly equal distribution of proteins into 0.2 and 0.3 M salt eluting fractions. These conditions were chosen empirically after prior runs eluting the lower and higher salt concentrations. Progesterone added to the estrogen treatment resulted in a relative decrease in the 0.2 M NaCl fraction.

It is possible to compare these results with those obtained from the same analysis performed on the *in vivo* material by determining the area under the elution profiles and calculating the percentage of the proteins that are basic, or in the two different NaCl eluting pools of acidic proteins. Table 2 shows the results for these experiments. Proliferative phase fluid composition resembles that of serum while the secretory fluids appear to contain more basic proteins, perhaps at the expense of the 0.2 M NaCl pool.

The distribution of media proteins from the estrogen treatment resembles that of the proliferative fluid samples. Estrogen- and progesterone-treated cells release proteins with a distribution pattern similar to that seen in secretory phase fluids,

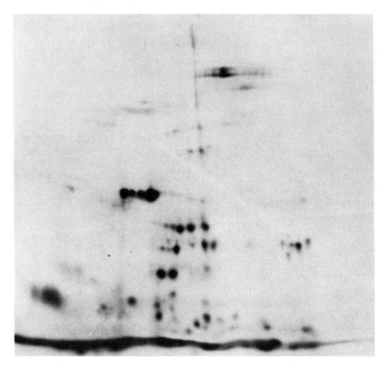

FIG. 4. Fluorogram (3-week exposure) of a two-dimensional gel electrophoretic analysis of media proteins from the control (unstimulated) monolayer culture of human endometrium. Isoelectric focusing was from right to left (basic → acidic) and the second dimension slab gel was homogenous 10% acrylamide in sodium dodecyl sulfate (25 mA/gel).

i.e., relatively more basic protein and a lower 0.2 M salt pool of acidic protein. A more rigorous analysis of these media proteins was accomplished by two dimensional electrophoretic analysis followed by fluorography of the radio-labeled protein spots.

A fluorogram of the proteins recovered from the media of control (unstimulated) cultures is shown in Fig. 4. By comparison, treatment of cells with DES yields a different pattern (Fig. 5). The circles are areas where proteins have been lost relative to the control culture and the arrows indicate spots unique to the estrogen treated cell media. The culture exposed to DES and progesterone results in further protein changes (Fig. 6). Here, as above, the open circles are proteins that are missing relative to the control culture. The filled circles are areas of proteins that are present in the DES treated culture but disappear with addition of progesterone. The arrows are proteins found only in the DES plus progesterone treated culture.

DISCUSSION

The studies reported here are a continuation of a project in which the proteins secreted by the human endometrium in response to progesterone will be identified.

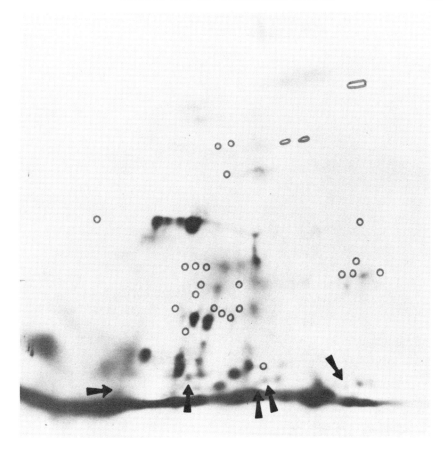

FIG. 5. Fluorogram (3-week exposure) of a two dimensional gel electrophoretic analysis of media protein from diethylstilbestrol treated endometrial cell culture. *Arrows* indicate protein spots found only in this treatment. The *circles* mark proteins found in the control culture but missing with estrogen treatment. All other conditions as in Fig. 4.

TABLE 2. *Percent distribution of proteins in luminal fluids, sera, and tissue culture media*

| | | Acidic | |
Sample	Basic	0.2 M NaCl	0.3 M NaCl
Serum	5.4	47.6	47.0
Proliferative fluid	6.4	50.6	43.1
DES-treated culture	2.4	46.8	50.3
Secretory fluid	11.6	38.9	49.5
DES-PRO treated culture	21.1	20.4	56.5

DES = diethylstilbestrol; PRO = progesterone.

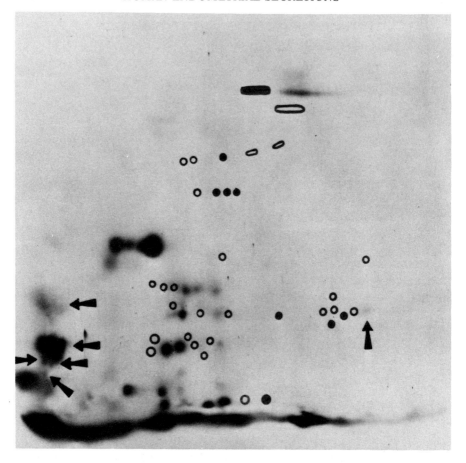

FIG. 6. Fluorogram (3-week exposure) of a two-dimensional gel electrophoretic analysis of media proteins from endometrial cultures treated with diethylstilbestrol and progesterone. The *arrows* mark proteins found only with the addition of progesterone. The *open circles* mark proteins missing with progesterone treatment but present in the control cultures. The *filled circles* mark proteins missing here but present in the media from estrogen-treated cultures. All other conditions as in Fig. 4.

Our earlier studies described the presence of a pool of proteins, termed peak III, recovered from secretory phase luminal washes subjected to Sephadex G200 column chromatography (13). These proteins are still an area of intense research in our laboratory. The focus of the present study is to catalogue the acidic proteins that are recovered from the uterus as a preparation for a direct comparison with those recovered from hormonally stimulated monolayer cell cultures of human endometrium. We recognize that whatever protein is recovered from the *in vivo* samples and determined to be specific for the secretory phase should also be demonstrable as a progesterone-dependent protein *in vitro* before it can be firmly identified as a product that is controlled by the action of progesterone.

The Gravlee jet wash device is adequate for our purposes of sample collection, as it is not significantly damaging to the endometrium. The luminal wash samples do not resemble the blood samples as they would if trauma were a problem. Further, qualitative differences are seen between serum and luminal fluids from different phases of the menstrual cycle with protein staining techniques after two-dimensional electrophoresis of the acidic proteins. Although there are proteins in the uterine fluids that derive from serum, as might be expected, the fluids are not identical and the cyclic changes suggest a hormonal influence on luminal fluid composition. The problem of dealing with a mixture of serum-derived and endometrium-derived proteins is overcome by experiments on endometrial cells in culture *in vitro* studied in the absence of added protein. It is interesting that the proteins formed from radiolabeled amino acids and secreted into the medium resemble those found *in vivo*, both by the relatively simple breakdown into basic and acidic protein pools by ion-exchange chromatography and by the patterns seen on the two-dimensional gels. Further, the proteins recovered in the tissue culture experiments differed depending upon whether progesterone, DES, or both were added to the medium.

CONCLUSIONS

In summary, differences are evident in the composition of proteins recovered from the lumen of the uterus during different phases of the normal menstrual cycle. In addition, alterations in the protein content of media collected from control and hormone-treated cultures are also observed. This model system makes it possible to compare *in vivo* and *in vitro* experimental data so that the endometrial contribution to the luminal fluids can be assessed and located and proteins that prove to be progesterone-dependent *in vitro* may also be located in the *in vivo* samples.

ACKNOWLEDGMENTS

This work was supported by the American Cancer Society Grant #PDT 138, Vincent Research Fund, and the Boston Biomedical Research Foundation. The authors wish to thank Ms. Karen Russo and Ms. Lisa Maiuri for their assistance in the preparation of this manuscript and Ms. H. Jane Anthony for technical assistance during this project.

REFERENCES

1. Bonner, W. M., and Laskey, R. A. (1974): A film detection method for tritium labeled proteins and nucleic acids in polyacrylamide gels. *Eur. J. Biochem.*, 46:83–88.
2. Dorrington, J. H., Rotter, N. F., and Fritz, I. B. (1974): The effects of FSH on cell preparations of the rat testis. In: *Hormone binding and target cell activation in the testis*, edited by M. L. Dufau and A. R. Means. Plenum Press, New York.
3. Esber, H. J., Payne, I. J., and Bogden, A. E. (1973): Variability of hormone concentrations and ratios in commercial sera used for tissue culture. *J. Natl. Cancer Inst.*, 50:559–562.
4. Gravlee, L. C. (1969): Jet-irrigation method for the diagnosis of endometrial carcinoma. *Obstet. Gynecol.*, 32:168–173.
5. Janne, O., Kontula, K., Luukkainen, T., and Vihko, R. (1975): Oestrogen-induced progesterone receptor in human uterus. *J. Steroid Biochem.*, 6:501–509.

6. Liszczak, T. M., Richardson, G. S., MacLaughlin, D. T., and Kornblith, P. L. (1977): Ultrastructure of human endometrial epithelium in monolayer culture with and without steroid hormones. *In Vitro*, 13:344–356.

7. Lowry, O. H., Roseborough, N. J., Farr, A. L., and Randall, R. J. (1951): Protein measurement with Folin phenol reagent. *J. Biol. Chem.*, 193:265–275.

8. MacLaughlin, D. T., and Richardson, G. S. (1979): The specificity of the endometrial response to estrogens and progestins. In: *Steroid Receptors and the Management of Cancer, Vol. 1*, edited by E. B. Thompson and M. E. Lippman, pp. 161–172. CRC Press, New York.

9. Noyes, A. T., Hertig, A. T., and Rock, J. (1950): Dating the endometrial biopsy. *Fertil. Steril.*, 1:3–25.

10. O'Farrell, P. H. (1975): High resolution two-dimensional electrophoresis of proteins. *J. Biol. Chem.*, 250:4007–4021.

11. Paul, J. (1973): *Cell and Tissue Culture*. Edinburgh, London.

12. Spellman, C. M., Fottrell, P. R., Baynes, S., O'Dwyer, B. M., and Clinch, J. D. (1973): A study of some enzymes and isoenzymes of carbohydrate metabolism in the human endometrium during the menstrual cycle. *Clin. Chem. Acta*, 48:259.

13. Sylvan, P. E., MacLaughlin, D. T., Richardson, G. S., Scully, R. E., and Nikrui, N. (1981): Human uterine luminal fluid proteins associated with secretory phase endometrium: Progesterone-induced proteins? *Biol. Reprod.*, 24:423–429.

14. Tseng, L., and Gurpide, E. (1975): Induction of human endometrial estradiol dehydrogenase by progestins. *Endocrinology*, 97:825–833.

15. Tseng, L., Gusberg, S. B., and Gurpide, E. (1977): Estradiol receptor and 17β dehydrogenase in normal and abnormal endometrium. *Ann. NY Acad. Sci.*, 286:190–198.

16. Waddell, W. I. (1956): A simple ultraviolet spectrophotometric method for the determination of protein. *J. Lab. Clin. Med.*, 48:311–314.

17. Wilson, E. (1967): Induction of malate dehydrogenase by oestradiol-17β in the human endometrium. *Nature (Lond.)*, 215:758–759.

Steroids and Endometrial Cancer,
edited by V. M. Jasonni, et al.
Raven Press, New York © 1983.

Estrogen and Progestin Effects on Epithelium and Stroma from Pre- and Postmenopausal Endometria: Application to Clinical Studies of the Climacteric Syndrome

*R. J. B. King and **M. I. Whitehead

*Hormone Biochemistry Department, Imperial Cancer Research Fund,
London WC2A 3PX; and **Department of Obstetrics and Gynecology,
King's College Hospital Medical School, London SE5 8RX, United Kingdom*

Adenocarcinoma of the human endometrium is derived from the epithelium; therefore, the behavior of epithelial cells is relevant both to the genesis and response of such tumors. Thus, it is surprising that little attention has been devoted to the analysis of epithelial cells as distinct from whole endometrium, which also includes stromal elements. We have developed methods to separate and culture epithelium and stroma (24,25) and to analyze separately their biochemistry with special reference to the changes brought about by estrogen plus progestin (17,21,22). The choice of these two classes of female sex hormones was based on two factors. First, they determine to a large extent the behavior of the endometrium during the normal menstrual cycle. More importantly for the topic of this chapter, both estrogens and progestins have been implicated in the genesis and treatment of endometrial cancer. Prolonged estrogen action, unopposed or inadequately opposed by intermittent progestin action, has long been held to be a risk factor for endometrial cancer, regardless of whether the hormone imbalance is of natural (4,11,32) or exogenous (6,32) origin. Further, progestins are widely used in the management of endometrial cancer (2).

Endometrial cancer is most commonly detected in postmenopausal women but, given the long time period from initiation to the production of clinically detectable tumor, it is probable that many such tumors are of premenopausal origin. Estrogens usually are considered to be tumor promoters rather than initiators, although an additional preparative action seems likely (15). These putative actions of estrogen extend the period of interest into both the pre- and post-menopausal phases of a woman's life. We have therefore compared the endocrine behavior of epithelium and stroma from pre- and postmenopausal women, as it is not known if the sensitivity to steroids changes after the climacteric.

The postmenopausal endometria were obtained from women receiving exogenous progestins and/or estrogens. For reasons discussed elsewhere in this volume and by us (23,40), the somewhat empirical nature of these treatments gives cause for concern with respect to both the estrogenic and progestogenic components, estrogens because of their hepatic and tumorigenic effects and progestins because of potential cardiovascular complications. We have therefore adapted our methodologies so that the endometrial potencies of commercially available hormone preparations can be evaluated with a view to the development of safer forms of hormone replacement therapy.

The choice of biochemical parameters to be assayed was determined by the current models of how female sex steroids affect DNA synthesis. Estrogen action is mediated by the estrogen receptor machinery, which includes the transfer of receptor into the nucleus, so we measured both soluble (REC) and nuclear (REN) estradiol receptor (25), the total receptor content (RET) being obtained as the sum of REC and REN. Synthesis of DNA was monitored by [³H]thymidine ([³H]TdR) autoradiography (2). Because an additional feature of estrogen stimulation is the increase in soluble progesterone receptor (RP), this was also assayed (23). All of these parameters can be taken as indices of estrogen action, but provided the estrogenic environment remains relatively constant, some also indicate progestin effects. Thus, progestins inhibit estrogen-induced DNA synthesis (8,20), and both total and nuclear estradiol receptor content (1,7). The mechanisms involved in the latter response are incompletely understood and have been discussed elsewhere (9,19,26,34); however, the general feeling is that progestins exert at least part of their antiestrogenic effects by inhibition of receptor synthesis and by inducing the enzyme estradiol dehydrogenase. Hence, we have used estradiol dehydrogenase as an additional index of progestational activity together with another enzyme, isocitric dehydrogenase. The function of the latter enzyme is uncertain, but it is progestin-sensitive and appears to correlate with the secretory response to progestins (14,22).

ANALYSIS OF EPITHELIUM AND STROMA

Patients and Methods

Premenopausal endometria were obtained at hysterectomy for nonmalignant disorders, and postmenopausal samples were obtained by suction curettage as previously described (12,23). All of the biochemical methods have been published (20,22,23). The methods for separating epithelium and stroma have been described elsewhere (17,22,24,25).

Estradiol Receptors

In all types of sample no quantitative differences between epithelium and stroma were observed for RET (Fig. 1a), REN (Fig. 1b), REC (Fig. 1c) or the percentage of receptor in the nucleus (Fig. 1d). The K_D of REC for [³H]estradiol was 4×10^{-10}M in epithelium and 1×10^{-10}M in stroma; no type II sites were detected (21).

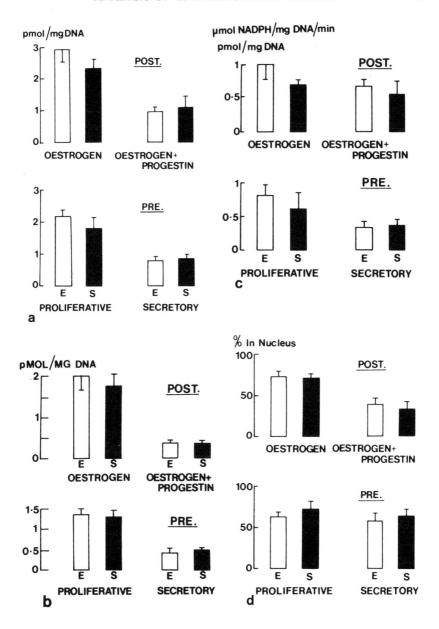

FIG. 1. a: Total estradiol receptor; **b:** nuclear estradiol receptor; **c:** soluble estradiol receptor; **d:** estradiol receptor. Estradiol receptor content of epithelium (E) and stroma (S) from postmenopausal (POST) and premenopausal (PRE) endometria. The postmenopausal women were taking the stated hormones at the time of curettage. The menstrual cycle stage of the premenopausal samples was assessed by light microscopy. Results are given as mean ± SEM for at least four analyses.

Similarly, only type I nuclear sites were detected in intact endometrium or separated epithelium and stroma (21).

The quantities of REN, REC, and RET were the same in premenopausal proliferative, as in estrogen-treated, postmenopausal epithelium, and stroma. The same conclusion applied to the comparison of premenopausal secretory phase samples with specimens from postmenopausal women treated with estrogen plus progestin. Regardless of menopausal status, progestins decreased both RET and REN in epithelium and stroma. The suppression of RET was primarily due to reduction of REN in both pre- and postmenopausal samples. This results in a diminished proportion of RET in the nucleus of progestin treated postmenopausal samples, although this result was not obtained with premenopausal endometria (Fig. 1d). This is the only difference in receptor quantitation between pre- and postmenopausal samples that we have encountered and its physiological relevance is dubious as we have shown that after *in vivo* injection of 'H estradiol into premenopausal women, a lower percentage of the endometrial 'H estradiol was in the nuclei of secretory than proliferative phase samples (3). A similar progestin effect on the nuclear content of estradiol receptors in premenopausal intact endometrium was noted in superfusion (37) and receptor quantitation experiments (1).

Our conclusion from these experiments is that the control of estradiol receptor concentration is similar in epithelium and stroma and that these controls are not affected by menopausal status. The evidence as to what those controls might be suggests that several methods of regulation occur. The constitutive levels of RE (18) can be increased by estrogen and decreased by progestin as has been previously demonstrated for intact endometrium (1,7,27,29,31). The progestin effects involve at least two mechanisms, direct inhibition of receptor synthesis and reduction of intracellular estradiol due to its metabolism by estradiol dehydrogenase (9,19,34). Progestins lower RE levels induced by a number of estrogens, including those like ethinyl estradiol that are not substrates for estradiol dehydrogenase (11,19,26). Hence the latter enzyme cannot be the sole regulatory factor. The strong evidence for estradiol dehydrogenase function derives from metabolic experiments (9,10,19,33) and inverse correlations between enzyme activity and REN and DNA synthesis (20). However, certain features of its action need further clarification. All of the evidence cited in support of its biological function was obtained with intact, human endometrium. Our data (see below) indicate that the enzyme is induced by progestins in epithelium but not stroma; yet the receptor change occurs in both cell fractions. Potential explanations for the anomalous stromal result are that estradiol metabolism may occur so rapidly in the epithelium that insufficient hormone is available for the stromal cells (19) or that enzyme activity does change in the stroma but is not detected by our method. Using a different method for separating epithelium and stroma, Liu and Tseng (28) did find progestin-induced changes in stromal dehydrogenase albeit of a much lower magnitude than that seen in epithelium. Further, large changes in estradiol dehydrogenase activity are not required to affect biological response (20). However, discussion of the biological function of this enzyme should take note of the observation that it is induced by estrogen and not progestin in rat uterine epithelium (31) at a time when receptor levels remain high (5).

Progesterone Receptor

No quantitative difference between pre- and post-menopausal samples were observed (Fig. 2a). Soluble RP levels were decreased by progestins in both epithelium and stroma. This result would be anticipated simply because of the transfer of RP into the nuclear compartment, which we have not quantitated. However, published data by other groups (26,27,29) suggest that progestins also cause a net decrease in RP content. The K_D of RP is about 4×10^{-9} M in both epithelium and stroma (21), but there is less RP in stroma than epithelium. This quantitative difference might be related to different progestin effects in the two compartments (17,22).

DNA Synthesis

There were no differences between the comparable pre- and postmenopausal samples (Fig. 2b). Synthesis of DNA was high in both epithelium and stroma in estrogenized endometria and was suppressed by progestin in both fractions.

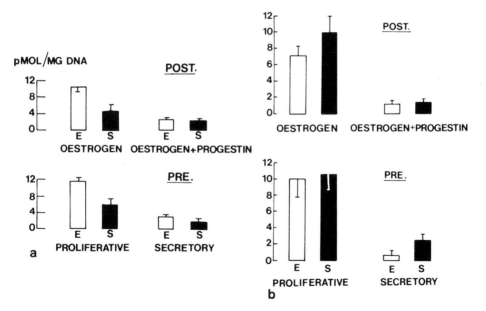

FIG. 2. a: Soluble progesterone receptor content of epithelium and stroma. **b:** Autoradiographic assessment of DNA synthesis in epithelium and stroma after [³H]thymidine ([³H]TdR) labeling of intact endometrium. *Ordinates:* Epithelium = % of glandular epithelial nuclei labeled with [³H]TdR; stroma = no. stromal cell (all types) nuclei labeled with [³H]TdR/high power microscopic field. Abbreviations and details are given in the legend to Fig. 1.

Enzyme Changes

There were no significant differences between the pre- and postmenopausal samples for either isocitric (Fig. 3a) or estradiol dehydrogenase (Fig. 3b). Both dehydrogenases were markedly elevated in epithelium but not stroma after progestin exposure.

EPITHELIAL AND STROMAL CHANGES IN RELATION TO ANALYSES OF INTACT ENDOMETRIUM

In many cases, it is neither practical nor possible to separate an endometrial sample into its component cell types. Our results with the fractionated samples indicate that analyses of intact endometrium can yield useful information about the behavior of both epithelium and stroma. As both REN and RET partition equally between epithelium and stroma and are influenced by progestins equally in both compartments, it follows that their assay in intact endometrium provides information about both epithelium and stroma. Conversely, estradiol and isocitric dehydrogenase activities are confined mainly to the epithelium so that activities measured in intact endometrium reflect progestin effects on the epithelium.

Interpretation of RP data are more problematical. The lower RP content of stroma as compared with epithelium means that the concentration of RP in intact endometrium in part depends on the proportion of epithelium to stroma in the specimen. This is not a major problem if, for example, one wishes to compare the effects of

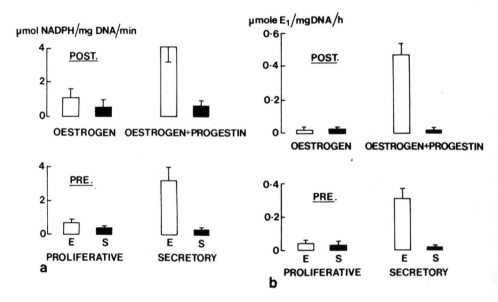

FIG. 3. **a:** Isocitric dehydrogenase. **b:** Estradiol dehydrogenase; dehydrogenase activities of epithelium and stroma. Abbreviations and details are given in the legend to Fig. 1. E_1 = estrone formed from the substrate, estradiol.

different estrogen preparations under constant treatment conditions (see below) but can present problems in comparing different types of hyperplasia in which cell proportions are markedly different (13,23,25,27,29,33).

CONCLUSIONS

With one possible exception (percent of RE in nucleus), we have found no differences between the behavior of epithelium and stroma to the hormone environment of the premenopausal menstrual cycle and to the postmenopausal endometrium exposed to the stimulus of exogenous estrogens and progestins.

Clinical Applications

For reasons given in the introduction, we wished to study the effect of different types, doses, duration, and routes of administration of various estrogen and progestin preparations on the postmenopausal endometrium. We particularly wished to gain information about hormone effects on the epithelial cells because of the potential neoplastic transformation of those cells. From the data discussed in the previous section, analysis of intact endometrium can be used for this purpose provided that the test preparations do not influence markedly the proportions of epithelium to stroma. Over the time scale used in our studies, this condition appears to be met, although very prolonged use of some estrogens does produce a greater incidence of hyperplasia than other preparations (35,38). Details of patients and hormone preparations used will be found in references 23 and 39.

Estrogens

Our data for REN and RP are summarized in Fig. 4. Regardless of type of estrogen or the route of administration, all subjected the endometrium to a potent estrogenic stimulus at least equal to that seen in the proliferative phase of a normal menstrual cycle. These and additional results are discussed in greater detail elsewhere (17,23), but it is not surprising that prolonged administration of these estrogens unopposed by a progestin can result in endometrial hyperplasia (35,36,38). Given the association between the more severe types of hyperplasia and neoplasia (15), the increased risk of cancer is also understandable.

Progestins

Maximal progestin effects on the estrogenized endometrium are obtained after 6 days oral administration of compounds such as norethisterone (17) and norgestrel (unpublished results). These effects are maintained up to at least 10 days of treatment. Hence, we have chosen 6 days as our routine test period for monitoring different progestin (Fig. 5). Clearly, all doses of the progestins tested are producing near maximal effects on the epithelium, and we have not yet attained a dose–response relationship for any of the parameters measured.

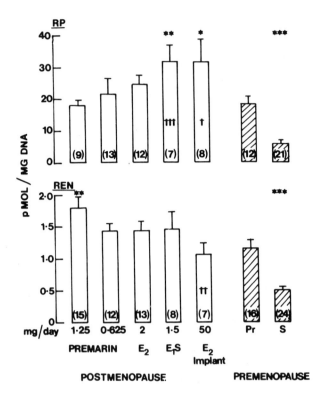

FIG. 4. Nuclear estradiol receptor (REN) and soluble progesterone receptor (RP) content of endometria from postmenopausal women treated with the stated estrogens. Premarin = conjugated equine estrogens. E_2 = estradiol valerate; E_1S = piperazine estrone sulphate; E_2 implant = subcutaneous estradiol implant; Pr = proliferative phase; S = secretory phase. Results are expressed as mean ± SEM (no. observations). Comparison with premenopausal, proliferative phase samples by Student's t-test, $*P < 0.05$; $**P < 0.01$; $***P < 0.001$. Comparison of 1.25 mg Premarin samples with other postmenopausal treatments by Student's t-test, $†P < 0.05$; $††P < 0.01$; $†††P < 0.001$. (From King et al., ref. 17, with permission.)

The data presented in Fig. 5 were obtained with 1.25 mg/day Premarin. The progestins were just as efficacious against 0.625 mg/day Premarin (39). Further details and discussion of the progestin effects will be found in references 17 and 40.

SUMMARY

We feel that these types of analysis provide a relatively simple but powerful method for determining endometrial potencies of clinically useful hormone preparations. All of the preparations thus far analyzed, whether estrogen or progestin, are maximally stimulating the endometrial epithelial and stromal cells, and there is a potential for using even lower doses of progestin with the attendant diminished risk of unwanted side effects.

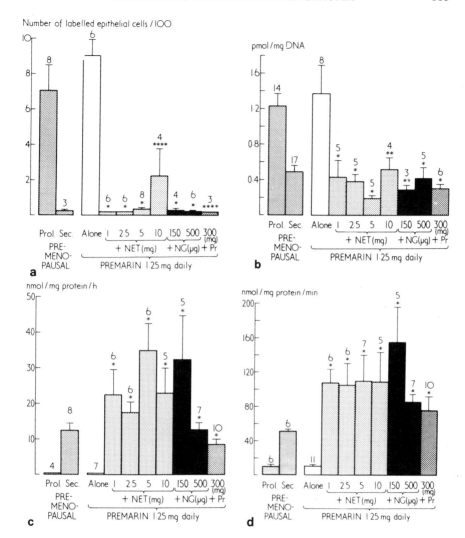

FIG. 5. a: Labelling index; **b:** nuclear estrogen receptor; **c:** estradiol 17β dehydrogenase; **d:** isocitrate dehydrogenase. Effect of progestins on Premarin-stimulated, postmenopausal endometria. NET = norethisterone; NG = D/L norgestrel; Pr = progesterone. The stated doses were taken by mouth daily for 6 days. Data from premenopausal proliferative (Prol) and secretory (Sec) phase samples are included for comparison. Results are expressed as mean ± SEM (no. observations). Statistical comparisons of Premarin alone versus Premarin plus the stated dose of progestin using Student's t-test; *$P < 0.02$; **$P < 0.005$; ***$P < 0.01$; ****$P < 0.02$. (From Whitehead et al., ref. 40, with permission.)

ACKNOWLEDGMENTS

We acknowledge the help of Professor R. W. Taylor (St. Thomas' Hospital, London) in supplying many of the premenopausal samples and our clinical and nursing colleagues at King's College Hospital and the Chelsea Hospital for Women, London, for the postmenopausal samples.

REFERENCES

1. Bayard, F., Damilano, S., Robel, P., and Baulieu, E. E. (1978): Cytoplasmic and nuclear estradiol and progesterone receptors in human endometrium. *J. Clin. Endocrinol. Metab.*, 46:635–648.
2. Bönte, J., and Kohorn, E. I. (1978): The response of hyperplastic dysplastic and neoplastic endometrium to progestational therapy. In: *Hormonal Biology of Endometrial Cancer, Vol. 42*, edited by G. S. Richardson and D. T. MacLaughlin, UICC Technical Reports, pp. 155–184. Geneva.
3. Brush, M. G., Taylor, R. W., and King, R. J. B. (1967): The uptake of $(6,7-{}^3H)$ oestradiol by the normal human reproductive tract. *J. Endocrinol.*, 39:599–607.
4. Brush, M. G., Milton, P. J. D., Swain, M. C., and Moore, J. W. (1975): Endometrial cystic hyperplasia—a premalignant state or a complex endocrine disorder? In: *Gynaecological Malignancy* edited by M. G. Brush and R. W. Taylor, pp. 155–178. Baillière Tindall, London.
5. Clark, J. H., and Peck, E. J. (1979): *Female Sex Steroids, Vol. 14, Monographs on Endocrinology*, pp. 158–160. Springer Verlag, Berlin.
6. Cramer, D. W., and Knapp, R. C. (1979): Review of epidemiologic studies of endometrial cancer and exogenous estrogen. *Obstet. Gynecol.*, 54:521–526.
7. Croker, S. G., Milton, P. J. D., and King, R. J. B. (1974): Uptake of $(6,7-{}^3H)$ oestradiol-17β by normal and abnormal human endometrium. *J. Endocrinol.*, 62:145–152.
8. Ferenczy, A., Bertrand, G., and Gelfand, M. M. (1979): Proliferation kinetics of human endometrium during the normal menstrual cycle. *Am. J. Obstet. Gynecol.*, 133:859–867.
9. Gurpide, E. (1978): Enzymatic modulation of hormonal action at the target tissue. *J. Toxicol. Environ. Health*, 4:249–268.
10. Gurpide, E., and Maeks, C. (1981): Influence of endometrial 17β-hydroxysteroid dehydrogenase activity on the binding of estradiol to receptors. *J. Clin. Endocrinol. Metab.*, 52:252–253.
11. Gusberg, S. B. (1976): The individual at high risk for endometrial carcinoma. *Am. J. Obstet. Gynecol.*, 1:535–542.
12. Holt, E. M. (1970): Outpatient diagnostic curettage. *J. Obstet. Gynaecol. Br. Emp.*, 77:1043–1046.
13. Jänne, O., Kauppila, A., Kontula, K., Syrjälä, P., Vierikko, P., and Vihko, R. (1980): Female sex steroid receptors in human endometrial hyperplasia and carcinoma. In: *Steroid Receptors and Hormone Dependent Neoplasia*, edited by J. L. Wittliff and O. Dapunt, pp. 37–44. Masson Publishing, New York.
14. Jelinek, J., Jelinkova, M., Hagenfeldt, K., Landgren, B. M., and Diczfalusy, E. (1978): Effect of two progestins on human endometrial enzymes and trace elements. *Acta Endocrinol.*, 88:580–588.
15. King, R. J. B. (1981): Effects of female sex hormones on human endometrium in relation to neoplasia. In: *Mechanism of Steroid Action*, edited by G. P. Lewis and M. Ginsburg, pp. 49–58. MacMillan, London.
16. King, R. J. B., Beard, V., Gordon, J., Pooley, A. S., Smith, J. A., Steggles, A. W., and Vertes, M. (1971): Studies on estradiol binding in mammalian tissues. In: *Advances in the Biosciences 7*, edited by G. Raspé, pp. 21–44. Pergamon Press, Viesweg.
17. King, R. J. B., Lane, G., Siddle, N., Taylor, R. W., Townsend, P. T., and Whitehead, M. I. (1981): Assessment of oestrogen and progestin effects on epithelium and stroma from pre- and postmenopausal endometria. *J. Steroid Biochem.*, 15:175–181.
18. King, R. J. B., and Mainwaring, W. I. P. (1974): In: *Steroid-Cell Interactions*, pp. 225–226. Butterworths, London.
19. King, R. J. B., Townsend, P. T., Siddle, N., and Whitehead, M. I. (1983): Mechanisms of progestin action on hormone endometrium. In: *Hormone Cell Interactions in Reproductive Tissues*, edited by J. Wittliff and O. Dapunt. Masson Publishing, New York *(in press)*.
20. King, R. J. B., Townsend, P. T., and Whitehead, M. I. (1981): The role of estradiol dehydrogenase in mediating progestin effects on endometrium from postmenopausal women receiving estrogens and progestins. *J. Steroid Biochem.*, 14:235–238.
21. King, R. J. B., Townsend, P. T., Siddle, N., Whitehead, M. I., and Taylor, R. W. (1982): Regulation of estrogen and progesterone receptor levels in epithelium and stroma from pre- and post menopausal endometrium. *J. Steroid. Biochem.*, 16:21–29.

22. King, R. J. B., Townsend, P. T., Whitehead, M. I., Young, O., and Taylor, R. W. (1981): Biochemical analyses of separated epithelium and stroma from endometria of premenopausal and postmenopausal women receiving estrogen and progestins. *J. Steroid Biochem.*, 14:979–987.
23. King, R. J. B., Whitehead, M. I., Campbell, S., and Minardi, J. (1979): Effect of estrogen and progestin treatment on endometria from postmenopausal women. *Cancer Res.*, 39:1094–1101.
24. Kirk, D., and Irwin, J. C. (1980): Normal human endometrium in cell culture. In: *Methods in Cell Biology, Vol. 21B,* edited by C. C. Harris, B. F. Trump, and G. D. Stoner, pp. 51–77. Academic Press, New York.
25. Kirk, D., King, R. J. B., Heyes, J., Peachey, L., Hirsch, P. J., and Taylor, R. W. (1978): Normal human endometrium in cell culture. *In Vitro*, 13:651–662.
26. Kreitmann, B., Bugat, R., and Bayard, F. (1979): Estrogen and progestin regulation of the progesterone receptor concentration in human endometrium. *J. Clin. Endocrinol. Metab.*, 49:926–929.
27. Levy, C., Robel, P., Gautray, J. P., De Brux, J., Verma, U., Descomps, B., Baulieu, E. E., and Eychenne, B. (1980): Estradiol and progesterone receptors in human endometrium: Normal and abnormal menstrual cycles and early pregnancy. *Am. J. Obstet. Gynecol.*, 136:646–651.
28. Liu, H. C., and Tseng, L. (1979): Estradiol metabolism in isolated human endometrial epithelial glands and stromal cells. *Endocrinology*, 104:1674–1681.
29. Martin, P. M., Rolland, P. H., Gammerre, M., Serment, H., and Toga, M. (1979): Estradiol and progesterone receptors in normal and neoplastic endometrium: Correlations between receptors, histopathological examinations and clinical responses under progestin therapy. *Int. J. Cancer*, 23:321–329.
30. Patinawin, S., Wahawisan, R., and Gorrell, T. A. (1980): Histochemical localization of 17β-hydroxysteroid dehydrogenase activity in rat uterus. *J. Steroid Biochem.*, 13:1277–1281.
31. Pollow, K., Schmidt-Gollwitzer, M., and Pollow, B. (1980): Progesterone- and estradiol-binding proteins from normal human endometrium and endometrial carcinoma: A comparative study. In: *Steroid Receptors and Hormone-Dependent Neoplasia,* edited by J. L. Wittliff and O. Dapunt, pp. 69–94. Masson Publishing, New York.
32. Richardson, G. S. (1978): The patient with endometrial cancer. In: *Hormonal Biology of Endometrial Cancer, Vol. 42,* edited by G. S. Richardson and D. T. MacLaughlin, UICC Technical Reports, pp. 11–35. Geneva.
33. Rodriquez, J., Sen, K. K., Seski, J. C., Menon, M., Johnson, T. R., and Menon, K. M. J. (1979): Progesterone binding by human endometrial tissue during the proliferative and secretory phases of the menstrual cycle and by hyperplastic and carcinomatous endometrium. *Am. J. Obstet. Gynecol.*, 133:660–665.
34. Schmidt-Gollwitzer, M., Genz, T., Schmidt-Gollwitzer, K., Pollow, B., and Pollow, K. (1978): Correlation between oestradiol and progesterone receptor levels, 17 βhydroxysteroid dehydrogenase activity and endometrial tissue levels of oestradiol oestrone and progesterone in women. In: *Endometrial Cancer,* edited by M. G. Brush, R. J. B. King, and R. W. Taylor, pp. 227–241. Baillière Tindall, London.
35. Sturdee, D. W., Wade-Evans, T., Paterson, M. E. L., Thom, M., and Studd, J. W. W. (1978): Relations between bleeding pattern, endometrial histology, and oestrogen treatment in menopausal women. *Br. Med. J.*, 1:1575–1577.
36. Thom, M. H., White, P. J., Williams, R. M., Sturdee, D. W., Paterson, M. E. L., Wade-Evans, T., and Studd, J. W. W. (1979): Prevention and treatment of endometrial disease in climacteric women receiving oestrogen therapy. *Lancet*, 2:455–457.
37. Tseng, L., and Gurpide, E. (1972): Nuclear concentration of estradiol in superfused slices of human endometrium. *Am. J. Obstet. Gynecol.*, 114:995–1001.
38. Whitehead, M. I. (1978): The effects of oestrogens and progestogens on the postmenopausal endometrium. *Maturitas*, 1:87–98.
39. Whitehead, M. I., Townsend, P. T., Pryse-Davies, J., Ryder, T., Lane, G., Siddle, N., and King, R. J. B. (1981): Actions of progestins on the morphology and biochemistry of the endometrium of postmenopausal women receiving low dose oestrogen therapy. *Am. J. Obstet. Gynecol.*, 142:791–795.
40. Whitehead, M. I., Siddle, N. C., Townsend, P. T., Lane, G., and King, R. J. B. (1983): The use of progestins and progesterone in the treatment of climacteric and postmenopausal symptoms. In: *Progesterone and Progestins,* edited by P. Mauvais-Jarvis, pp. 277–296. Raven Press, New York.

Steroids and Endometrial Cancer,
edited by V. M. Jasonni, et al.
Raven Press, New York © 1983.

Estrogen Production in Endometrial Cancer

V. H. T. James, M. J. Reed, and Elizabeth J. Folkerd

*Department of Chemical Pathology, St. Mary's Hospital Medical School,
London, W2 1PG United Kingdom*

After the menopause, the incidence of endometrial and breast cancer increases considerably. Despite extensive epidemiological and endocrinological investigations, it is still unclear what major factors are involved in this apparent increased risk of malignancy in the older female. However, the menopause is characterized by highly significant changes in the endocrine environment; in particular, estrogen hormone production diminishes and eventually becomes insignificant, whereas androgen production may increase (12). This process, however, is a slow transition from the characteristic cyclic pattern of the normal menstrual cycle, through a period of uncoordinated steroid production, until eventually the ovary contributes little to estrogen production. It is tempting, therefore, to look at the altered hormone balance and the complementary evidence from excessive or altered estrogen exposure and to seek to deduce from this some endocrine participation in the development of these malignancies. The evidence appears superficially more convincing in the case of endometrial cancer; in spite of reservations expressed by some groups (3,18), there are now several well-documented reports (1,8,17,28) that implicate estrogen use as a factor in the genesis of endometrial cancer.

As yet, no entirely convincing evidence has been produced for altered estrogen metabolism in women with endometrial cancer. Extensive studies have been made of indirect estrogen production, and particular emphasis has been given to estrone and the production of this steroid from androstenedione. A series of studies over several years, particularly those of Siiteri and MacDonald (16,24), have given us a valuable insight into the mechanisms of estrone production in the human female. These data have essentially led to the view that the major determinant in the control of estrone production in women is weight, as the two factors are positively related. In addition, androstenedione conversion to estrone appears to be age-related, and older women (i.e., postmenopausal) show roughly double the conversion rate of younger women (9). As both weight and age are risk factors for endometrial cancer, the hypothesis of the role of altered conversion and increased production of estrone in endometrial cancer is attractive (25). However, women with endometrial cancer when properly matched for weight were not found to differ from healthy controls when estrogen metabolism was investigated (16,21).

Although the data do not support the idea of a central role for increased estrone production in endometrial cancer, it would be premature to abandon the concept that altered estrogen is possibly a major factor. First, it is estradiol rather than estrone that is currently thought to be involved directly in the mechanism of estrogen action at the cellular level; hence, it is clearly more pertinent to study estradiol metabolism. Further, the action of steroids at the tissue level is influenced by a variety of factors, particularly plasma protein binding. The local indirect production of estrogens in a metabolically active tissue (e.g., adipose tissue) may produce significantly increased concentrations of estrogens, including estradiol. All these factors require study, as in many respects our knowledge of estrogen metabolism is minimal.

Our studies have therefore been aimed in three directions: (a) to attempt to describe estrogen more completely, particularly estradiol production in older women; (b) to examine the indirect or peripheral production of estrogen in body tissues and to define the factors that influence this production; and (c) to examine the significance of binding proteins in regulating estrogen exposure. In this chapter, we report some of our studies of the first two of these.

MATERIALS AND METHODS

The techniques employed for the investigation of steroid kinetics and for the *in vitro* studies have been described in detail elsewhere (4,5,10,22).

RESULTS

Figure 1 shows the estrogen clearance rates, measured by the double-isotope infusion technique, in six women with endometrial cancer and five with endometrial hyperplasia. All subjects were either postmenopausal or, in three cases, perimenopausal. Table 1 gives the clinical and biochemical details. The normal ranges shown in Fig. 1 are derived from literature values. When compared with the subjects' ideal body weight, there was a significant correlation for the metabolic clearance of estrone (MCR $-$ El, $r = 0.84$, $p < 0.01$). Although a correlation was also found between the metabolic clearance rate of estradiol (MCR $-$ E2) and ideal body weight ($r = 0.54$), further studies are required to confirm the significance of this observation. Using the metabolic clearance rates and the plasma concentrations of endogenous steroid, production rates of estrone and estradiol were calculated. The results are shown in Table 2 and Fig. 2. The normal range of estrogen production is derived from literature values. From the measured conversion of estrone to estradiol, it is possible to calculate the proportion of the estradiol production rate that can be accounted for by conversion of estrone. These results are shown in Table 2.

The results of the *in vitro* studies are shown in Figs. 3 and 4. Subcutaneous adipose tissue was obtained from tissue removed at surgery from a series of patients undergoing surgery for nonendocrine and nonmalignant conditions. Five patients with endometrial cancer and one with endometrial hyperplasia were also studied.

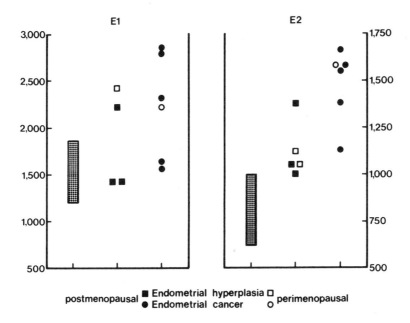

FIG. 1. Clearance rates of estrone and estradiol in women with endometrial hyperplasia or endometrial cancer. Ranges for normal postmenopausal women are indicated by the *shaded bars* (data from ref. 14). (From James et al., ref. 10, with permission.)

TABLE 1. *Endometrial cancer study*

Subject	Conditions	Age (yr)	LMP/YPM	Wt (kg)	LH[a] (IU/liter)	FSH[b] (IU/liter)	Progesterone (ng/ml)
1	EH	54	Persistent bleeding 3 months	71	34	42	0.16
2	EH	71	21	93	—	—	0.20
3	EH	45	Continuous loss 6 months	74	4	7	0.18
4	EH	50	Irregular periods LMP 22 days	54	2	2	0.49
5	EH	56	LMP 14 months and 2 months ago	51	21	41	0.17
6	EC	47	1	65	49	46	0.15
7	EC	50	2	60	36	29	0.19
8	EC	70	6	70	33	43	0.30
9	EC	51	1	70	7	11	0.34
10	EC	67	13	73	—	—	0.33
11	EC	78	23	74	—	—	0.47

[a]Normal ranges premenopausal, 10 ± 5 IU/liter; postmenopausal, >25 IU/liter.
[b]Normal ranges premenopausal, 5 ± 4 IU/liter; postmenopausal, >25 IU/liter.
EH = endometrial hyperplasia; EC = endometrial cancer; LMP = last monthly period; YPM = years postmenopausal.

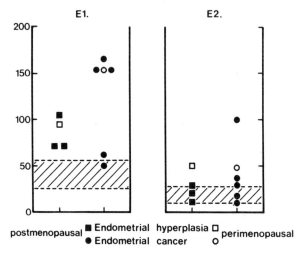

FIG. 2. Production rates of estrone and estradiol in women with endometrial hyperplasia or endometrial cancer. Ranges for normal postmenopausal women are indicated by the *shaded areas* (data from ref. 20).

TABLE 2. *Production rates of estrone (PR-E1) and estradiol (PR-E2), conversion of estrone to estradiol ([ρ] E1E2) and the percentage of estradiol derived from estrone (PRE2-E1)*

Subject	Condition	PR-E1 (μg/24 hr)	[ρ] E1E2 (%)	PR-E2 (μg/24 hr)	PRE2-E1 (%)
1	EH	72.2	3.8	30.7	8.9
2	EH	104.0	4.7	22.2	22.0
3[a]	EH	—	—	60.6	—
4	EH	96.2	4.1	51.7	7.6
5	EH	71.0	4.0	11.1	25.6
6	EC	61.2	3.3	101.4	2.0
7	EC	55.0	5.3	29.2	10.0
8	EC	165.4	8.1	35.8	37.4
9	EC	158.7	3.9	48.8	12.7
10	EC	158.3	3.0	19.6	24.2
11	EC	156.9	6.1	12.5	76.6

[a]The conversion of testosterone to estradiol was measured in this subject.
EH = endometrial hyperplasia; EC = endometrial cancer.

The results are shown in Figs. 3 and 4. Figure 3 shows the relationship between the conversion of androstenedione to estrone and age and the results from the patients with endometrial disease. Figure 4 shows the conversion of estrone to estradiol by adipose tissue as measured *in vitro* related to age in the control patients and also in those with endometrial disease.

DISCUSSION

The use of radiolabeled steroid tracer techniques pioneered by Baird et al. (2) currently offers the sharpest insight into steroid metabolism *in vivo*. Despite obvious

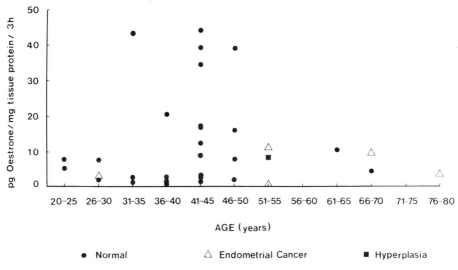

FIG. 3. Correlation between age and the *in vitro* conversion of androstenedione to estrone by adipose tissue taken from normal women and women with endometrial cancer or hyperplasia (data from ref. 5).

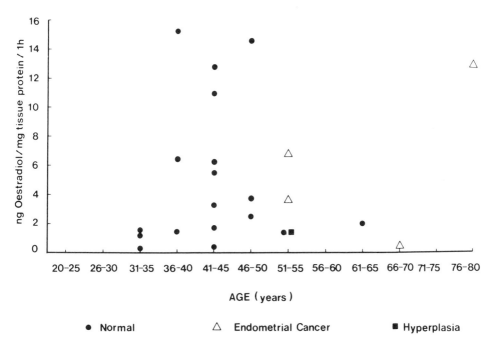

FIG. 4. Correlation between age and the *in vitro* conversion of estrone to estradiol by adipose tissue taken from normal women and women with endometrial cancer or hyperplasia (data from refs. 4 and 5).

practical limitations and the possible problems of kinetic model, this method has provided some of the most important data currently available in several areas of clinical endocrinology. To our knowledge, there are no data on estradiol clearance, production, and interconversion in patients with endometrial cancer; indeed, even control data for women in the postmenopausal age group are very limited.

Our data for metabolic clearance rate measurements in the patients studied here are shown in Fig. 1. Several of the women had elevated clearance of estrone, which may be explicable in two patients because they were perimenopausal. In the case of estradiol, almost all patients, those with hyperplasia and those with cancer, had relatively high clearance rates. The cancer patients demonstrated particularly elevated clearances. Although there are apparently no other published studies for comparison, it is of interest that Kirschner et al. (13), studying postmenopausal women with breast cancer, also found elevated clearance rates for both estrone and estradiol.

The reason for the increased rate of clearance is not known. In the case of steroids, which are firmly bound to plasma protein, a relationship between clearance rate and the unbound steroid concentration has been reported (26), but in patients with endometrial cancer, neither we nor others have found differences from normal. In our study, there was a significant relationship between estrone clearance and ideal body weight, which merits further study.

Estrogen production rates were calculated from plasma levels and clearance (Fig. 2). In agreement with others estrone production rates were elevated as compared to control subjects, and when compared with ideal body weight, a significant correlation ($r = 0.65$) was found. Thus, the significance of an increase in estrone production has to be considered against the effect of weight, and in the case of some of our patients, their menopausal status. Further, the major role for estrone may be essentially as a prehormone for estradiol, and the measurement of estradiol production would seem to be a more relevant indicator. In the patients studied here, estradiol production was, with one exception, essentially similar to that reported by Pratt and Longcope (20). The single patient with an elevated level was within 1 year of her menopause, which may explain the relatively high estradiol production. It may also be significant when considered in relation to the lack of opposition by progesterone in this patient.

Thus, in the relatively few patients studied so far, the production rate of estrone was elevated in some, but the influence of weight is clearly important, whereas the production rate of estradiol was not elevated consistently. Although the metabolic clearance rate was increased, the plasma levels tended to be low, resulting in normal rates of production.

It seems anomalous that although estrone production was elevated, estradiol production was not, as estrone is undoubtedly a major precursor for estradiol. As shown in Table 2, the proportion of estradiol that could be accounted for in this way varied from as little as 2 to 77%. The proportion exceeded 40% in only one patient.

Besides peripheral conversion of estrone to estradiol, the potential sources of estradiol are the ovary and the adrenal cortex, by direct secretion. It is extremely difficult to assess the role of these tissues in terms of their contribution to the total estrogen production. Investigations carried out during surgery (27) suffer from the disadvantage that the surgical intervention itself may alter the factor governing steroid secretion, e.g., adrenocorticotropic hormone (ACTH) in the case of the adrenal. Further, the demonstration of a gradient between the concentration of steroid in the venous effluent of, e.g., the ovary (15), as compared with peripheral levels is not interpreted easily without knowledge of the rate of blood flow, which in the postmenopausal ovary may be severely reduced (11). Thus, although there are positive data in regard to both ovarian and adrenal secretion of estradiol in postmenopausal women, it is not possible to assess their quantitative importance. Unless the kinetic model used to study estrogen secretion is badly at fault, it would appear that direct secretion of estradiol may make a significant contribution to the total production of estradiol in the postmenopausal woman.

Although, as determined by isotopic studies, there was no indication in the group of patients studied of excessive production of estradiol (in contrast to estrone), it should be remembered that the technique employed is unable to distinguish any differences in estrogen production between various tissues, and it can indicate only the overall level of production. Because a substantial proportion of estrogen is produced indirectly by conversion of androstenedione to estrone and hence to estradiol, and because we have shown that the metabolic activity of adipose tissue from different body sites differs considerably (5,7), it follows that there may be considerable regional variations in estrogen production throughout body tissues. Thus, local estrogen production may be relatively elevated in one tissue compared with another. For this reason, we have attempted to relate the *in vitro* production of estrogen to those factors that have been shown to be significant by isotopic *in vivo* techniques. Thus, the conversion of androstenedione to estrone has been shown to be weight-related (16,24), with obese subjects showing enhanced conversion, and age-related (9), increasing in older women. In patients with endometrial cancer, no difference from normal has been found, although in contrast, Schindler et al. (23) demonstrated enhanced aromatase activity *in vitro* in adipose tissue from endometrial cancer patients.

Several authors have demonstrated the capacity for aromatization in various body tissues, including adipose tissue (19). Factors influencing aromatase activity remain unclear; the extent to which adipose tissue varies in this regard and the effect of various parameters, such as age, weight, etc., are attracting attention only now.

We have studied the relationship between excess body weight and aromatase and have found only a weak correlation ($r = 0.32$) in normal subjects (5). In addition, in contrast to the *in vivo* kinetic studies, there is little evidence for any change in activity in older versus younger women. This may be due to the relatively small number of older women studied so far. However, it does appear that there is possibly some enhancement of activity in the women of perimenopausal age. A somewhat similar pattern was seen when 17β-hydroxysteroid dehydrogenase activity in adipose tissue was investigated in a further series of patients. The conversion of estrone to estradiol, as shown in Fig. 4, also reached a peak in the perimenopausal age group. We have been unable to find evidence that adipose tissue in the small group of patients with endometrial cancer that we have studied was more active in terms of aromatase or dehydrogenase activity.

Recently, Forney et al. (6) reported the results of a similar study in which they examined the *in vitro* aromatase activity of slices of adipose tissue from control subjects and from patients with endometrial cancer. They concluded that the rate of conversion of androstenedione to estrone measured *in vitro* in this way correlated significantly with the calculated mass of adipose tissue, but not with age. More importantly, they also found that the mean rate of estrone production by adipose tissue from women with endometrial hyperplasia and endometrial cancer was significantly greater than that from women of equivalent weight. Their conclusions thus differ somewhat from ours. We were unable to find a convincing relationship to excess body weight. However, it should be noted that the correlation observed by Forney et al. (6) was not strong (i.e., $r = 0.25$) when calculated for the controls and was higher in the cancer patients ($r = 0.72$). Since correlation data are highly sensitive to outlying results, their finding, though interesting, requires confirmation from a larger study. We agree with Forney et al. (6) in regard to the data on age, and it is interesting to note that inspection of their data also suggests a slight increase in activity in tissue from women of perimenopausal age, although these authors did not comment on this. Finally, we were unable to confirm the earlier report of Schindler et al. (23) and Forney et al. (6) that tissue from patients with endometrial disease was more active than control tissue; although we observed higher conversion of estrone to estradiol in some of our patients, there are insufficient data to draw any conclusions.

Therefore, the problem of the role of altered steroid metabolism in the genesis of endometrial cancer remains unresolved. Our finding of an increased clearance of estrogen in the patients, taken together with a similar finding by others in breast cancer, suggests enhanced tissue metabolism or tissue response to estrogen and the implications and the mechanism deserve further study. The observation of a possible increase in aromatase and dehydrogenase activity of adipose tissue from women of perimenopausal age is intriguing and needs substantiation. The increase in aromatization reported by Forney et al. (6) in their cancer patients is also potentially an important finding, if confirmed.

In conclusion, it seems likely that the important areas for further study will be those related to estradiol production and clearance and tissue response, as it is this hormone rather than estrone that appears to be fundamentally implicated in the mechanism of hormone action, both in normal and in neoplastic tissue.

ACKNOWLEDGMENT

This work was supported by a grant from the Cancer Research Campaign.

REFERENCES

1. Antunes, C. M. F., Stolley, P. D., Rosenheim, N. B., Davies, J. L., Tonascia, J. A., Brown, C., Burnett, L., Rutledge, M. A., Pokempner, M., and Garcia, R. (1979): Endometrial cancer and estrogen use. *N. Engl. J. Med.*, 300:9–13.
2. Baird, D. T., Horton, R., Longcope, C., and Tait, J. F. (1969): Steroid dynamics under steady-state conditions. *Recent Prog. Horm. Res.*, 25:611–656.
3. Feinstein, A. R., and Horwitz, R. I. (1978): A critique of the statistical evidence associating estrogens with endometrial cancer. *Cancer Res.*, 38:4001–4005.
4. Folkerd, E. J., and James, V. H. T. (1982): Studies on the activity of 17β-hydroxysteroid dehydrogenase in human adipose tissue. *J. Steroid Biochem.*, 16:439–543.
5. Folkerd, E. J., Reed, M. J., and James, V. H. T. (1982): Oestrogen production in adipose tissue from normal women and women with endometrial cancer *in vitro*. *J. Steroid Biochem.*, 16:297–302.
6. Forney, J. P., Milewich, L., Chen, G. T., Garlock, J. L., Schwarz, B. E., Edman, C. D., and MacDonald, P. C. (1981): Aromatization of androstenedione to oestrone by human adipose tissue *in vitro*. Correlation with adipose tissue mass, age, and endometrial neoplasia. *J. Clin. Endocrinol. Metab.*, 53:192–199.
7. Frost, P. G., Reed, M. J., and James, V. H. T. (1980): The aromatization of androstenedione by human adipose and liver tissue. *J. Steroid Biochem.*, 13:1427–1431.
8. Hammond, C. B., Jelovsek, F. R., Lee, K. L., Creasman, W. T., and Parker, R. T. (1979): Effects of long-term estrogen replacement therapy: II. Neoplasia. *Am. J. Obstet. Gynecol.*, 133:537–547.
9. Hemsell, D. L., Grodin, J. M., Brenner, P. F., Siiteri, P. K., and MacDonald, P. C. (1974): Plasma precursors of estrogen. II. Correlation of the extent of conversion of plasma androstenedione to oestrone with age. *J. Clin. Endocrinol. Metab.*, 38:476–479.
10. James, V. H. T., Reed, M. J., and Folkerd, E. J. (1981): Studies of oestrogen metabolism in postmenopausal women with cancer. *J. Steroid Biochem.*, 15:235–246.
11. Janson, P. O., and Jansson, I. (1977): The acute effect of hysterectomy on ovarian blood flow. *Am. J. Obstet. Gynecol.*, 127:349–352.
12. Judd, H. L., Judd, G. E., Lucas, W. E., and Yen, S. S. C. (1974): Endocrine function of the postmenopausal ovary: Concentration of androgens and estrogens in ovarian and peripheral vein blood. *J. Clin. Endocrinol. Metab.*, 39:1020–1024.
13. Kirschner, M. A., Cohen, F. B., and Ryan, C. (1978): Androgen-estrogen production rates in postmenopausal women with breast cancer. *Cancer Res.*, 38:4029–4035.
14. Longcope, C. (1971): Metabolic clearance and blood production rates in postmenopausal women. *Am. J. Obstet. Gynecol.*, 111:778–781.
15. Longcope, C., Hunter, R., and Franz, C. (1980): Steroid secretion by the postmenopausal ovary. *Am. J. Obstet. Gynecol.*, 138:564–568.
16. MacDonald, P. C., Edman, C. D., Hemsell, D. L., Porter, J. C., and Siiteri, P. K. (1978): Effect of obesity on conversion of plasma androstenedione to oestrone in women with and without endometrial cancer. *Am. J. Obstet. Gynecol.*, 130:448–455.
17. Mack, T. M., Pike, M. C., Henderson, B. E., Pfeffer, R. J., Gerkins, V. R., Arthur, M., and Brown, S. E. (1976): Estrogens and endometrial cancer in a retirement community. *N. Engl. J. Med.*, 294:1262–1267.
18. MacRae, K. D. (1981): Health risks of oestrogen therapy. *J. Endocrinol.*, 89:145P–148P.
19. Nimrod, A., and Ryan, K. J. (1975): Aromatization of androgens by human abdominal and breast fat tissue. *J. Clin. Endocrinol. Metab.*, 40:367–372.
20. Pratt, J. H., and Longcope, C. (1978): Estriol production rates and breast cancer. *J. Clin. Endocrinol. Metab.*, 46:44–47.
21. Reed, M. J., Hutton, J. D., Baxendale, P. M., James, V. H. T., Jacobs, H. S., and Fisher, R. P. (1979): The conversion of androstenedione to oestrone in women with endometrial cancer. *J. Steroid Biochem.*, 11:905–911.
22. Reed, M. J., Hutton, J. D., Beard, R. W., Jacobs, H. S., and James, V. H. T. (1979): Plasma hormone levels and oestrogen production in a postmenopausal woman with endometrial carcinoma and an ovarian thecoma. *Clin. Endocrinol.*, 11:141–150.
23. Schindler, A. E., Ebert, A., and Friedrich, E. (1972): Conversion of androstenedione to oestrone by human fat tissue. *J. Clin. Endocrinol. Metab.*, 35:627–630.
24. Siiteri, P. K., and MacDonald, P. C. (1973): Role of extraglandular estrogen in human endocri-

nology. In: *Handbook of Physiology, Vol. II*, edited by R. O. Greep and E. B. Astwood, pp. 615–629. American Physiological Society, Washington, D.C.

25. Siiteri, P. K., Schwarz, B. E., and MacDonald, P. C. (1974): Estrogen receptors and the estrone hypothesis in relation to endometrial and breast cancer. *Gynecol. Oncol.*, 2:228–238.
26. Vermeulen, A., Verdonck, L., Van der Straeten, M., and Orie, N. (1969): Capacity of the testosterone-binding globulin in human plasma and influence of specific binding of testosterone on its metabolic clearance rate. *J. Clin. Endocrinol. Metab.*, 29:1470–1480.
27. Wasada, T., Akamine, Y., Kato, K-J., Ibayashi, H., and Namura, Y. (1978): Adrenal contribution to circulating oestrogens in women. *Endocrinol. Jpn.*, 25:123–128.
28. Weiss, N. S., and Sayvetz, T. A. (1980): Incidence of endometrial cancer in relation to the use of oral contraceptives. *N. Engl. J. Med.*, 302:551–554.

Steroids and Endometrial Cancer,
edited by V. M. Jasonni, et al.
Raven Press, New York © 1983.

Effects of Progestins on Endometrial Adenocarcinoma

E. Gurpide, C. F. Holinka, and L. Deligdisch

Division of Reproductive Biology and Pathology, Departments of Obstetrics and Gynecology, Mount Sinai School of Medicine, New York, New York 10029

For several years, our research on endometrial cancer has been carried out in parallel with studies of histologically normal endometrium. We pursued two general aims: (a) to identify biochemical differences between neoplastic and normal endometrium; and (b) to develop practical tests to distinguish patients with endometrial cancer who may respond to hormone-related therapy from those who are unlikely responders. Achievement of the first goal could allow further investigation into the nature of the transformation process. Availability of a predictive test for responsiveness to progestins or antiestrogens could influence the management of patients, as less than one-half of those treated respond to hormonal therapy (16).

Figure 1 illustrates our use of endometrial specimens. Tissue fragments, obtained by curettage or after hysterectomy, were examined histologically for dating according to the criteria of Noyes et al. (25) in premenopausal patients, or for evaluation of the degree of differentiation of the tumor in patients with endometrial adenocarcinoma. Biochemical studies on these specimens include measurements of estradiol and progesterone receptor levels, enzymatic activities, and prostaglandin production. We also examined these parameters in glandular and stromal fractions obtained by collagenase digestion of the tissue and separation of the glands from the filtrate consisting of dispersed cells (29,30). Monolayers of epithelial cells are derived from isolated glands incubated in HAM-F10 medium containing 10% fetal bovine serum; stromal cell cultures are obtained by transferring the stromal fraction to plastic dishes and allowing the fibroblast-like cells to attach for 30 min, changing the medium to eliminate erythrocytes and other suspended cells. Epithelial cultures can usually be maintained for only one passage, but stromal cell cultures have been maintained consistently for over 40 passages.

Effects of estradiol and progesterone on endometrial tissue and cells have been investigated at different levels, i.e., *in vivo* by administration of the ovarian hormones to the patient before removal of the endometrial specimen, or *in vitro* by adding the hormones to the medium used for cell cultures or for incubations of fragments of tissue and isolated glands under organ culture conditions.

Morphologic observations are carried out in parallel with biochemical measurements, since it is clear that histology serves to detect hormonal effects on the

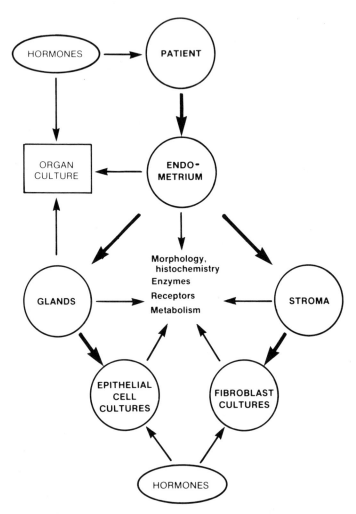

FIG. 1. Diagram showing the origin of samples used in endometrial studies. Effects of hormones are tested by examination of tissue obtained at different phases of the menstrual cycle or after hormonal treatment of the patient and *in vitro* after addition of hormones to the medium used for organ culture of minced tissue and glands or for culturing epithelial and stromal cells.

endometrium, such as changes corresponding to the passage from estrogen-dominated to progesterone-dominated hormonal environment during the menstrual cycle.

HISTOLOGIC EVALUATION OF RESPONSE OF ENDOMETRIAL CARCINOMA TO PROGESTINS

Several publications have indicated that progestins can produce in endometrial adenocarcinoma histologic changes characteristic of the transition from proliferative to secretory endometrium, e.g., formation of subnuclear glycogen vacuoles, verifiable by the periodic acid-Schiff (PAS)-diastase technique, and a quiescence of the epithelial cells that is accompanied by a lowering of the nuclear-cytoplasmic ratio. These changes have been observed *in vivo* after administration of progestins to patients (2,9,13,18) and *in vitro* during incubations of neoplastic tissue in medium containing progestins (12,19). Because the hormonal effects are detected in only some of the specimens of endometrial adenocarcinoma, it is conceivable that a response could identify patients who would benefit from progestin therapy. Obviously, such a correlation can be established only in trials comparing short-term effects of progestins with subsequent clinical responses to hormonal therapy, objectively evaluated by standard criteria.

In preliminary studies, we sought to correlate histologic responses to progestins with levels of progesterone receptors in the tumor, since previous reports by Ehrlich et al. and other groups (5,22,39) have shown that the presence of receptors in recurrent endometrial cancer is a useful indicator of responsiveness to treatment.

Although comparisons of progesterone receptor levels in primary and metastatic endometrial cancer have been reported in only a few cases, the available data indicates good agreement (32), for example, in breast cancer (24). Therefore, correlation of histologic responses and levels of progesterone receptors in the primary tumor may validate the application of a histologic test for the prediction of the outcome of progestin therapy for recurrences that may develop eventually in the same patient.

Table 1 shows results obtained *in vivo* by oral administration of medroxyprogesterone acetate (MPA, Provera®) for 2 to 3 days to postmenopausal patients with endometrial adenocarcinoma (12). Specimens obtained by curettage before administration of MPA were used for the estimation of progesterone receptor levels and histologic examination. Receptor concentrations were measured in the cytosol fraction of the tissue homogenate by incubation with 20 nM tritiated progesterone plus 2 μM cortisol in the presence or absence of a 100-fold excess of unlabeled progesterone, followed by separation of unbound hormone with dextran-coated charcoal, according to the method described by Bayard et al. (3). Glycogen accumulation was detected by the appearance of glycogen vacuoles in the glandular epithelium

TABLE 1. In vivo *responses of postmenopausal endometrial adenocarcinoma to MPA*

Cytosolic progesterone receptor (fmoles/mg protein)	Grade	Glycogen accumulation (histology)
~0	1	None
80	3	None
160	3	None
190	1	None
360	2	+
380	1	+
2,400	2	+ +

of specimens obtained after hysterectomy at the end of the period of administration of the progestin.

Responses were observed only when the levels of receptor exceeded values in the 200 to 350 fmoles/mg protein range. The strongest response was noted in the specimen with the highest level of progesterone receptor. The absence of responses in the poorly differentiated specimens was evident in the few glandular elements present in the tissue, which did not show subnuclear vacuoles. It was of interest to note that the tumor infiltrated in the myometrium did not show any response to progestins, even in the three cases in which such a histologic response was present in the superficial adenocarcinoma.

Studies on responsiveness *in vitro* were carried out by incubating fragments of endometrial carcinoma taken after hysterectomy of postmenopausal patients. In every case, a portion of the specimen was used immediately for progesterone receptor determinations, another for histologic examination, and the rest for organ culture. The portion of the tissue to be incubated was cut into small pieces with ophthalmic scissors and placed on lens paper disks on stainless steel grids distributed in polystyrene dishes, 35 mm in diameter (Falcon Plastics, Los Angeles), containing approximately 2 ml of medium (HAM F-10 with 10% fetal calf serum, 10 mg/ml insulin, 5 mg/ml glucose, and 1% of an antibiotic-antimycotic mixture, GIBCO, Grand Island, New York). The medium in some of the dishes contained 0.5 μg/ml MPA. The dishes were placed in a CO_2-air incubator and kept for 2 days at 37°C in a humidified atmosphere. Specimens were sectioned and stained with hematoxylin-eosin or PAS following standard procedures (33).

The results shown in Table 2 indicate that responsiveness *in vitro* is related to the levels of cytosolic progesterone receptor; responses were observed when the levels exceeded 300 fmoles/mg protein. This value is similar to the cutoff level found in *in vivo* experiments (Table 1) but higher than the 50 fmoles/mg protein proposed by Young and Ehrlich (39) or the levels of sensitivity of the receptor assay (less than 10 fmoles/mg protein) proposed by other groups.

TABLE 2. In vitro *responses of postmenopausal endometrial adenocarcinoma to MPA*

Cytosolic progesterone receptor (fmoles/mg protein)	Grade	Glycogen accumulation (histology)
~0	3	None
180	3	None
190	1	None
240	1	None
280	2	None
340	2	+ +
580	1	+
800	1	+
1,320	1	+ +
1,580	1	+

Therefore, it appears that histologic testing of a single specimen taken from the excised uterus might provide evidence for responsiveness to progestins and information about levels of progesterone receptor in the tissue. The simplicity of the test, which involves techniques routinely used in pathology laboratories, justifies further evaluation of its merit.

Heterogeneity in the responses within the tissue was evident in these experiments. Glands showing clear subnuclear vacuolization could be found side by side with glands without vacuoles or with unresponsive papillary projections.

ENZYMATIC ACTIVITIES

Three enzymatic activities of particular interest in endometrial cancer have been studied in our laboratories, i.e., 17β hydroxysteroid dehydrogenase (17βHSD), peroxidase, and ornithine decarboxylase (ODC).

As described elsewhere, 17βHSD activity, mainly localized in the glandular epithelium, is stimulated by progestins, both *in vivo* and *in vitro* (31,36). The regulatory influence of progestins on 17βHSD is reflected by the low activities of proliferative endometrium and endometrial adenocarcinoma not exposed to progesterone (37). The increased activity of the enzyme during the luteal phase provokes an elevation of the rate constant of conversion of estradiol to estrone and a decline in the intracellular concentration of estradiol (7,34). Only a small fraction of estrone is reduced to estradiol; the remainder is further metabolized to estrone sulfate (4) or leaves the cell (8). The increased metabolism of estradiol to estrone under the influence of progesterone is evident from superfusions of proliferative and secretory endometrium with labeled estradiol and estrone (38) and from comparisons of endometrial and plasma levels of these compounds during the menstrual cycle (6,27). The stimulating effect of progesterone on 17βHSD activity, together with its depressing action on estrogen receptor concentration, may account for the antiestrogenicity of progestins. Estrone, formed from estradiol in the endometrium, does not appear to be estrogenic per se, as it is not receptor-bound, or only to a much lesser extent than estradiol, in endometrial nuclei (7,17,35).

The effectiveness of progestin treatment on endometrial cancer may or may not be related to these antiestrogenic effects of progesterone. It is clear, however, that progestins can stimulate 17βHSD *in vivo* in endometrial cancer (26,37). Measurements of the enzymatic activity can therefore be used as an endpoint to evaluate *in vivo* responsiveness of the carcinoma to short-term treatment with a progestin (9). However, in contrast to the results obtained with normal proliferative endometrium, no *in vitro* stimulation of the enzymatic activity has been achieved with endometrial adenocarcinoma, even in those specimens that showed histologic responses to MPA during incubation (12). Therefore, stimulation of 17βHSD *in vitro* under the conditions used in our laboratories is not a suitable test of responsiveness of endometrial adenocarcinoma to progestins.

The reasons underlying the different *in vitro* inducibility of 17βHSD in proliferative normal endometrium and endometrial cancer have not been identified. One possibility considered was that stromal cells, which are relatively fewer in endometrial cancer than in normal tissue, might participate in the elicitation of the response. However, it was shown that 17βHSD activity could be stimulated by MPA during incubations of isolated glands from proliferative normal endometrium (11). Interestingly, epithelial cell cultures derived from responsive glands did not increase their 17βHSD activity when MPA was added to the medium (12). It was therefore not surprising to find no effects of MPA on the enzymatic activity of monolayer cultures of cancer cells. This loss of effects of progestins on 17βHSD of endometrial cancer in organ culture and in epithelial cell cultures derived from specimens of both normal and neoplastic endometrium responsive under *in vivo* conditions is of considerable biologic interest.

Induction or stimulation of 17βHSD in human endometrium and in rhesus monkeys (20) is achieved with progestins but not with estrogens. In contrast, *in vivo* experiments carried out in rats (1,40) and rabbits (15) showed that estrogens but not progestins stimulate this uterine enzymatic activity. Such contradictory species specificity in the stimulation of uterine enzymes by ovarian hormones is not limited to 17βHSD (11).

Uterine peroxidase in rats and mice can be elevated over a hundredfold by administration of estrogens (14,21). No evidence of estrogen stimulation of peroxidase was found when this enzymatic activity was measured in human endometrium throughout the menstrual cycle (10). Levels, in fact, were slightly higher during the luteal phase than during the estrogen dominated follicular phase. As Fig. 2 shows, peroxidase activity was significantly higher in specimens of endometrial cancer than in normal endometrium. Attempts to modify this enzymatic activity *in vitro*, by incubation of tissue fragments or cells in culture with estrogens, have been unsuccessful as the activity is lost under culture conditions.

Ornithine decarboxylase (ODC) is another enzyme reported to be elevated in endometrial cancer (23). Although the enormous range of activity within similar types of tissue makes these differences not statistically significant, the participation of the enzyme in the formation of growth-promoting polyamines (28) adds interest to the observation. Results from experiments carried out in our laboratories show, however, that active proliferation of cells is not necessarily associated with measurable levels of ODC. Activity of this enzyme was negligible in cultures of stromal cells at confluence and during a period of proliferation identified by cell counting and measurements of rates of [^{3}H]thymidine incorporation into DNA. In contrast, cultures of an endometrial adenocarcinoma cell line (HEC-1B) showed significant activity during proliferation but not at confluence. The activity in this and other cell lines could be promptly (4–6 hr) induced in confluent cultures by renewing the serum-containing medium or by replacing it with a 10 μM solution of asparagine in buffer (11). These stimulatory maneuvers were ineffective in stromal cell cultures.

CONCLUSIONS

A correlation between histologic responses to progestins of postmenopausal endometrial adenocarcinoma and levels of cytosolic progesterone receptors was found

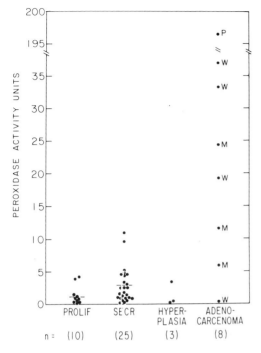

FIG. 2. Peroxidase activity in normal proliferative and secretory endometrium and in specimens derived from hyperplastic and neoplastic endometrial tissue. (From Holinka and Gurpide, ref. 11, with permission.)

in both *in vivo* and *in vitro* experiments. The lowest concentration of receptor associated with responses was about 300 fmoles/mg protein. Stimulation of $17\beta HSD$ could be used as an endpoint for responses to progestins *in vivo* but not *in vitro*.

Peroxidase activities were usually much higher in specimens of endometrial cancer than in normal endometrium. In contrast to observations in rodents, there is no indication that peroxidase activity is stimulated by estrogens; the activity was lost under *in vitro* conditions.

Ornithine decarboxylase was not found to be an infallible marker for cell proliferation, since culture of endometrial stromal cells grew actively in the absence of detectable ODC activity.

The clear association of histologic responses to progestins and levels of progesterone receptors suggests that *in vitro* incubations of tissue fragments with progestins and histologic detection of glycogen accumulation can serve as the basis for a practical test to predict responsiveness of endometrial adenocarcinoma to hormonal treatment.

ACKNOWLEDGMENTS

We are grateful to the surgeons in the Department of Obstetrics and Gynecology, Mount Sinai School of Medicine, and to Dr. Robert Wallach, Beth Israel Medical Center, New York, for their collaboration in the collection of specimens. These studies were supported by Grant CA 15648 from the National Cancer Institute and Grant HD-07197 from the National Institutes of Health.

REFERENCES

1. Amr, S., Faye, J. C., Bayard, F., and Kreitmann, O. (1980): Induction of rat endometrial estradiol 17β dehydrogenase activity by estradiol and progesterone. *Biol. Reprod.*, 22:159–163.
2. Anderson, D. G. (1965): Management of advanced endometrial adenocarcinoma with medroxyprogesterone acetate. *Am. J. Obstet. Gynecol.*, 92:87–99.
3. Bayard, F., Damilano, S., Robel, P., and Baulieu, E. E. (1978): Cytoplasmic and nuclear estradiol and progesterone receptor in human endometrium. *J. Clin. Endocrinol. Metab.*, 46:635–648.
4. Buirchell, B. J., and Hähnel, R. (1975): Metabolism of estradiol 17β in human endometrium during the menstrual cycle. *J. Steroid Biochem.*, 6:1489–1494.
5. Creasman, W. T., McCarty, K. S., Barton, T. K., and McCarty, K. S. Jr. (1980): Clinical correlates of estrogen- and progesterone binding proteins in human endometrial adenocarcinoma. *Obstet. Gynecol.*, 55:363–370.
6. Guerrero, R. B., Landgren, M., Montiel, R., Cekan, Z., and Diczfalusy, E. (1975): Unconjugated steroids in the human endometrium. *Contraception*, 11:169–177.
7. Gurpide, E. (1978): Enzymatic modulation of hormonal action at the target tissue. *J. Toxicol. Environ. Health*, 4:249–268.
8. Gurpide, E., and Welch, M. (1969): Dynamics of uptake of estrogens and androgens by human endometrium. *J. Biol. Chem.*, 244:5159–5169.
9. Gurpide, E., Tseng, L., and Gusberg, S. B. (1977): Estrogen metabolism in normal and neoplastic endometrium. *Am. J. Obstet. Gynecol.*, 129:809–816.
10. Holinka, C. F., and Gurpide, E. (1980): Peroxidase activity in glands and stroma of human endometrium. *Am. J. Obstet. Gynecol.*, 138:599–603.
11. Holinka, C. F., and Gurpide, E. (1981): Hormone-related enzymatic activity of normal and cancer cells of human endometrium. *J. Steroid Biochem.*, 15:183–192.
12. Holinka, C. F., Deligdisch, L., Deppe, G., Fleming, H., Namit, C., de la Pena, M. M., and Gurpide, E. (1981): Evaluation in in vivo and in vitro responses of endometrial adenocarcinoma to progestins. In: *Hormones and Cancer*, edited by W. W. Leavitt, pp. 365–376. Plenum Press, New York.
13. Howard, J. A., Cornes, J. S., Jackson, W. D., and Bye, P. (1974): Effect of a systemically administered progestogen on histopathology of endometrial carcinoma. *Br. J. Obstet. Gynecaecol.*, 81:786–790.
14. Jellinck, P. H., and Lyttle, C. R. (1973): Estrogen-induced uterine enzymes in the control of estradiol action. *Adv. Enzyme Regul.*, 11:17–33.
15. Jutting, G. (1970): Hormonale Enzyminduktion in Myometrium Beispiel einer Östrogenwirkum am Erfolgsorgan. *Acta Endocrinol. [Suppl.] (Copenh)*, 145:9–46.
16. Kelly, R. M., and Baker, W. H. (1965): The role of progesterone in human endometrial cancer. *Cancer Res.*, 25:1190–1192.
17. King, R. J. B., Dyer, G., Collins, W. P., and Whitehead, M. I. (1980): Intracellular estradiol, estrone and estrogen receptor levels in endometria from postmenopausal women receiving estrogens and progestins. *J. Steroid Biochem.*, 13:377–382.
18. Kistner, R. W., Griffiths, C. T., and Craig, J. M. (1965): The use of progestational agents in the management of endometrial cancer. *Cancer*, 18:1563–1579.
19. Kohorn, E. I. (1976): The limitations of progesterone sensitivity testing of endometrial carcinoma using organ culture. In: *Human Tumours in Short-Term Culture*, edited by P. P. Dendy, pp. 245–253. Academic Press, New York.
20. Kreitmann, O., Kreitmann-Gimbal, B., Bayard, F., and Hodgen, G. D. (1980): 17β Hydroxysteroid dehydrogenase in monkey endometrium: Characterization of enzyme activity and effects of estradiol alone or in combination with progesterone. *Steroids*, 34:693–703.
21. Lyttle, C. R., and De Sombre, E. R. (1977): Uterine peroxidase as a marker for estrogen action. *Proc. Natl. Acad. Sci. USA*, 74:3162–3166.
22. Martin, P. M., Rolland, P. H., Gammerre, M., Serment, H., and Toga, M. (1979): Estradiol and progesterone receptors in normal and neoplastic endometrium: correlations between receptors, histopathological examinations and clinical responses under progestin therapy. *Int. J. Cancer*, 23:321–329.

23. Mortel, R., Levy, C., Wolff, J. P., Nicolas, J.-C., Robel, P., and Baulieu, E. E. (1981): Female sex steroid receptors in postmenopausal endometrial carcinoma and biochemical response to an antiestrogen. *Cancer Res.*, 41:1140–1147.
24. McGuire, W. L., Horwitz, K. B., Zava, D. T., Garola, R. E., and Chamness, G. C. (1978): Hormones in breast cancer: Update 1978. *Metabolism*, 27:487–501.
25. Noyes, R. H., Hertig, A. T., and Rock, J. (1950): Dating the endometrial biopsy. *Fertil. Steril.*, 1:3–25.
26. Pollow, K., Boquoi, E., Lübbert, H., and Pollow, B. (1975): Effect of gestagen therapy upon 17β hydroxysteroid dehydrogenase in human endometrial adenocarcinoma. *J. Endocrinol.*, 67:131–132.
27. Pollow, K., Schmidt-Gollwitzer, M., and Pollow, B. (1980): Progesterone and estradiol binding proteins from normal human endometrium and endometrial carcinoma: a comparative study. In: *Steroid Receptors and Hormone-Dependent Neoplasia*, edited by J. L. Wittliff and O. Dapunt, pp. 69–94. Masson Publishing Inc., New York.
28. Russell, D. H., and Durie, B. G. M. (1978): Polyamines as biochemical markers of normal and malignant growth. In: *Progress in Cancer Research Therapy, Vol. 8*, Raven Press, New York.
29. Satyaswaroop, P. G., Bressler, R. S., de la Pena, M. M., and Gurpide, E. (1979): Isolation and culture of human endometrial glands. *J. Clin. Endocrinol. Metab.*, 48:639–641.
30. Satyaswaroop, P. G., Fleming, H., Bressler, R. S., and Gurpide, E. (1978): Human endometrial cancer cell cultures for hormonal studies. *Cancer Res.*, 38:4367–4375.
31. Scublinsky, A., Marin, C., and Gurpide, E. (1976): Localization of estradiol 17β dehydrogenase in human endometrium. *J. Steroid Biochem.*, 7:745–747.
32. Syrjälä, P., Kontula, K., Jänne, O., Kauppila, A., and Vihko, R. (1978): Steroid receptors in normal and neoplastic human uterine tissue. In: *Endometrial Cancer*, edited by M. G. Brush, R. J. B. King, and R. W. Taylor, pp. 242–251. Bailliere Tindall, London.
33. Thompson, S. W. (1966): Selected histochemical and histopathological methods. C. C Thomas, Springfield, Illinois.
34. Tseng, L., and Gurpide, E. (1972): Changes in the *in vitro* metabolism of estradiol during the menstrual cycle. *Am. J. Obstet. Gynecol.*, 114:1002–1011.
35. Tseng, L., and Gurpide, E. (1973): Effect of estrone and progesterone on the nuclear uptake of estradiol by slices of human endometrium. *Endocrinology*, 93:245–252.
36. Tseng, L., and Gurpide, E. (1975): Induction of human endometrial estradiol dehydrogenase by progestins. *Endocrinology*, 97:825–833.
37. Tseng, L., Gusberg, S. B., and Gurpide, E. (1977): Estradiol receptor and 17β dehydrogenase in normal and abnormal human endometrium. *Ann. NY Acad. Sci.*, 286:190–198.
38. Tseng, L., Stolee, A., and Gurpide, E. (1972): Quantitative studies on the uptake and metabolism of estrogens and progesterone by human endometrium. *Endocrinology*, 90:390–404.
39. Young, P. C. M., and Ehrlich, C. E. (1979): Progesterone receptors in human endometrial cancer. In: *Steroid Receptors and the Management of Cancer, Vol. 1*, edited by E. B. Thompson and M. E. Lippman, pp. 135–159. CRC Press Inc., Florida.
40. Wahawisan, R., and Gorell, T. A. (1980): Steroidal control of rat uterine 17β hydroxysteroid dehydrogenase activity. *Steroids*, 36:115–129.

Steroids and Endometrial Cancer,
edited by V. M. Jasonni, et al.
Raven Press, New York © 1983.

Adrenal Androgens and Endometrial Cancer

J. Poortman, R. Andriesse, G. H. Donker, and J. H. H. Thijssen

*Department of Endocrinology, University Hospital, State University of Utrecht,
Utrecht, The Netherlands*

Studies on the etiology of human endometrial cancer have shown that there are a number of risk factors for this disease. These risk factors can be associated with changes in the production rate and metabolism of steroid hormones. Such changes may lead to changes in the endocrine environment in the body, which are thought to be involved in the induction and/or growth promotion of endometrial cancer cells.

For many years, there was a general belief that a change in the endocrine milieu leading to an increased estrogenic activity, especially in postmenopausal women, was causally related to the disease. Such increased activity can be derived from a higher production rate of estradiol and estrone and/or from a decreased metabolic clearance rate of estradiol and estrone. The resulting effect is an elevated peripheral plasma level of these compounds with continuously increased action of these estrogens in their target tissues.

Convincing data, however, have been published that exclude this possibility. MacDonald et al. (5) have shown that there are no differences either in the estrogen production rate or in the conversion rate of androstenedione to estrone between women with and without endometrial cancer after careful matching for age and body weight. Judd et al. (3) have found that there are no differences in the serum levels of estrone and estradiol between cancer patients and matched controls.

Another mechanism resulting in an increased estrogenic activity is a diminished opposition by steroid hormones that modulate the effects of estrogens. Some years ago, we postulated that adrenal androgens could play such a role (7). We found that C-19 steroids were able to inhibit the binding of estradiol to its specific receptor, which is an essential step in the process of biological activity. A diminished production rate of C-19 steroids could then lead to a decreased inhibition, which in turn leads to an increased estrogenic stimulation at the target cell (10). In view of this hypothesis, we investigated the plasma levels and blood production rates of some of these C-19 steroids in postmenopausal endometrial cancer patients and in healthy control women. Some data have already been published (2,8).

MATERIALS AND METHODS

Subjects

Three postmenopausal women with an atypical adenomatous hyperplastic endometrium and eight postmenopausal women with an endometrial carcinoma participated in this study. Diagnosis was made after a diagnostic curettage and proven after hysterectomy. Five of the carcinoma patients had an adenocarcinoma, stage 1; three were stage 2, including one patient with an endometrial acanthoma. The characteristics of the five normal volunteers are described in a previous paper (8). All patients and volunteers participating in this study gave their informed consent.

Measurement of Metabolic Clearance Rate

The metabolic clearance rate (MCR) measurements were done by a constant infusion technique. Tritium and carbon-14 labeled precursors and products were infused for 10 to 12 hr to reach a steady state. The metabolic clearance rate can be calculated from the infusion rate and the radioactivity level reached for a particular steroid. The daily production rate is calculated as the product of MCR and the mean daily plasma level of a particular steroid. The techniques used and the calculation procedures have been described in detail (6,8).

Plasma Level of Endogenous Androgens

In a different study group consisting of 30 normal control women, three women with atypical adenomatous hyperplasia of the endometrium and 18 endometrial cancer patients (12 stage 1 and six stage 2) of postmenopausal age, we measured the level of circulating androgens. Plasma concentration of testosterone (T), 5-androstene-3β,17β-diol (Adiol), androstenedione (A), dehydroepiandrosterone (DHEA), and its sulfate (DHEA-S) were measured by radioimmunoassay using specific antisera. The measurement of DHEA-S was done in diluted plasma with a highly specific antiserum against DHEA-S. For the assay of DHEA and Adiol, the plasma extracts were purifed by Celite chromatography, as described by Abraham et al. (1). Characteristics of these assays, including specificity, precision, inter- and intrassay variation, have been published recently (4).

RESULTS

Plasma Levels of Androgens

A summary of the endogenous levels of T, A, Adiol, DHEA, and DHEA-S found in 30 normal postmenopausal women, in six hyperplasia patients, and in 18 endometrial cancer patients is given in Table 1.

The relative small number of samples and the large standard deviation found for some of the estimations made it difficult to draw definite conclusions. However,

TABLE 1. *Plasma androgens in endometrial cancer*

	Normal (N = 30)	Atypical adenomatous hyperplasia (N = 6)	Cancer (N = 18)
DHEA-S (μmoles/liter)	2.22	1.41	2.35
± SD	1.67	0.88	1.46
DHEA (nmoles/liter)	9.22	8.70	10.83
± SD	7.72	5.24	9.99
Adiol (nmoles/liter)	1.27	1.34	1.86
± SD	0.76	0.77	1.30
Testosterone (nmoles/liter)	0.75	1.15	0.86
± SD	0.45	1.09	0.34
Androstenedione (nmoles/liter)	2.28	3.83	2.55
± SD	1.16	2.99	1.24

DHEA-S = dehydroepiandrosterone-sulfate; DHEA = dehydroepiandrosterone; Adiol = 5-androstene-3β,17β-diol.
Mean ± SD.

there appeared to be no gross abnormalities in these androgen levels between controls and cancer patients. In the cancer patients, the mean value for Adiol was somewhat elevated as compared to the normal group and the hyperplasia group. The group of hyperplasia patients showed a relative low level of DHEA-S: The six plasma levels found were all below the mean value of the normal group and below the mean value of the cancer group.

For DHEA-S, DHEA, and Adiol we found a clear negative correlation between the plasma level and the age of the subject. The decline in plasma level with age was stronger for the early postmenopausal group between age 50 and 60 than for the older age group above age 60 (Fig. 1). It could be seen also that the cancer patients and the hyperplasia patients were randomly scattered compared to the normal group. For T and A, we did not find such an age-dependent decline in plasma level (Fig. 2).

These data are consistent with the observation that there is a decline in the adrenal cortical function with age, especially concerning the androgen secretion and production. DHEA and DHEA-S are entirely derived from adrenal secretion and interconversion, Adiol is a peripheral product of DHEA and DHEA-S metabolism. Testosterone and androstenedione are derived mainly from the stromal compartment of the postmenopausal ovary. This stromal activity in androgen production shows no clear decline with age.

Blood Production Rates, Fractional Conversion Rates, and Relative Contributions

The results for the daily production rate are all derived from 10 to 12 hr infusions. The fractional conversion rates were calculated with the assumption of a metabolic

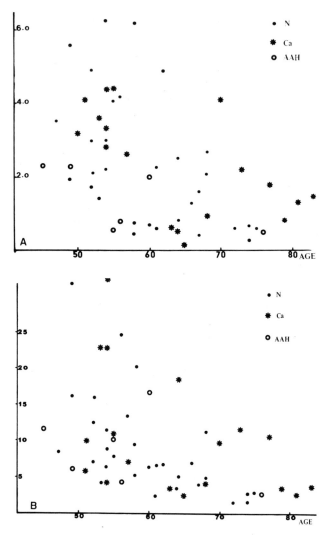

FIG. 1. A: Relation between age of the subject and the plasma level of dehydroepiandrosterone-sulfate (DHEA-S) (μmole/liter);   **B:** dehydroepiandrosterone (DHEA) (nmole/liter); and
C *(top of facing page)*: 5-androstene-3β,17β-diol (Adiol) (nmole/liter), in 30 normal postmenopausal women, six postmenopausal women with an atypical adenomatous hyperplastic endometrium, and 18 women with endometrial cancer.

clearance rate of Adiol of 800 liters per day and of identical clearance rates for
DHEA-S and 5-androstene-3β,17β-diol-3-mono-sulfate.

The data obtained are summarized in Table 2. From these data, we calculated
the relative contribution of a precursor hormone to a product. These relative contributions are given in Table 3. From the daily production rate of each hormone

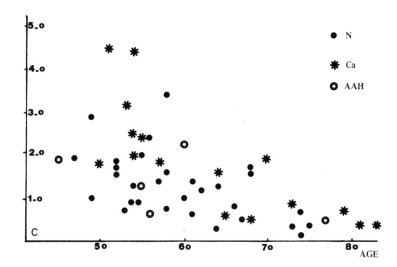

and the relative contribution of a precursor, we calculated the fraction of the daily production that is derived from this peripheral metabolism. In Table 3 these metabolic contributions are indicated as a percentage of the total production.

Tables 2 and 3 show clearly that the differences found between the three groups studied are very limited. There is one interesting observation: for both patients with a hyperplasia and patients with endometrial cancer, we found that the conversion to the sulpho-conjugated compounds is decreased as compared to the normal women. The fractional conversion rates of DHEA-S to Adiol-S, of DHEA to Adiol-S, and of DHEA to DHEA-S are all much lower than found for the normal women (see Table 2).

CONCLUSIONS

The results presented in this chapter do not support the concept that a decreased production rate or decreased plasma levels of androgens are associated with endometrial cancer. This finding is surprising with respect to the older studies in which a decreased excretion rate of androgen metabolites was reported (9,11). It is very difficult to indicate which factors are responsible for this discrepancy. Even by calculating an androgen index as the sum of all androgens measured (sum of DHEA-S + DHEA + T + A + Adiol), we found no differences between our control population and the cancer group.

For some of the conversion rates, we find rather large differences. However, at present we do not know the biological consequences of these changes.

There is still another consideration. We have studied patients with an established malignancy. It must be kept in mind that in a case in which the steroid hormonal environment is involved in the growth control of endometrium, small changes in

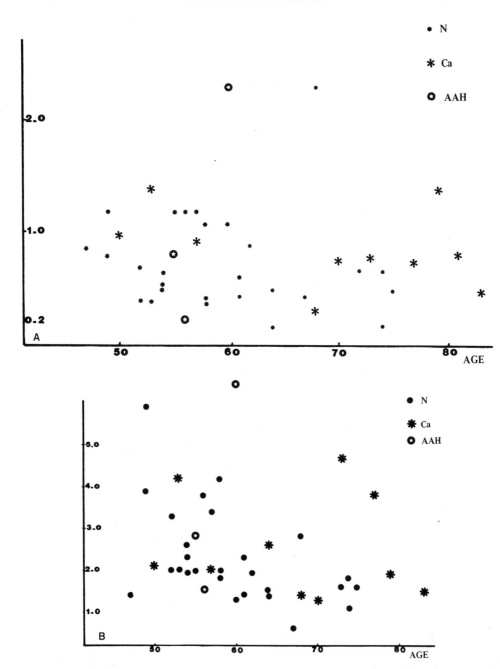

FIG. 2. **A:** Relation between age of the subject and the plasma level of testosterone (Test) (nmole/liter) and **B**: androstenedione (Adione) (nmole/liter) in 30 normal postmenopausal women, six postmenopausal women with an atypical adenomatous hyperplastic endometrium, and 18 postmenopausal women with endometrial cancer.

TABLE 2. *Daily production rate of DHEA-S and DHEA (mg/day)
and the fractional conversion rates*

	Normals (N = 4)	Atypical adenomatous hyperplasia (N = 3)	Endometrial cancer (N = 9)
PRDHEA-S (mg)	16.3	15.2	19.6
PRDHEA (mg)	2.8	4.0	2.2
ρDHEA-S→DHEA	0.15	0.12	0.11
ρDHEA→DHEA-S	0.55	0.47	0.36
ρDHEA-S→Adiol	0.012	0.015	0.016
ρDHEA→Adiol	0.05	0.08	0.12
ρDHEA-S→Adiol-S	0.111	0.058	0.046

DHEA-S = dehydroepiandrosterone-sulfate; DHEA = dehydroepiandrosterone; Adiol = 5-androstene-3β,17β-diol; PR = production rate.

TABLE 3. *Relative contribution of precursors to metabolic products*

	Normal (N = 4)	Atypical adenomatous hyperplasia (N = 3)	Endometrial carcinoma (N = 9)
DHEA-S→DHEA (mg)	2.44 (87%)	1.90 (47%)	1.90 (86%)
DHEA-S→DHEA-S	1.53 (9%)	1.74 (12%)	0.96 (5%)
DHEA-S→Adiol	0.21 (45%)	0.20 (44%)	0.30 (65%)
DHEA→Adiol	0.13 (28%)	0.35 (76%)	0.058 (12%)

DHEA-S = dehydroepiandrosterone-sulfate; DHEA = dehydroepiandrosterone; Adiol = 5-androstene-3β,17β-diol.

the balance between androgens and estrogens might precede by many years the clinical detection of a malignancy. At the time of diagnosis of this malignancy, the hormonal differences may be masked by other factors, including stress and metabolic activity of the tumor itself.

REFERENCES

1. Abraham, G. E., Maroulis, G. B., and Manlimos, F. S. (1977): Comparison between urinary 17-ketosteroids and serum androgens in hirsute patients. *Obstet. Gynecol.*, 49:454–461.
2. Andriessé, R., Thijssen, J. H. H., Donker, G. H., and Poortman, J. (1980): Adrenal androgens and endometrial carcinoma. In: *Adrenal Androgens*, edited by A. R. Genazzani, H. H. Thijssen, and P. K. Siiteri, pp. 355–366. Raven Press, New York.
3. Judd, H. L., Davidson, B. J., Frumar, A. M., Shamonki, I. M., Lagasse, L. D., and Ballon, S. C. (1980): Serum androgens and estrogens in postmenopausal women with and without endometrial cancer. *Am. J. Obstet. Gynecol.*, 136:859–870.
4. van Landeghem, A. A. J., Poortman, J., Deshpande, N., Di Martino, L., Tarquini, A., Thijssen,

J. H. H., and Schwarz, F. (1981): Plasma concentration gradient of steroid hormones across human mammary tumours *in vivo. J. Steroid. Biochem.*, 14:741–747.

5. MacDonald, P. C., Edman, G. D., Hemsell, D. L., Porter, J. C., and Siiteri, P. K. (1978): Effect of obesity on conversion of plasma androstenedione to estrone in postmenopausal women with and without endometrial cancer. *Am. J. Obstet. Gynecol.*, 130:448–455.

6. Poortman, J., Thijssen, J. H. H., and Schwarz, F. (1973): Androgen production and conversion to estrogens in normal postmenopausal women and in selected breast cancer patients. *J. Clin. Endocrinol. Metab.*, 37:101–109.

7. Poortman, J., and Thijssen, J. H. H. (1978): The role of androgens in the aetiology of endometrial cancer: A hypothesis. In: *Endometrial Cancer*, edited by M. G. Brush, R. J. B. King, and R. W. Taylor, pp. 375–382. Baillière Tindall, London.

8. Poortman, J., Andriesse, R., Agema, A., Donker, G. H., Schwarz, F., and Thijssen, J. H. H. (1980): Adrenal androgen secretion and metabolism in postmenopausal women. In: *Adrenal Androgens*, edited by A. R. Genazzani, J. H. H. Thijssen, and P. K. Siiteri, pp. 219–239. Raven Press, New York.

9. Sall, S., and Calanog, A. (1972): Steroid excretion patterns in postmenopausal women with benign and neoplastic endometrium. *Am. J. Obstet. Gynecol.*, 114:153–161.

10. Thijssen, J. H. H., Poortman, J., and Schwarz, F. (1975): Androgens in postmenopausal breast cancer: Excretion, production and interaction with estrogens. *J. Steroid. Biochem.*, 6:729–734.

11. de Waard, F., Thijssen, J. H. H., Veeman, W., and Sander, P. C. (1968): The steroid hormone excretion pattern in women with endometrial carcinoma. *Cancer*, 22:988–996.

Steroids and Endometrial Cancer,
edited by V. M. Jasonni, et al.
Raven Press, New York © 1983.

Endocrine Implications of Endometrial Estrogen Sulfurylation

S. C. Brooks, C. Christensen, S. Meyers, J. Corombos, and B. A. Pack

Department of Biochemistry, Wayne University School of Medicine, Detroit, Michigan 48201

The concept that *in situ* metabolism of 17β-estradiol (E_2) may have a role in controlling the activity of this hormone in target tissues has not been widely appreciated. Recent reports from our group (8,9,16–18,20) and from the laboratories of Gurpide (12,24,25) and Tseng (15,26,27) have documented uterine estrogen metabolism and suggested an influence of these enzymic conversions on the steroid's uterine effects. It had become apparent from the work of Gurpide and his colleagues that uterine E_2 dehydrogenase activity varied significantly during the menstrual cycle, being significantly higher in secretory tissue (24). These investigators proceeded to show that this oxido-reduction enzyme was stimulated by progestins *in vivo* (25). Data from our studies with rat uteri likewise demonstrated a variation of E_2 oxidation (to estrone, E_1) during the estrous cycle (16). E_2 dehydrogenase was absent from immature rat uterus or from the uteri of ovariectomized rats (16).

Using porcine uterus, Pack and Brooks first reported in 1974 the existence of uterine estrogen sulfurylation activity (17). This enzymic function was shown to be appreciable in secretory endometrium; immature and estrous tissues were nearly devoid of estrogen sulfotransferase activity.

STEROID SULFURYLATION

First discovered in 1957 (21), "active sulfate" was shown to consist of a high energy phosphosulfate group esterified (through the phosphate) to the 5'-position of 3'-phosphoadenosine. This compound, commonly termed PAPS, is able to transfer sulfate to numerous acceptors, each class of compounds to be sulfurylated requiring a specific enzyme for the transfer of sulfate from PAPS. Steroid sulfotransferases make up a class of such enzymes and include 3β-hydroxysteroid (3) and estrogen (1,2,4) sulfotransferases. Depending on the tissue of origin, each of these enzymes have been shown to have varying specificities. These catalysts isolated from liver characteristically display very low specificity toward substrates (7). On the other hand, those arising in endocrine organs are highly specific for the steroid structure of their substrates (e.g., estrogen sulfotransferase from the adrenal gland will not react with neutral steroids or with phenol, 4 and 23).

Both E_2 and E_1 are secreted from the ovaries as free steroids and as sulfate esters (11). This combination of plasma estrogens and their esters is in equilibrium with hepatic tissue where the estrogens may be oxidized, reduced, or hydroxylated. In addition, these estrogens are conjugated to glucuronic acid and/or sulfate, whereas the preformed sulfates can be hydrolyzed by hepatic enzymes. For the most part, estrogen glucosiduronates and diconjugates are excreted. However, free estrogens or their 3-sulfates are readily taken into target tissues (uterus), the sulfates being hydrolyzed in the process (16). Once within porcine or human endometrial cells, E_2 and E_1 are in equilibrium (E_2 dehydrogenase) and either estrogen may be sulfurylated (9,18). Porcine uterus has been shown to contain both 3β-hydroxysteroid and estrogen sulfotransferase of high specificity (S. C. Brooks et al., *manuscript in preparation*).

PROGESTERONE REQUIREMENT FOR UTERINE ESTROGEN SULFURYLATION

The cyclic sulfurylation by porcine uterine tissue reported earlier (17,18) was unique to the activity of estrogen sulfotransferase. Uterine sulfatase (the hydrolytic enzyme) activity remained unchanged throughout the porcine estrous cycle. Further, neutral steroids (e.g., dehydroepiandrosterone) were sulfurylated actively and equally during the various phases of the estrous cycle (17). Such sulfurylation, although not of estrogens, demonstrated that uterine PAPS was not limiting at any time during the estrous cycle in the pig.

Interestingly, in both porcine (17) and human (10,20) endometrium, estrogen sulfotransferase activity mimics the plasma progesterone (Pg) pattern throughout the reproductive cycle. In fact, if porcine uteri are examined following implantation of the blastocyst, the resulting prolonged elevation of plasma Pg is accompanied by a continuation of estrogen sulfurylation (18). These observations suggest the Pg induction of uterine estrogen sulfotransferase. In order to obtain more direct evidence for the involvement of Pg in the induction or activation of an enzyme specific for estrogen sulfurylation, the following experiments were performed with the uteri from ovariectomized pigs.

Three-hundred-pound mature domestic pigs were ovariectomized and housed in individual pens for 21 days before initiating the steroid protocol. At this time and after 7 days of corn oil injections (5 ml/day), the endometria of these uteri were devoid of estrogen sulfotransferase activity and contained very low levels of cytoplasmic Pg receptor. Following 4 or 7 days of E_2 injections (i.m., 250 μg/day E_2 in 2 ml corn oil), Pg receptor levels were elevated in the uteri from sacrificed pigs, but estrogens were not sulfurylated by this E_2 stimulated tissue. However, when ovariectomized pigs were treated with Pg (25 mg/day in 5 ml corn oil) in addition to the E_2 in the last 3 days of a 7-day regimen, significant levels of estrogen sulfurylation appeared coincident with the depression of cytoplasmic Pg receptor

(S. C. Brooks et al., *manuscript in preparation*). Although depressed by ovariectomy, 3β-hydroxysteroid sulfotransferase activity was not influenced by either of the administered steroids.

More directly, it was also possible to harvest the uteri from ovariectomized pigs thus treated with E_2 for 4 days (to induce Pg receptor) and expose these endometrial minces to hormones in organ culture. When cultured in a media containing 10% serum from adrenalectomized–castrated calves, this estrogen stimulated tissue displayed estrogen sulfurylation only in those dishes supplemented with 10^{-8}M E_2 plus 10^{-6}M Pg (Table 1). Seven- to 8-month-old gilts were ovariectomized 21 days prior to initiating the *in vivo* estrogen administration. Each pig was injected (i.m.) with 250 μg E_2 in 2 ml corn oil per day for 4 days. At the termination of this treatment the pigs were sacrificed, uteri removed, the horns clamped and sterilized in ice cold 70% ethanol for 1 hr. Each horn was then washed with buffer, opened, the endometrium cut off and minced in MEM containing gentamycin (40 μg/ml). Small pieces (<5 mg ea) were placed on sterile gauze in a petri dish containing 15 ml of Earles MEM supplemented with insulin (10 μg/ml), gentamycin (20 μg/ml), 5 ml fungizone solution and made 10% with adrenalectomized-castrated calf serum (gift of B. Katzenellenbogen, University of Illinois). Each petri dish contained 100 mg of minced endometrium, which was cultured in a temperature (37°), CO_2 (5%), and humidity (90%) controlled environment. Steroid hormones were added in 100 μl ethanol and control media contained an equal amount of ethanol. After 3 days, endometrial pieces were removed, washed with ice cold saline and placed in ½ ml sulfate-free Krebs-Ringer bicarbonate buffer with 50 nM [2,4,6,7-^{3}H]-estradiol-17β (specific activity 100 Ci/mmole) and 10^{-4}M $Na_2{}^{35}SO_4$ (specific activity 1 Ci/mmole). Incubations were carried out for 2 hr as described previously (17). After extraction of estrogens and their conjugates (17), the free estrogens were separated from sulfates and glucosiduronates on instant thin layer chromatography (SA, Gelman) by developing (3×) with $CHCl_3$:MeOH (97:3). The origin was then eluted with ethanol, evaporated and re-chromatographed on silica gel (SG, Gelman) sheets with $CHCl_3$:acetone:acetic acid (110:35:6). After cutting strips into 1-cm segments and eluting (ethanol), aliquots of the eluant were monitored for radioactivity. Total

TABLE 1. In vitro *effect of E_2 and/or Pg on porcine endometrial estrogen conjugation*

Duration of endometrial culture (days)	Hormones added	Estrogen conjugation (pmole/hr/0.1 g tissue)	
		Sulfurylation	Glucosiduronation
0	—	0.39 ± 0.15	0.11
3	none	0.99 ± 0.37	0.65 ± 0.09
3	10^{-8} M E_2	1.07 ± 0.17	0.70 ± 0.14
3	10^{-8} M E_2 + 10^{-6} M Pg	7.02 ± 1.43	0.37 ± 0.05

counts per minute in the peak for each conjugate (unlabeled standards were co-chromatographed) indicated extent of each ester formed. Estrogen sulfates displayed an R_f of 0.75 and the esters with glucuronic acid migrated 0.25 the distance of the front. The optimum level of Pg required to induce estrogen sulfurylation in these organ cultures was 10^{-6}M (limited solubility in media prohibited greater concentrations). However, significant stimulation was apparent with Pg concentrations of 10^{-9} M and 10^{-7} M (Fig. 1). E_2, of course, was administered concurrently to maintain Pg receptor. Physiological levels of Pg in plasma approach 10^{-7} M.

A more dramatic dependence of endometrial estrogen sulfuryaltion on the presence of Pg in organ culture is shown by the data in Fig. 2. Here the estrogen sulfotransferase activity of endometrial cells from hormone-treated (E_2 and Pg), ovariectomized pigs was maintained in culture for one week by the inclusion of E_2 (10^{-8} M) and Pg (10^{-6} M). This enzymic activity, however, was lost in cultures with no steroids or with E_2 alone. In these experiments, estrogen sulfurylation displayed an absolute dependence on Pg, whether this steroid was added or removed from E_2 supplemented cultures midway through the experiment. Recently, a similar

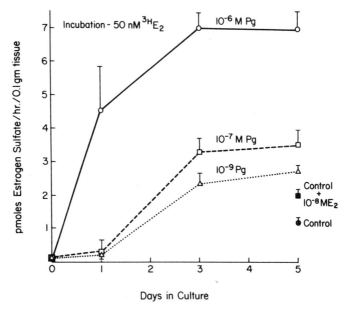

FIG. 1. *In vitro* effect of progesterone (Pg) concentration on estrogen sulfotransferase in uteri from ovariectomized (OXV) pigs injected with E_2. Experimental procedures were the same as those described in Table 1 except that serum from OVX pigs was utilized in cultures in place of that from adrenalectomized-castrated calves. Media was renewed every 2 days. Radioimmunoassay of E_2 and Pg in OVX serum showed both steroids to be present at low levels (E_2, 2.5×10^{-11} M and Pg, 0.7×10^{-9} M). Therefore, control cultures and those with E_2 alone (10^{-8} M) displayed some estrogen sulfurylation. Increasing Pg levels (10^{-9} M; 10^{-7} M; and 10^{-6} M) in the presence of 10^{-8} M E_2 brought about increasing synthesis of estrogen sulfates. Standard deviation of triplicate cultures is shown.

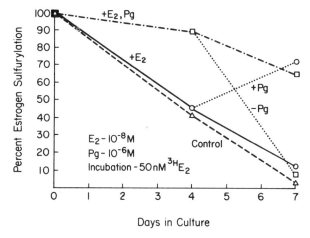

Days in Culture

FIG. 2. Effect of addition or withdrawal of progesterone (Pg) on porcine uterine estrogen sulfotransferase in organ culture. Experimental procedures were the same as those described in Fig. 1 except that the ovariectomized (OVX) pigs were primed with E_2 (250 µg/day) for 4 days followed by the injection of E_2 (250 µg) and Pg (25 mg) per day for 3 days. Endometria cultured without added hormones (△---△) lost estrogen sulfotransferase activity after 1 week in culture. At the same time, the presence of both E_2 and Pg (□-•-□) preserved 65% of the sulfurylation activity. Although those endometria cultured with only E_2 (o——o) lost significant sulfotransferase activity by 4 days, this activity was restored with 3 additional days in culture in the presence of E_2 and Pg (o••••o). Conversely, the removal of Pg (□••••□) from cultures at 4 days demonstrated that E_2 alone was not capable of maintaining estrogen sulfurylation.

dependence of estrogen sulfurylation on Pg was reported by Tseng and Liu (26) in human endometrial cultures.

Although only a trace appeared in incubations of fresh uterine tissue shortly following removal, significant formation of estrogen glucosiduronate did occur following organ culture of endometrial minces. The esterification of estrogen to glucuronic acid, unusual for uterus, was not influenced by either of the administered hormones (Table 1).

INTERRELATIONSHIP OF E_2 OXIDATION AND ESTROGEN SULFURYLATION IN UTERI

Examination of E_2 uterine metabolism over a period of 2 hr has shown the early (within 0.5 hr) formation of [³H]E_1 from [³H]E_2. The level of free [³H]E_1 in these incubations reached a plateau near 15% of the added [³H]E_2 after 1 hr (17). However, sulfurylation continued linearly for the entire incubation period. Estrone sulfate (E_1S) always comprised the major portion of the sulfate fraction, the remainder being 17β-estradiol-3-sulfate (E_2-3S). This predominance of estrone sulfate is to be expected, as earlier experiments in our laboratory (23) had clearly demonstrated the lower K_m (higher affinity) and higher V_{max} of E_1 for the bovine adrenal estrogen sulfotransferase. This being the case, it is easier to understand the set of relationships depicted in Table 2.

TABLE 2. *Uterine metabolism of* E_2

Tissue	E_2-3S	b ←	E_2	aª ⇌	E_1	bᵇ →	E_1-S	Total oxidationᶜ
Porcine uterus (pmoles)								
Immature	0		8.7		1.3		0	1.3
Proliferative	0		8.4		1.6		0	1.6
Secretory	1.7		3.3		1.7		3.3	5.0
Human endometrium (pmoles)				←				
Proliferative	0		4.5		5.5		0	5.5
Secretory	1.4		1.5		4.2		3.9	8.1

ªa = E_2 dehydrogenase.
ᵇb = Estrogen sulfotransferase.
ᶜTotal oxidation is the sum of E_1 and its sulfate (E_1S).
Reprinted from S. C. Brooks et al. (9), with permission.

In incubations of immature or proliferative uteri with a physiological level of E_2 (10^{-9} M), the equilibrium state of E_2 dehydrogenase produces a consistent quantity of E_1 from E_2 (approximately 17% in porcine and 55% in human uteri, Table 2). Once ovulation occurs and the endometrium is exposed to Pg, the appearance of estrogen sulfotransferase has a dramatic effect on this equilibrium favoring oxidation. This influence of sulfurylation on the oxido-reduction equilibrium is brought about by the fact that estrogen sulfotransferase binds more tightly to the E_1 formed in the equilibrium with E_2. Therefore, E_1 is more rapidly removed from the equilibrium as E_1S. Total oxidation of E_2, represented by E_1 + E_1S, is then much greater in secretory endometrium than would be possible by the activity of E_2 dehydrogenase alone. It remains now to be demonstrated whether the activity of E_2 dehydrogenase itself is elevated in secretory uteri.

Employing a recently developed inhibitor, specific for estrogen sulfotransferase (4-nitroestrone 3-methyl ether) (22) it has been possible to examine directly the *in vitro* activity of E_2 dehydrogenase in porcine secretory endometrium. In these experiments, estrogen sulfurylation was inhibited 85%. Moreover, without significant estrogen sulfurylation, secretory endometrium was capable of oxidizing 37% of the added $[^3H]E_2$ to $[^3H]E_1$, in addition to some 0.67 pmoles of $[^3H]E_1$ found as $[^3H]E_1$S (Table 3). These data represent greater than a threefold increase in E_2 dehydrogenase activity in the Pg influenced tissue. Oxidation, however, was facilitated by the activity of estrogen sulfotransferase in the uninhibited control tissue where total oxidation (E_1 + E_1S) was 25% greater. At the same time, it is important to note that most of the estrogen present in the incubated secretory endometrium was found as estrogen sulfates (E_2-3S and E_1S) (Table 3).

POSSIBLE ROLE OF ESTROGEN SULFURYLATION IN UTERUS

The remaining fate of E_2 in uterine tissue is its high affinity binding to the specific E_2 receptor. Since E_1 binds with less affinity to this protein and the 3-sulfurylated estrogens are unable to bind, it is quite possible that these Pg-influenced metabolic

TABLE 3. *Effect of the inhibition of estrogen sulfurylation on the oxidation of E_2 to E_1 by porcine uteri*

Incubation[a]	Estrogens recovered (pmoles)				
	E_2	E_1	E_2-3S	E_1S	$E_1 + E_1$S
Control	2.6	1.2	2.2	4.2	5.4
+ 40 μM 4 NO_2E_1–30Me[b]	5.5	3.7	0.29	0.67	4.37

[a]Two hr, 37°C, 400 mg secretory uterine minces, 4 nM $[^3H]E_2$ in 2.5 ml buffer.
[b]4-Nitroestrone 3-methyl ether.

functions are important in the *in situ* control of E_2 endometrial activity. This premise is of special importance in endometrial adenocarcinoma, a disease believed to result from an unusually high degree of E_2 activity within endometrial cells.

Well-documented functions of E_2 in target tissues are the induction of Pg receptor and the replenishment of its own receptor (13,14). On the other hand, Pg while controlling the secretory differentiation of the endometrium, also has the role of "down regulating" (depressing the cellular level of) E_2 receptor (14). The mechanism by which this "down regulation" is carried out is unknown presently. It is conceivable, however, that the regulatory function of Pg may be accomplished through the induction of enzymes that convert E_2 to metabolites that cannot bind to (estrogen sulfates) or have less affinity (E_1) for receptor. In this Pg-induced absence of the estrogen-receptor complex, nuclear translocation will not occur and the receptor will not be replenished, therefore displaying "down regulation." This phenomenon would be possible if the Pg receptor has a long enough half-life or if small amounts of E_2 receptor can replenish the Pg receptor. Furthermore, the described binding of estrogen to the sulfotransferase in the presence of receptor would require a higher concentration of and a significant affinity for the enzyme. Tseng and Mazella (27) have reported a K_m of 5 nM for uterine estrogen sulfotransferase. The above concept is represented in Fig. 3, which also depicts another possibility (14): the turn off of E_2 receptor synthesis by direct chromatin interaction of Pg receptor complex.

Examining the levels of cytoplasmic and nuclear estrogen receptors throughout the porcine estrous cycle has yielded the data presented in Fig. 4 (19). At estrus, the high plasma E_2 translocates nearly all receptor to the nucleus. Shortly thereafter, the nuclear concentration of E_2 receptor drops to a consistent but biologically important level (5), which is maintained for approximately one week. This pattern of nuclear E_2 receptor is similar to that observed *in vitro* where the more permanent nuclear concentration of E_2 receptor was considerably less than the level resulting from the initial influx of E_2 receptor (6).

The cytoplasmic E_2 receptor level rises sharply immediately following ovulation and the induction by Pg of estrogen sulfotransferase (Fig. 4). Sulfurylation of estrogens, having prohibited the binding of E_2 to receptor and the nuclear translocation of E_2 receptor complex, results in decreased receptor replenishment and therefore a loss of the binding protein as determined by its half-life. Without the

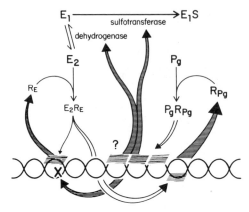

FIG. 3. Suggested role of progesterone (Pg) in the activation or induction of estrogen dehydrogenase and/or sulfotransferase in endometrial cells. R_E = estrogen receptor; E_2R_E = complex; R_{Pg} = progestrone receptor.

translocation of cytoplasmic E_2 receptor, the nuclear receptor disappears by one week following the initiation of estrogen sulfurylation (Fig. 4). In general, whenever estrogen sulfurylation activity is high, nuclear E_2 receptor levels are low. This is also true in postimplantation porcine uteri (18) and in secretory human endometrium (20).

CONCLUSIONS

As well as being bound by its receptor, E_2 is destined to be metabolized by specific uterine enzymes with which it may come into contact. Two uterine enzymes have been identified that may enter into an *in situ* metabolic "deactivation" of E_2. The products of E_2 dehydrogenase (E_1) and estrogen sulfotransferase (estrogen sulfates) do not bind to the classical estrogen receptor at physiological concentrations. Furthermore, Pg is essential to the stimulation of the dehydrogenase and the induction of an estrogen sulfurylating enzyme. In concert with the dehydrogenase, oxidation of E_2 to E_1 is facilitated by the lower K_m of E_1 with the sulfotransferase, which promotes the preferential removal of oxidized product from the E_2 dehydrogenase equilibrium. Without appreciable E_2 binding in secretory endometrium, little receptor complex will interact with chromatin, resulting in minimal replenishment of E_2 receptor. The result of this Pg-initiated combination of events would be represented by a decrease or "down regulation" of cellular E_2 receptor. Control of estrogenicity by Pg has been demonstrated in highly differentiated endometrial adenocarcinoma, but it is not possible to induce estrogen sulfotransferase activity in the undifferentiated neoplasm (10).

ACKNOWLEDGMENTS

These investigations were supported in part by U.S. Public Health Service Research Grant No. CA-22828 from the National Cancer Institute and Grant Nos. HD-8735 and HD-14775 from the National Institute of Child Health and Human

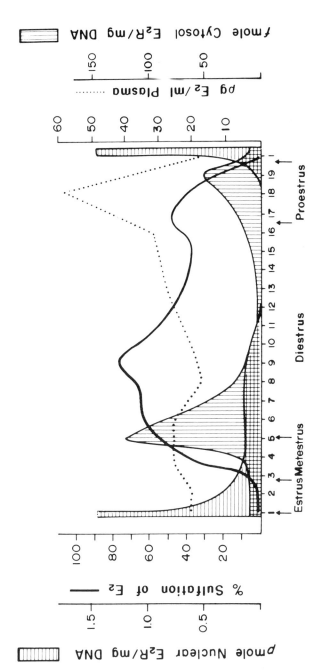

FIG. 4. Days of porcine estrous cycle. Composite plot showing relationship between gilt plasma E_2 levels (····), uterine estrogen sulfurylation (——), cytosolic E_2 receptor (▥), and nuclear E_2 receptor (▦) throughout the porcine estrous cycle. (From Pack and Brooks, ref. 17, with permission.)

Development. In addition, the authors wish to thank Mia Coppens and the Department Humane Biologie, Afdeling Biochemie, Katholieke Universiteit Leuven, for the excellent typing of the manuscript.

REFERENCES

1. Adams, J. B. (1967): Enzymic synthesis of steroid sulphates: V. On the binding of estrogens to estrogen sulphotransferase. *Biochim. Biophys. Acta*, 146:522–528.
2. Adams, J. B., and Chulavatnatol, M. (1967): Enzymic synthesis of steroid sulphates: IV. The nature of the two forms of estrogen sulphotransferase of bovine adrenals. *Biochim. Biophys. Acta*, 146:509–521.
3. Adams, J. B., and Edwards, A. M. (1968): Enzymic synthesis of steroid sulphates: VII. Association-dissociation equilibria in the steroid alcohol sulphotransferase of human adrenal gland extracts. *Biochim. Biophys. Acta*, 167:122–140.
4. Adams, J. B., and Poulos, A. (1967): Enzymic synthesis of steroid sulphates: III. Isolation and properties of estrogen sulphotransferase of bovine adrenal glands. *Biochim. Biophys. Acta*, 146:493–508.
5. Anderson, J. N., Peck, Jr., E. J., and Clark, J. H. (1973): Nuclear receptor estrogen complex: Relationship between concentration and early uterotrophic responses. *Endocrinology*, 92:1488–1495.
6. Anderson, J. N., Peck, Jr., E. J., and Clark, J. H. (1975): Estrogen induced uterine responses and growth: Relationship to receptor estrogen binding by uterine nuclei. *Endocrinology*, 96:160–167.
7. Banerjee, R. K., and Roy, A. B. (1966): The sulfotransferases of guinea pig liver. *Mol. Pharmacol.*, 2:56–66.
8. Brooks, S. C., Rozhin, J., Pack, B. A., Horn, L., Godefroi, V. C., Locke, E. R., Zemlicka, J., and Singh, D. V. (1978): Role of sulfate conjugation in estrogen metabolism and activity. *J. Toxicol. Environ. Health*, 4:293–300.
9. Brooks, S. C., Horn, L., Pack, B. A., Rozhin, J., Hansen, E., and Goldberg, R. (1980): Estrogen metabolism and function in vivo and in vitro. In: *Estrogens in the Environment*, edited by J. A. McLachlan, pp. 147–167. Elsevier North Holland, New York.
10. Buirchell, B. J., and Hähnel, R. (1975): Metabolism of estradiol-17β in human endometrium during the menstrual cycle. *J. Steroid Biochem.*, 6:1489–1494.
11. Giorgi, E. P. (1967): Determination of free and conjugated oestrogens in fluid from human ovaries. *J. Endocrinol.*, 37:211–219.
12. Gurpide, E. (1978): Enzymatic modulation of hormonal action on the target tissue. *J. Toxicol. Environ. Health*, 4:249–268.
13. Horwitz, K. B., and McGuire, W. L. (1978): Estrogen control of progesterone receptor in human breast cancer: Correlation with nuclear processing of estrogen receptor. *J. Biol. Chem.*, 253:2223–2228.
14. Hseuh, A. J. W., Peck, Jr., E. J., and Clark, J. H. (1975): Progesterone antagonism of the oestrogen receptor and oestrogen-induced uterine growth. *Nature* (London), 254:337–339.
15. Liu, H. C., and Tseng, L. (1979): Estradiol metabolism in isolated human endometrial epithelial glands and stromal cells. *Endocrinology*, 104:1674–1681.
16. Pack, B. A., and Brooks, S. C. (1970): Metabolism of estrogens and their sulfates in rat uterine minces. *Endocrinology*, 87:924–933.
17. Pack, B. A., and Brooks, S. C. (1974): Cyclic activity of estrogen sulfotransferase in the gilt uterus. *Endocrinology*, 95:1680–1690.
18. Pack, B. A., Brooks, C. L., Dukelow, W. R., and Brooks, S. C. (1979): The metabolism and nuclear migration of estrogen in porcine uterus throughout the implantation process. *Biol. of Reprod.*, 20:545–551.
19. Pack, B. A., Christensen, C., Douraghy, M., and Brooks, S. C. (1978): Nuclear and cytosolic estrogen receptor in gilt endometrium throughout the estrous cycle. *Endocrinology*, 103:2129–2136.
20. Pack, B. A., Tovar, R., Booth, E., and Brooks, S. C. (1979): The cyclic relationship of estrogen sulfurylation to the nuclear receptor level in human endometrial curettings. *J. Clin. Endocrinol. Metab.*, 48:420–424.

21. Robbins, P. W., and Lipman, F. (1957): Isolation and identification of active sulfate. *J. Biol. Chem.*, 229:837–851.
22. Rozhin, J., Huo, A., Zemlicka, J., and Brooks, S. C. (1977): Studies on bovine adrenal estrogen sulfotransferase: Inhibition and possible involvement of adenine-estrogen stacking. *J. Biol. Chem.*, 252:7214–7220.
23. Rozhin, J., Soderstrom, R. L., and Brooks, S. C. (1974): Specificity studies on bovine adrenal estrogen sulfotransferase. *J. Biol. Chem.*, 249:2079–2087.
24. Tseng, L., and Gurpide, E. (1974): Estradiol and 20α-dehydroprogesterone dehydrogenase activities in human endometrium during the menstrual cycle. *Endocrinology*, 94:419–423.
25. Tseng, L., and Gurpide, E. (1979): Stimulation of various 17β- and 20α-hydroxysteroid dehydrogenase activities by progestins in human endometrium. *Endocrinology*, 104:1745–1748.
26. Tseng, L., and Liu, H. C. (1981): Stimulation of arylsulfotransferase activity by progestins in human endometrium *in vitro*. *J. Clin. Endocrinol. Metab.*, 53:418–421.
27. Tseng, L., and Mazella, J. (1980): Cyclic change of estradiol metabolic enzymes in human endometrium during the menstrual cycle. In: *Proceedings of 8th Brook Lodge Conference on Problem of Reproductive Physiology*, edited by F. A. Kimball, p. 211. Spectrum Publishing, Inc. New York.

Steroids and Endometrial Cancer,
edited by V. M. Jasonni, et al.
Raven Press, New York © 1983.

Metabolic Aspects of Estrone Sulfate in Postmenopausal Women

V. M. Jasonni, C. Bulletti, A. P. Ferraretti, F. Franceschetti,
G. F. Bolelli, M. Bonavia, and C. Flamigni

*Department of Reproductive Physiopathology, St. Orsola's General Hospital,
University of Bologna, 40138 Bologna, Italy*

Estrone sulfate (E_1S) is the estrogen present in plasma at the highest levels in nonpregnant women as well as in normal men (1,4,11,16,19). It may represent an important reserve of active hormones, as it can be converted to estrone (E_1) by arylsulfatases, which are present in several tissues, such as hypothalamus, cerebral cortex, and endometrium (6,15); the E_1S may enter into endometrial cells, where it is converted to E_1 (26).

However, the reverse reaction can occur: The liver is probably the major site of sulfurylation (12), and *in vitro* studies have shown that the sulfotransferase activity is present in the endometrium and is greatly stimulated during the secretory phase (22).

Few data are available in the literature concerning plasma E_1S in postmenopausal women (8,23). The present study was undertaken to examine endogenous E_1S metabolism in postmenopausal women with endometrial cancer and appropriately matched control subjects.

MATERIALS AND METHODS

Subjects

Ten postmenopausal women with histologically proven adenocarcinoma of the endometrium and 28 control subjects, 20 of normal weight and eight overweight, were studied. All cancer patients had fractional curettages that established the diagnosis. The cancer patients had at least 6 months of amenorrhea prior to the bleeding that was associated with present illness. All control subjects had at least 1 year of amenorrhea prior to the study.

Cancer and control subjects ranged 1 to 15 years' postmenopause; all patients in both groups had elevated gonadotropins, and all had been off exogenous estrogens for at least 1 month prior to the study. The excess fat was calculated for each patient from the tables supplied by the Metropolitan Life Insurance Co.

Reagents

All solvents for plasma extraction (diethyl ether; Merck) and chromatography (benzene, methanol, ethanol; C. Erba) were of reagent grade and were used without further purification.

Phosphate ethylenediaminotetraacetate (EDTA) buffer (0.05 M, pH 7.5, + 0.1% gelatine + 0.1% sodium azide) and acetate buffer (0.2 M, pH 4.2) were made in sterile double-distilled water and stored at 4°C.

Arylsulfatase (Helix Pomatia Type H1; Sigma), stored at −20°C, was dissolved prior to use (250 U/ml) in acetate buffer and charcoal treated to minimize the blank values (27).

Sephadex LH-20 (Pharmacia), activated "celite" analytical filter aid (BDH), charcoal (Norit A; Sigma), dextran T 70 (Pharmacia), and scintillation fluid, Pico-Fluor 30 (Packard Instruments), were used as supplied.

Radioactive Steroids

[2,4,6,7,-³H]Estrone and estradiol-17β were delivered by Radiochemical Center, Amersham, specific activity 102 Ci/mmole; [6,7-³H]extrone sulfate, potassium salt, specific activity 43 Ci/mmole, was purchased from New England Nuclear Corp. All labeled steroids were purified by chromatography on Sephadex LH-20 columns and stored in stock solutions in ethanol at −20°C.

Estrogen Standard

Estrone and estradiol-17β (Sigma) were used without further purification and stored in ethanol solutions at −20°C. Estrone sulfate was purified by Sephadex LH-20 column.

ANALYTICAL PROCEDURE

Plasma E_1S and E_1 Assay

To each plasma sample (1 ml) [6,7-³H]E_1S (200 dpm) in saline solution was added to count for procedural losses. The plasma samples were extracted twice with diethyl-ether (10 ml) to remove free estrogens. Each extract was treated with 250 units of charcoal-treated arylsulfatase, diluted 1:2 with saline buffer (pH 4.2), and left overnight at 37°C. The liberated estrone was extracted twice with diethyl-ether (20 ml). The ether phases were pooled and evaporated to dryness and cromatographed on Sephadex LH-20 columns, according to Olivo et al. (20).

The estrone fraction was dried under nitrogen and dissolved in 1 ml of 0.05 M phosphate buffer, pH 7.4. To determine recovery for estrone a 0.5 ml aliquot of this phase was assayed for radioactivity. The losses ranged between 40 and 50%.

Duplicate aliquots of 100 μl, 50 μl, and 25 μl were used for radio immunoassay (RIA). The RIA was performed as previously reported (7), using an antiserum obtained in our department.

An enzyme blank was measured in a similar manner, using 1 ml of buffer and 250 units of enzyme; the assay blank values ranged usually below 5 pg/ml. The intra- and interassay variations were below 10 and 15%, respectively.

The glucuronide contamination was assayed adding 1 μg of E_1 glucuronide to five samples and carried out through the extraction and hydrolysis; the contamination was lower than 0.5%.

Plasma E_1S-^3H and E_1-^3H Assay

E_1S (1 μg) in saline solution was added to plasma samples (10 ml) to correct for losses. The procedures of extraction, hydrolysis, and separation were those previously described for the assay of unlabeled E_1S.

ANALYSIS OF DATA

Constant Infusions

The infusions were performed with labeled and unlabeled E_1S in the same four healthy postmenopausal women in order to determine the validity of the constant infusions using unlabeled E_1S. In all the other subjects the constant infusions were performed with unlabeled E_1S.

A priming dose of E_1S was used prior to the constant infusions in order to achieve the steady state as rapidly as possible. The size of the priming dose in relationship to the amount infused was calculated as described by Tait and Burstein (25). For each individual infusion, from the third hour to the end of infusion, the concentrations in plasma of E_1S were related to time of sampling by linear regression analysis (14).

Values of metabolic clearance rate, plasma production rate, instant conversion ratio, and the fraction of plasma production rate of the product derived from E_1S infused were calculated according to Longcope and Tait (14).

Basal Levels

The plasma basal levels of E_1S and E_1 are expressed as the mean of six determinations performed on six different samples of plasma: blood samples were drawn from each subject at 20-min intervals for 2 hr through an indwelling venous catheter, beginning at 8:00 a.m. on two consecutive mornings. Plasma was separated within 15 min and stored at $-20°C$ until assayed.

RESULTS

Plasma E_1S and E_1 levels in postmenopausal women with and without endometrial cancer are reported in Fig. 1. In the tumor patients, the mean concentrations ($\pm$ SE) were 617.5 $\pm$ 67.8 and 46.6 $\pm$ 4.8 pg/ml for E_1S and E_1, respectively. In the control subjects, the mean levels ($\pm$ SE) were 318.4 $\pm$ 19.9 and 35.6 $\pm$ 2.7 pg/ml for the same respective hormones.

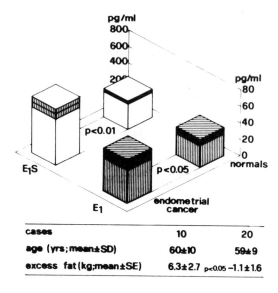

FIG. 1. Plasma E_1S and E_1 levels in postmenopausal women with and without endometrial cancer. Age (mean ± SD) and excess fat (mean ± SE) are also reported.

cases	10	20
age (yrs; mean±SD)	60±10	59±9
excess fat (kg;mean±SE)	6.3±2.7 $_{p<0.05}$	–1.1±1.6

The E_1S and E_1 plasma levels were found significantly higher in the tumor patients than in the control subjects ($p < 0.05$); however, the excess fat was also significantly higher in cancer group than in the control subjects ($p < 0.05$).

In order to determine the influence of body weight on E_1S levels, 28 postmenopausal women without endometrial cancer, verified by endometrial biopsy, to exclude the presence of the silent endometrial cancer, were investigated.

Analysis of a possible relationship between the weight and E_1S plasma levels revealed positive correlation between E_1S levels and excess fat; the same result was obtained, even considering the cancer patients.

Analysis of a possible relationship between E_1S plasma levels and age was also performed. In order to avoid the influence of body weight and of endometrial cancer, 20 postmenopausal women with normal weight and without adenocarcinoma of the endometrium were studied. No positive or negative correlation between E_1S levels and age was found.

These results disagree with those of Franz et al. (8), who found negative correlation between age and E_1S levels; these conflicting data might be due to a relatively small number of cases we have studied. However, in a recent study of Noel et al. (18), no correlation between E_1S plasma levels and age was found in postmenopausal women.

In postmenopausal women, the relationship between the endogenous estrogen production and the adenocarcinoma of the endometrium has not been defined clearly. Several studies (2,3,10) have observed higher levels of E_1 and E_2 or enhanced conversion ratios of androstenedione to E_1 in women with this tumor as compared to normal subjects. However, other studies (5,17) have not confirmed these observations; in recent and extensive studies on androgens and estrogens (13) in postmenopausal women with and without endometrial cancer, it has been stated that estrogen levels are related to weight but not to endometrial cancer or to age.

Because the major source of E_1S in postmenopausal women as well as in both normal males (15) and fertile women (24) is apparently the peripheral conversion of E_1 and E_2, which are both circulating at higher levels in obese postmenopausal women than in postmenopausal women with normal weight, it is not surprising that E_1S plasma levels were found to be significantly higher in obese postmenopausal women.

In order to investigate the influence of weight on E_1S metabolism, kinetic studies of E_1S in obese and nonobese postmenopausal women were performed.

KINETIC STUDIES

Constant Infusions

Constant infusions with labeled and unlabeled E_1S were performed in two post-menopausal women previously studied with $[6,7-^3H]E_1S$ single injection.

The results obtained (Table 1) clearly demonstrate that (a) there appeared to be little change in the concentration of E_1S or $[6,7-^3H]E_1S$ after 20 hr of infusion and (b) both constant infusions, with labeled and unlabeled E_1S, gave similar metabolic clearance rate (MCR) values.

The E_1S MCR appeared to be independent of plasma concentration, increasing twofold the rate of E_1S infusion (Table 2); the MCR value does not change. The instant conversion ratio (CR) of E_1S into E_1 was not substrate dependent and the same CR obtained when the rate of infusion was increased twofold (Table 2).

This method for calculating the MCR E_1S appears valid, and constant infusions with unlabeled E_1S were performed in five obese postmenopausal women and in five postmenopausal women with normal weight; the results are summarized in Fig. 2.

The E_1S plasma production rate was found to be significantly higher in obese subjects, and the E_1S MCR, if considered per liter per square meter, was significantly lower.

These results could explain the higher E_1S plasma levels in obese postmenopausal women; in fact, the plasma E_1S concentration equals the E_1S production rate to the E_1S MCR ratio. The enhanced E_1S production rate is probably due to the higher estrogen levels present in obese subjects.

Recently, androstenedione 3-enol sulfate has been found in plasma (9), and it is possible that it may be metabolized directly to E_1S, as in placental microsomes (21). However, if androstenedione 3-enol sulfate plays a role in E_1S production, it is reasonable to suppose an enhanced peripheral conversion of this conjugated steroid to E_1S.

On the other hand, the lower E_1S MCR observed in the group of the obese subjects might be due to a slow release of E_1S from the peripheral tissues; in obese

TABLE 1. *Estrone sulfate infusion*

Patient	Infusion rate	Hours from start of infusion						Slope	MCR	MCR
		4	12	20	22	24	26			
Labeled	dpm/day × 10⁶			dpm/ml				%/100 min	1/day	1/day/m²
BM	767	2,180	1,875	2,226	2,053	1,949	2,027	−3.3	374	226
ML	764	1,880	1,781	2,023	1,703	1,941	1,904	1.4	408	215
Mean	765	2,030	1,828	2,124	1,878	1,945	1,965	—	391	220
Unlabeled	mg/day			ng/ml				%/100 min	1/day	1/day/m²
BM	9.0	23.7	23.8	24.1	22.9	25.4	24.1	2.2	377	228
ML	10.9	25.1	24.4	25.8	25.2	26.3	25.8	3.2	429	226
Mean	9.9	24.4	24.1	24.9	24.1	25.9	25.0	—	403	227

TABLE 2. *Mean (± SE) MCR of the infused E_1S*
in two postmenopausal women[a]

Subjects	E_1S infusion rate (mg/hr)	MCR (1/day)	$\Delta E_1/\Delta E_1S$
1	8	421	0.051
	16	425	0.053
2	8	448	0.062
	16	437	0.059

[a]The instant conversion ratio of E_1S into E_1 is expressed as percentage.

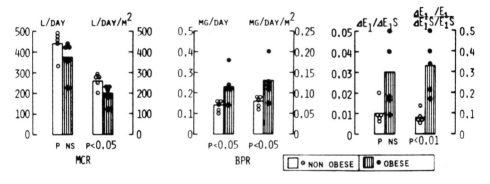

FIG. 2. In obese subjects, the plasma production rate of E_1S as well as the E_1S to E_1 contribution are significantly higher; on the contrary, the E_1S MCR, if expressed per liter per square meter, is significantly lower.

subjects, the rate of excretion of E_1 was found inversely related to the excess body weight (17).

The fraction of the plasma production rate of E_1 derived from E_1S was found to be higher in obese subjects, whereas the instant conversion ratio of E_1S to E_1 showed no significant differences between the two groups. The higher contribution of E_1S to E_1 found in obese subjects might be due to a higher level of equilibrium between these two steroids; however, further investigations are needed to confirm and to clarify this point.

CONCLUSIONS

Our data show that the E_1S levels are related to body weight but not to endometrial cancer, as it has been found for E_1 (13). The biological role of E_1S is still unknown; however, it may be considered as an important reservoir of active hormones; the endometrium metabolizes E_1S to E_1 and E_2 (26), as well as other tissues. Conversely, the reverse reaction may represent an inactivation of free estrogens that may play a role on estrogen balance; the sulfurylation of E_1 in the endometrium was found to be higher during the secretory phase than in the proliferative phase (22).

Obviously, further studies are needed to clarify the role of E_1S on estrogen balance; however, it seems evident that E_1S should be taken into consideration during the studies on estrogen metabolism.

ACKNOWLEDGMENT

Supported by grant CNR 80.01546.96.

REFERENCES

1. Brown, J. B., and Smith, B. S. (1977): Oestrone sulphate the major circulating oestrogen in the normal menstrual cycle? *J. Reprod. Fertil.*, 24:142.
2. Calanog, A., Sall, S., Gordon, G. G., Olivo, J., and Southren, A. L. (1976): Testosterone metabolism in endometrial cancer. *Am. J. Obstet. Gynecol.*, 124:60–63.
3. Calanog, A., Sall, S., Gordon, G. G., and Southren, A. L. (1977): Androstenedione metabolism in patients with endometrial cancer. *Am. J. Obstet. Gynecol.*, 129:553–556.
4. Carlström, K., and Sköldefors, H. (1977): Determination of total Oestrone in peripheral serum from non-pregnant humans. *J. Steroid Biochem.*, 8:1127–1128.
5. Edman, C. D., Aimon, E. J., and MacDonald, P. C. (1978): Identification of the estrogen product of extraglandular aromatization of plasma Androstenedione. *Am. J. Obstet. Gynecol.*, 130:439–447.
6. Fishman, J., and Hellman, L. (1973): Comparative fate of Estrone and Estrone sulphate in man. *J. Clin. Endocrinol. Metab.*, 36:160–164.
7. Flamigni, C., Melega, C., Jasonni, V. M., and Bolelli, G. F. (1973): Radioimmunoassay of plasma estrogens. *Riv. Ital. Ginecol.*, 54:291–317.
8. Franz, C., Watson, D., and Longcope, C. (1979): Estrone sulphate and Dehydoepiandrosterone sulphate concentrations in normal subjects and men with cirrhosis. *Steroids*, 34:563–573.
9. Goodall, A. B., and James, V. H. T. (1981): Observations on the nature and origin of conjugated androstenedione in human plasma. *J. Steroid Biochem.*, 14:465–471.
10. Hausnecht, R. V., and Gusberg, S. B. (1973): Estrogen metabolism in patients at high risk for endometrial carcinoma. *Am. J. Obstet. Gynecol.*, 116:981–984.
11. Hawkins, R. A., and Oakey, R. E. (1974): Estimation of Oestrone sulphate, Oestriol-17β and oestrone in peripheral plasma: Concentrations during the menstrual cycle and in man. *J. Endocrinol.*, 60:3–17.
12. Hobkirk, R., Mellor, J. D., and Nielsen, M. (1975): In vitro metabolism of 17β-estradiol by human liver tissue. *Can. J. Biochem.*, 53:903–910.
13. Judd, H. L., Davidson, B. J., Frumar, A. M., Shamoki, I. M., Lagane, L. D., and Ballon, S. C. (1980): Serum androgens and estrogens in post-menopausal women with and without endometrial cancer. *Am. J. Obstet. Gynecol.*, 136:859–871.
14. Longcope, C., and Tait, J. F. (1971): Validity of metabolic clearance and interconversion rates of estrone and 17β-estradiol in normal adults. *J. Clin. Endocrinol. Metab.*, 32:481–490.
15. Longcope, C. (1972): The metabolism of Estrone sulphate in normal males. *J. Clin. Endocrinol. Metab.*, 34:113–122.
16. Loriaux, D. L., Ruder, H. J., and Lipsett, M. B. (1971): The measurement of estrone sulphate in plasma. *Steroids*, 18:463–472.
17. MacDonald, P. C., Edman, C. D., Hemsell, D. L., Porter, J. C., and Siiteri, P. K. (1978): Effect of obesity on conversion of plasma androstenedione to estrone in post-menopausal women with and without endometrial cancer. *Am. J. Obstet. Gynecol.*, 130:448–455.
18. Noel, C. T., Reed, M. J., Jacobs, H. S., and James, V. H. T. (1981): The plasma concentration of oestrone sulphate in post-menopausal women: Lack of diurnal variation, effect of ovariectomy, age and weight. *J. Steroid Biochem.*, 14:1101–1105.
19. Nuñez, M., Aedo, A. R., Landgreen, B. M., Cekon, S. Z., and Diczfalusy, E. (1977): Studies on the pattern of circulating steroids in the normal menstrual cycle. *Acta Endocrinol. (Copenh.)*, 86:621–633.
20. Olivo, J., Vittek, J., Southren, A. L., Gordon, G. G., and Rafii, F. (1973): A rapid method for the measurement of androgen kinetics and conversion to estrogens using Sephadex LH-20 column chromatography. *J. Clin. Endocrinol. Metab.*, 36:153–159.

21. Oertel, G. W., Treiber, L., and Rindt, W. (1967): Direct aromatization of C_{19} steroid sulphates. *Experientia*, 23:91–98.
22. Pack, B. A., Tovar, R., Booth, E., and Brooks, S. C. (1979): The cyclic relationship of estrogen sulphurylation to the nuclear receptor level in human endometrial curettings. *J. Clin. Endocrinol. Metab.*, 48:420–424.
23. Roberts, K. D., Rochefort, J. G., Blean, G., and Chapdelaine, A. (1980): Plasma estrone sulphate levels in post-menopausal women. *Steroids*, 35:179–187.
24. Ruder, H. J., Loriaux, D. L., and Lipsett, M. B. (1972): Estrone sulphate: Production rate and metabolism in man. *J. Clin. Invest.*, 51:1020–1033.
25. Tait, J. F., and Burstein, S. (1964): In: *The Hormones, Vol. 5*, edited by G. Pincus, K. V. Thimann, and E. B. Astwood, p. 441. Academic Press, New York.
26. Tseng, L., Stolee, A., and Gurpide, E. (1972): Quantitative studies on the uptake and metabolism of estrogens and progesterone by human endometrium. *Endocrinology*, 90:390–404.
27. Wright, K., Collins, D. C., Musey, P. I., and Preedy, J. R. K. (1978): A specific radioimmunoassay for estrone sulphate in plasma and urine without hydrolysis. *J. Clin. Endocrinol. Metab.*, 47:1092–1098.

Steroids and Endometrial Cancer,
edited by V. M. Jasonni, et al.
Raven Press, New York © 1983.

In Vivo Influx into Tissue of Circulating Estradiol in Postmenopausal Women with and without Endometrial Cancer

*Howard L. Judd, *Joseph C. Gambone, **William M. Pardridge, and **Leo D. Lagasse

*Divisions of Reproductive Endocrinology and Gynecologic Oncology, Department of Obstetrics and Gynecology; and **Division of Endocrinology and Metabolism, Department of Medicine, University of California, Los Angeles, Los Angeles, California 90024*

Endogenous estrogen metabolism plays a role in the pathogenesis of endometrial cancer. This concept is based on the observations that obese postmenopausal women have increased endogenous estrone (E_1) and estradiol (E_2) production (8,11) and are at greater risk for the development of this tumor (10). Sex hormone binding globulin (SHBG) levels show a negative correlation with body size (1,4). This raises the question as to the role protein binding of circulating E_2 plays in the development of this tumor.

Circulating E_2 is known to exist approximately 2% free (dialyzable) and 98% protein bound (3,21). The protein-bound moiety is distributed between SHBG and albumin (21). There is no consensus as to whether albumin or SHBG bound E_2 are available for transport into tissue (1,2,7,16,19–21).

The question of whether E_2 is transported into peripheral tissues is really an issue of whether it dissociates from the plasma protein within the capillary transit time of an organ, as plasma proteins (e.g., albumin or SBHG) do not leave the capillary space on a single pass through peripheral tissues to any extent (6). Recently, direct measurements of *in vivo* capillary transport of protein-bound steroids have been reported using a model system of estimating the influx of labeled steroid through the rat brain capillary wall, i.e., the blood brain barrier (BBB) (15,16). In the present study, the *in vivo* effects of plasma proteins on the transport of labeled E_2 through the rat BBB were measured using serum taken from postmenopausal patients with and without endometrial cancer.

METHODS AND MATERIALS

Twenty-five postmenopausal women with histologically proven adenocarcinoma of the endometrium and an equal number of control subjects were studied prospectively. All cancer patients had experienced vaginal bleeding and were found to have their tumors by fractional curettage. The cancer patients were amenorrheic for at least 6 months prior to the bleeding, which was associated with their present illness. The control subjects were also amenorrheic for at least 6 months before they were studied. All patients in both groups had elevated gonadotropins and had been off exogenous estrogens for at least 4 weeks before the study. Each control patient was matched to one of the cancer patients for age and percent ideal weight (Table 1). This latter parameter was calculated by dividing the subject's actual weight by her ideal weight and multiplying by 100. Ideal weights were obtained from the Metropolitan Life Company.

Venous blood samples were drawn from the women through an indwelling catheter on two consecutive mornings at 15 min intervals for 1 hr, starting at 8:00 a.m. Serum total E_2 was measured on all samples and the mean concentration of these eight measurements was utilized to represent the hormone level in that patient. For all other parameters, samples were pooled and a measurement was made on the pooled specimen.

Serum total E_2 was measured by a previously published radioimmunoassay procedure (5). The SHBG level was quantitated by a modification of the Rosner method (17), and percent non-SHBG bound E_2 by a modification of the method of Stump et al. (18).

The BBB transport of (^{3}H) E_2 was measured with the carotid injection technique developed by Oldendorf (13,14) and modified by Pardridge et al. (15,16) for assessment of steroids. A common carotid artery was exposed in a barbiturate anesthetized male rat weighing 200 to 300 g (sodium pentobarbital, 45 mg/kg i.p.). An approximately 200-μl bolus (the exact volume is immaterial) of buffered Ringers solution (pH, 7.4, 5mM HEPES, N-hydroxyethyl piperazine-N-2-ethanesulfonic acid) was rapidly (less than 1 sec) injected into the carotid artery via a 27-gauge needle; the injection solution contained 0.82 to 2.5 μCi/ml of the ^{3}H-labeled E_2, 0.2 to 0.5 μCi/ml of the (^{14}C) butanol reference, and was 96% human serum. The dilution of serum to a 96% solution allowed for convenient labeling of the plasma protein. At 15 sec after injection, the rat was decapitated; this circulation period is long enough to allow complete flow of the bolus through the brain, but sufficiently

TABLE 1. *Physical characteristics of (N = 25) postmenopausal women with endometrial cancer and control subjects*[a]

	Cancer	Control	p Value
Age (years)	61 ± 2	59 ± 1	NS
Years since menopause	14 ± 2	9 ± 1	NS
Weight (pounds)	165 ± 10	165 ± 9	NS
Percent ideal weight	127 ± 7	126 ± 7	NS

[a]Mean ± SE; age and weight matched.
NS = not significant.

short to minimize recirculation of isotope or loss of labeled compound from brain due to efflux back to blood (13,14). Subsequent to decapitation, the cerebral hemisphere ipsilateral to the injection and rostral to the midbrain was removed from the cranium and solubilized in duplicate in 1.5 ml of Soluene-350[1]; an aliquot of the injection solution was prepared similarly for double-isotope liquid-scintillation counting. Isotope counts per min were converted to disintegrations per min by standard quench corrections, and the percent brain influx index (BII) was calculated (13).

$$BII = \frac{(^3H/^{14}C)\ brain}{(^3H/^{14}C)\ injection\ mixture} \times 100$$

The BII $= Et/Er$, where $E =$ the percent extraction of unidirectional influx of test *(Et)* and reference *(Er)* isotopes. For butanol, $Er = 90\%$ (15); therefore, the BII overestimates Et by approximately 10%.

Method proofs of this *in vivo* model system for evaluating effects of protein binding of steroids on capillary clearance have been published previously (15,16). Differences between cancer and control subjects and obese and slender cancer patients were analyzed using appropriate paired and group t tests.

RESULTS

Figure 1 shows the mean $\pm$ SE BII of E_2 and the level of the hormone available for brain influx in the serum from the cancer and control subjects. This latter parameter was determined by multiplying the total E_2 level by the BII measured in each woman. The means of BII were 40.7 ± 2.8 and 33.9 ± 2.6 in the cancer and control subjects, respectively, whereas the levels of E_2 available for brain influx were 7 ± 1 pg/ml and 5 ± 1 pg/ml for the same respective subjects. These differences were not statistically significant.

Figure 2 shows the linear correlations of BII of E_2 and the level of E_2 available for brain influx with the percent ideal weight of the cancer and control subjects. Positive correlations of both parameters with percent ideal weight were seen in both groups.

Figure 3 shows the mean total E_2 concentrations and the levels available for brain influx in the five most obese (percent ideal weight 179 ± 13) and the five most slender (percent ideal weight 86 ± 4) patients with endometrial cancer. The total concentrations and the levels available for brain influx were 1.92 and 3.7 times greater in the obese than the slender patients, respectively, and these hormonal differences were highly significant ($p < 0.005$).

Linear regressions of the reciprocal of BII of E_2 and SHBG concentrations were calculated and positive correlations ($r = 0.78$) were observed for the two groups of subjects (Fig. 4). Linear regressions were also calculated for BII of E_2 and percent non-SHBG bound E_2. This latter parameter represents the amount of E_2

---

[1]Packard Instrument Co., Downers Grove, Illinois.

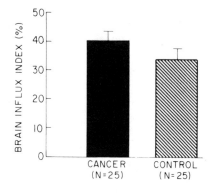

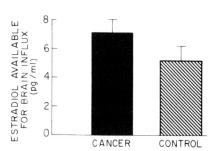

FIG. 1. Mean ± SE values of brain influx index of estradiol and estradiol available for tissue influx observed for 25 postmenopausal women with endometrial cancer and an equal number of control subjects matched to the cancer patients for age and percent ideal weight.

that is free or bound to albumin. Positive correlations were also observed in the cancer ($r = 0.86$) and the control ($r = 0.98$) subjects.

DISCUSSION

In the present study, an *in vivo* assay was employed to evaluate the effect of binding of E_2 by plasma proteins on the transfer of this estrogen across a capillary wall. Support that the BII reflects this was the striking correlations observed between the results of this *in vivo* assay (BII) and the *in vitro* measurements of a serum protein (SHBG) or the amounts of E_2 bound to serum proteins (percent non-SHBG bound E_2). The positive correlations of the reciprocal of the BII and SHBG in the cancer and control subjects were similar to those observed earlier by Pardridge et al. (16) in men and women. The very close correlations of BII with percent non-SHBG bound E_2 in the cancer ($r = 0.86$) and control ($r = 0.98$) subjects were very supportive of this *in vivo* model since both techniques are presumed to measure the same fraction of circulating E_2, i.e., dialyzable and albumin bound hormone (3,15,16).

Based on this *in vivo* assay of transport of E_2 across a capillary wall, the fraction of E_2 in the circulation of postmenopausal women that was available for influx into tissue corresponded to the dialyzable and the albumin bound portions. There was no difference of the BII or the level available for tissue influx of E_2 between the

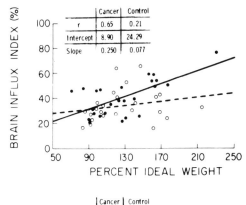

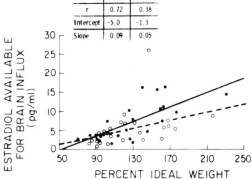

FIG. 2. Correlations of brain influx index of estradiol and estradiol available for tissue influx with percent ideal weight in cancer (——, ●) and control subjects (----, ○) (*N* = 25).

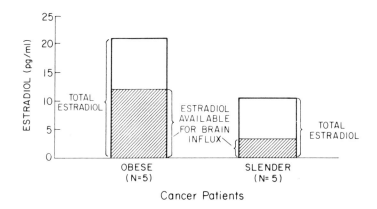

FIG. 3. Mean total E$_2$ concentrations and levels available for tissue influx in the five most obese (mean percent ideal weight 179) and the five most slender (mean percent ideal weight 86) patients with endometrial cancer.

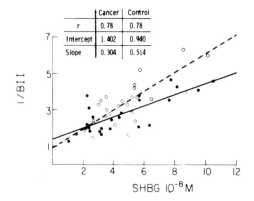

	Cancer	Control
r	0.78	0.78
Intercept	1.402	0.940
Slope	0.304	0.514

I/BII

SHBG IO⁻⁸M

FIG. 4. Correlations of the reciprocal of brain influx index (BII) with sex hormone-binding globulin (SHBG) levels and the BII with percent non-SHBG bound estradiol in both groups of patients.

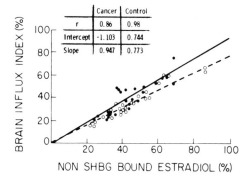

	Cancer	Control
r	0.86	0.98
Intercept	-1.103	0.744
Slope	0.947	0.773

BRAIN INFLUX INDEX (%)

NON SHBG BOUND ESTRADIOL (%)

cancer patients and their age and weight matched controls, suggesting there is no unique difference of transport of circulating E_2 into tissues of women who develop this tumor.

However, the BII and the total level of E_2 showed positive correlations with body size in both groups of subjects. For the BII, the correlation presumably reflected the lower concentrations of SHBG seen in the obese subjects, an observation made previously in both men and women (1,4). The mechanism responsible for lower concentrations of SHBG in obese subjects is unknown, but it is reversible with weight loss (12). The positive correlation of serum levels of total E_2 and body size reflects the enhanced conversion of androstenedione to E_1 that has been observed in obese postmenopausal women (11). Subsequently, a fraction of E_1 is converted to E_2 and accounts for most circulating E_2 in older women (9). The positive correlations of circulating E_1 and E_2 levels reported previously in postmenopausal women support this concept (8,20).

These dual effects of body size on E_2 metabolism are depicted in Fig. 3. In the most obese cancer patients, the mean total concentration of E_2 and the level available for brain influx were 22 pg/ml and 12 pg/ml, respectively, whereas the mean concentrations in the five most slender women were 11 pg/mg and 3 pg/ml for the same respective values. Thus, the obese women, whose mean percent ideal weight was 179, had total E_2 levels that were twofold higher, and levels of E_2 available for brain influx that were nearly fourfold greater than the mean concentrations observed in the slender patients, whose mean percent ideal weight was 86. These data suggest that obese postmenopausal women are at dual risk for the action of E_2 at the tissue level. They have higher total levels and proportionately greater bioavailable E_2 than slender subjects. These data provide further support for the concept that enhanced endogenous estrogen metabolism is the mechanism responsible for the increased risk of endometrial cancer in obese older women.

In the present study, the measurement of BII provided a useful *in vivo* model for the assessment of the influence of plasma proteins on the transport of E_2 across a capillary wall from serum samples drawn from patients with and without endometrial cancer. However, it must be recognized that the capillary bed studied was the BBB of the rat. It is possible that species and organ differences exist and that assessment of transport of E_2 across the rat's BBB may not necessarily reflect transport of the E_2 from the circulation into endometrial cells of human females. Studies are currently underway to assess possible species and organ differences of *in vivo* transport of circulating E_2 into tissues.

ACKNOWLEDGMENTS

This work supported by USPHS Grants Ca23093, RR00865, AM25744, and RCDA-AM-00783.

We would like to thank Ms. M. L. Lu and L. Obnial for their excellent technical assistance and the nursing staff in the Clinical Research Center for their devoted care.

REFERENCES

1. Anderson, D. C. (1974): Sex-hormone-binding globulin. *Clin. Endocrinol.*, 3:69–96.
2. Barton, R. M., and Westphal, U. (1972): Steroid hormone-binding proteins in blood plasma. *Metabolism*, 21:253–276.
3. Davidson, B. J., Gambone, J. C., Lagasse, L. D., Castaldo, T. W., Hammond, G. L., Siiteri, P. K., and Judd, H. L. (1980): Free estradiol in postmenopausal women with and without endometrial cancer. *J. Clin. Endocrinol. Metab.*, 52:404–408.
4. DeMoor, P., and Joossens, J. V. (1970): An inverse relation between body weight and the activity of the steroid binding β-globulin in human plasma. *Steroidologia*, 1:129–136.
5. DeVane, G. W., Czekala, N. M., Judd, H. L., and Yen, S. S. C. (1975): Circulating gonadotropins, estrogens, and androgens in polycystic ovarian disease. *Am. J. Obstet. Gynecol.*, 121:496–500.
6. Dewey, W. C. (1959): Vascular-extravascular exchange of I^{131} plasma proteins in the rat. *Am. J. Physiol.*, 197:423–431.
7. Giorgi, E. P., and Moses, T. F. (1975): Dissociation of testosterone from plasma protein during superfusion of slices from human prostate. *J. Endocrinol.*, 65:279–280.
8. Judd, H. L., Davidson, B. J., Frumar, A. M., Shamonki, I. M., Lagasse, L. D., and Ballon, S. C. (1980): Serum androgens and estrogens in postmenopausal women with and without endometrial cancer. *Am. J. Obstet. Gynecol.*, 136:859–871.
9. Judd, H. L., Shamonki, I. M., Frumar, A. M., and Lagasse, L. D. (1982): Origin of serum estradiol in postmenopausal women. *Obstet. Gynecol.*, 59:680–686.

10. Lucas, W. E. (1974): Causal relationships between endocrine-metabolic variables in patients with endometrial carcinoma. *Obstet. Gynecol. Surv.*, 29:507–528.

11. MacDonald, P. C., Edman, C. D., Hemsell, D. L., Porter, J. C., and Siiteri, P. K. (1978): Effect of obesity on conversion of plasma androstenedione to estrone in postmenopausal women with and without endometrial cancer. *Am. J. Obstet. Gynecol.*, 130:448–455.

12. O'Dea, J. P. K., Wieland, R. G., Hallberg, M. C., Llerena, L. A., Zorn, E. M., and Genuth, S. M. (1979): Effect of dietary weight loss on sex steroid binding, sex steroids, and gonadotropins in obese postmenopausal women. *J. Lab. Clin. Med.*, 93:1004–1009.

13. Oldendorf, W. H. (1970): Measurement of brain uptake of radio-labeled substances using a tritiated water internal standard. *Brain Res.*, 24:372–376.

14. Oldendorf, W. H., and Braun, L. D. (1976): ^{3}H tryptamine and ^{3}H-water as diffusible internal standards for measuring brain extraction of radio-labeled substances following carotid injection. *Brain Res.*, 113:219–223.

15. Pardridge, W. M., and Mietus, L. J. (1979): Transport of steroid hormones through the rat blood-brain barrier: Primary role of albumin-bound hormone. *J. Clin. Invest.*, 64:145–154.

16. Pardridge, W. M., Mietus, L. J., Frumar, A. M., Davidson, B. J., and Judd, H. L. (1980): Effects of human serum on transport of testosterone and estradiol into rat brain. *Am. J. Physiol.*, 239:E103–108.

17. Rosner, W. (1972): A simplified method for the quantitative determination of testosterone-estradiol-binding activity in human plasma. *J. Clin. Endocrinol. Metab.*, 34:983–988.

18. Stumpf, P. G., Nakamura, R. M., and Mishell, D. R. Jr. (1981): Changes in physiologically free circulating estradiol and testosterone during exposure to levonorgestrel. *J. Clin. Endocrinol. Metab.*, 52:138–143.

19. Vermeulen, A., Verdonck, L., Van der Straeten, M., and Orie, N. (1969): Capacity of the testosterone-binding globulin in human plasma and influence of specific binding of testosterone on its metabolic clearance rate. *J. Clin. Endocrinol. Metab.*, 29:1470–1480.

20. Vermeulen, A., and Verdonck, L. (1978): Sex hormone concentrations in postmenopausal women. *Clin. Endocrinol.*, 9:59–73.

21. Vermeulen, A. (1977): Transport and distribution of androgens at different ages. In: *Androgens and Anti-Androgens*, edited by L. Martin and M. Motta, pp. 53–65. Raven Press, New York.

Steroids and Endometrial Cancer,
edited by V. M. Jasonni, et al.
Raven Press, New York © 1983.

Actions and Potencies of Estriol in the Human

H. Kopera

*Institute of Experimental and Clinical Pharmacology, University of Graz,
A-8010 Graz, Austria*

Estriol was discovered in the urine of pregnant women in 1930 by Marrian, and by Doisy and co-workers. Butenandt, Doisy, and Marrian identified the structure. In humans, estriol is one of the metabolic end-products of estradiol; it does not bind to sex hormone binding globulin (SHBG), undergoes no metabolic changes other than conjugation, and is more rapidly eliminated than estradiol. Estriol levels are high in the menstrual cycle and increase progressively during pregnancy up to 12 to 40 mg/day before term. In pregnancy, most of the estriol is formed in the placenta by conversion of dehydro-epiandrosterone sulfate from the fetal adrenal.

PHARMACOLOGY

Estriol has been labeled as "impeded estrogen" (18); however, its behavior is "impeded" only with respect to particular target tissues and in dependence on the animal species and the experimental conditions. It antagonizes some estradiol effects. Estriol is bound to the nuclear receptor for such a short time that it does not cause full biologic response when administered in usual doses and form. Hence, estriol must be regarded as a short acting estrogen (3,8). In many pharmacological tests, estriol is weaker than other estrogens; nevertheless, it cannot be classified as a weak estrogen because of the competition between estradiol and estriol receptor complexes for nuclear retention sites, the short receptor binding, the importance of the form of administration, and the fact that several actions of estrogens show considerable variations of estrogenic effects in different tests.

In 1957, Puck et al. (40) demonstrated the clinical efficacy of estriol in the human and postulated a rather selective activity on the lower genital tract. This claim of a preferential effect of estriol on certain target organs is supported by the recent finding of a protein in the human vagina that binds estriol selectively (3).

Many questions concerning the various actions of estrogens (24) are insufficiently explored, and lack of data often prevents even speculations on the role played by an individual estrogen. Furthermore, most data on estriol originate from animal experiments and are of limited value for the human, particularly because this steroid is natural for man but less so for laboratory animals.

EFFECTS ON THE BRAIN

In rodents, estrogens exert profound effects on the brain thought to be present also in the human, as suggested by pathological situations and by estrogen therapy (25). However, nothing can be said as yet about relative potencies and involvement of the individual estrogens.

EFFECTS ON THE ENDOCRINE SYSTEM

Gonadotropins and prolactin are the only pituitary hormones that can be influenced by estrogens. Estriol seems to be a weak gonadotropin inhibitor; it suppresses gonadotropins only in the nonconjugated form, particularly after vaginal application (19,20,31,33,35,50). Serum prolactin values and thyrotropin-releasing factor (TRH)-stimulated prolactin either are elevated slightly or remain unchanged after estriol (19,20,33).

Whereas other estrogens induce significant elevations of serum concentrations of estrone and estradiol, oral and vaginal estriol administration is followed by a significant rise only of the serum estriol level (11,12,16,19,20,35,43). Higher concentrations of estrogens increase the thyroxine-binding capacity of serum through elevation of thyroxine-binding globulin (TBG). Estriol seems to lack this effect on thyroid hormone economy. The effects of estrogens on other endocrine glands, including parathyroid, thymus, adrenals, and the pancreas, are minimal.

EFFECTS ON BONE

Development, shaping, and growth of the skeleton, as well as maintenance of bone tissue, are significantly influenced by estrogenic hormones, which are responsible for the female bodily habit. Estrogen deficiency causes excessive growth in young girls and osteoporosis in adults. Consequently, estrogens are used for substitution therapy. The recommended doses for the treatment of excessively tall girls vary according to the estrogen administered. Estriol and conjugated estrogens require the highest dosage.

It should be undisputed that postmenopausal osteoporosis is causally related to estrogen deficiency; therefore, estrogens are used extensively for prophylaxis and treatment of this condition (15). Whether all estrogenic preparations are equally suitable still must be clarified. Present experience is insufficient to allow separation of qualitative from quantitative differences of the various estrogens with respect to their inhibitory effect on bone resorption (7,24), although there are indications that estriol might be less effective than other estrogens (34).

EFFECTS ON FATTY TISSUE AND SKIN

Estrogens influence the distribution of fatty tissue and thus the molding of the body contours. They are responsible for the growth of axillary and pubic hair; they affect hair follicles and the elasticity and color of hair; they improve the skin circulation, cause extracellular water retention, stimulate hyaluronidase, reduce sebum production, and promote skin pigment formation in certain areas. The concentration of estrogen receptors in the skin of castrated women can be raised (41), and reduced mitosis in the skin and epidermal atrophy following estrogen deprivation in postmenopausal women can be prevented by estriol dihemisuccinate (45).

EFFECTS ON BLOOD VESSELS, CIRCULATION, AND BLOOD

Increased fragility and permeability of small vessels and capillaries is reduced by estriol dihemisuccinate in animals (5) and in therapeutic practice (39). The steroid acts on the basal membrane of the vessel wall and on the mucopolysaccharides of the ground substance of the perivascular connective tissue (51). Larger vessels seem to dilate under estrogens, but comparisons with different estrogenic compounds have not been performed.

Estrogens exert a protective mechanism for the regulation of the systolic blood pressure and its reaction to artificial stress (10). This is in accordance with the increase of the mean blood pressure in estrogen-deprived women after menopause.

Some estrogens enhance thrombocyte aggregation and can affect fibrinolysis and coagulation factors causing changes which might result in untoward clinical effects. Estriol succinate seems to be without clinically relevant influence on haemostatic function (2,9,56,57).

EFFECTS ON WATER AND ELECTROLYTE BALANCE AND ON METABOLISM

Retention of water and sodium chloride caused by estrogens can be of clinical relevance in patients with heart or kidney diseases. A difference between the various estrogens has not been demonstrated.

Estrone, estradiol, and the artificial nonsteroidal estrogens exert some protein anabolic effect. They increase transport proteins resulting in elevation of globulin-bound hormones such as corticosteroids and thyroxine. Estrogens possibly lower blood cholesterol and the β/α-lipoprotein quotient, they increase triglycerides and high-density lipoprotein (HDL)-cholesterol (26).

Estriol was found to have no protein-inducing effect and lacks an influence on hormone-binding globulins such as TBG, SHBG, and corticosteroid-binding globulin (CBG) (4,20,35,52). Likewise, estriol produces few of the estrogenic effects on fat metabolism. It is reported to counteract untoward changes of fat metabolism in estrogen deficiency states (42,47).

Some differences of the effects of estriol as compared to those of other estrogens on mixed function monooxydase activities have been demonstrated in animal tissues (1). In contradistinction to the other natural estrogens estriol does not stimulate the enzyme isocitrate dehydrogenase in the placenta, which is important for the metabolism of estrogens; it even inhibits the respective stimulatory effect of estrone and estradiol (27).

EFFECTS ON THE GASTROINTESTINAL AND URINARY TRACT

Whereas few data indicate an influence of estrogens on gastric secretion or mucus production, these hormones are of great importance for the normal functioning of the urinary tract. Hormone deficiency as seen after the menopause is thought responsible for changes resulting in complex bladder symptoms (stress and urge incontinence, nycturia, dysuria, and frequency), ectropion, atrophy, and infections. Surgery and hormonal substitution with estrogens such as estriol are very beneficial (22,46,49,55).

EFFECTS ON THE REPRODUCTIVE ORGANS

The influences of estrogens on the reproductive system have been studied extensively. However, incomparability of the trials makes it inappropriate to calculate accurately the relative estrogenic potencies of the various preparations, although some conclusions concerning quantitative and a few with regard to qualitative differences can be drawn with fair approximation.

Fallopian Tube and Mammary Gland

The available data are insufficient to differentiate between the estrogenic substances with respect to their effects on the fallopian tube (increased motility) and the mammary gland (stimulation via the pituitary and suppression through direct effect).

Ovary

Direct effects, such as increasing the sensitivity to gonadotropins or supporting survival of the corpus luteum, as found in animals, are of hardly any importance in the human. However, inhibition of growth of the follicles and of ovulation—indirect estrogenic effects through suppression of follicle-stimulating hormone (FSH) release—is very pronounced in man. Measurement of the antiovulatory activity revealed impressive differences in potency, ethinylestradiol being about 100 times more potent than estradiol and presumably even much more so than estriol (36).

Uterus

Despite considerable variations between the results of the various trials with estrogens fairly reproducible orders of potency can be assumed, and perhaps some qualitative differences might be deduced as well.

Estrogens increase the blood supply and stimulate the growth of the myometrium. With the uterine weight as measurement of the potency of estrogens, estriol, given in the same manner as other estrogens, is usually the least potent substance.

The proliferative effect of estriol on the endometrium is by far the weakest of all estrogens; even excessive doses fail to produce regular proliferation and a normal withdrawal bleeding (28) (Table 1). Such differences are of clinical relevance when uterine bleeding is taken into account. Strong endometriotropic estrogens will be

TABLE 1. *Endometrial threshold and proliferation doses of commonly used oral estrogens*

Estrogen	Threshold dose (mg/14 days)	Full proliferation dose (mg/14 days)
Ethinylestradiol	0.2	2
Mestranol	0.3	3
Quinestrol	0.3	2–4
Diethylstilbestrol	2.5	20–30
Dienestroldiacetate	3–5	40–60
Estradiolvalerianate	6–10	60
Conjugated estrogens	5–12	60
Estriol	20[a]	120–150[b]

[a]Very variable; sometimes even higher.
[b]Irregular, atypical proliferation, mostly in the basal layer. Weak withdrawal effect.
(From ref. 28).

preferable whenever shedding is desirable. However, if endometrial proliferation followed by withdrawal or breakthrough bleeding must be avoided, estrogens with a weak proliferative effect will be the drug of choice. Estriol given in the recommended dosage schemes is not likely to cause appreciable endometrial proliferation (12); in fact, it was found to have such a weak effect on the endometrium that it can only be detected by electron microscopy (11,38). High doses of estriol produce some endometrial proliferation that rarely results in uterine bleeding, a phenomenon that cannot be explained satisfactorily (17).

In contrast to the lack of a strong effect on the corpus uteri, estriol in the usual dosage is very effective on the cervix uteri, vagina, and vulva when administered orally, parenterally, and particularly when applied locally (14,20,29,35,44,59). Similarly, there are no differences in therapeutic efficacy of estriol to other estrogens in most climacteric complaints and postmenopausal disturbances, provided these are not excessive (23,28,30,37,58).

EFFECTS ON MALIGNANT TUMORS

Animal experiments indicate that estriol differs from other estrogens not only by lacking cocarcinogenicity but also by acting as an anticarcinogen. This was demonstrated in rats with chemically induced mammary carcinoma (32,54). Obviously, such findings and similar observations in the human (6,53) appear to be of particular importance, more so as the presently heavily discussed cocarcinogenic effects of other natural and artificial estrogens cannot be refuted completely. So far, estriol therapy has indicated little hazard of cancer development (13,30,48). Indeed, estriol is less likely than estrone and estradiol to induce proliferative changes in target organs of cancer-prone women because it undergoes minimal metabolism, does not bind to SHBG and, under certain circumstances, has an antiestradiol action at the receptor site (21,32). Clearly, a major breakthrough in the medical use of estrogens would occur if anticancer properties of estriol found in animals could be confirmed for humans.

CONCLUSIONS

The available experimental and clinical data suggest that some of the qualities of estriol may be regarded as disadvantages in comparison to estrone and estradiol (Table 2). However, estriol has an appreciable number of other properties and features resembling advantages above estrone and estradiol that can outweigh such possible disadvantages (Table 3). The sum of the quantitative and probable qualitative pharmacological differences of estriol adds up to make it an estrogen distinguishable from other natural and artificial estrogens. This is reflected in the most relevant clinical effects of commonly used estrogenic substances (Table 4).

It also indicates that the therapeutic use of estriol preparations is particularly recommendable for: (a) the treatment of disorders of the lower genital tract; (b) prolonged treatment of conditions such as climacteric and postclimacteric complaints and disturbances; (c) subjects in whom central, endometriotropic, or metabolic effects of estrogens should be avoided; and (d) subjects with relative contraindications for estrogens.

TABLE 2. *Disadvantages of estriol vs. estrone and estradiol*

Weaker effect on
    Severe menopausal complaints
    Psychic postmenopausal complaints
    Calcium loss (?)
Weaker inhibitory effect on
    Gonadotropins
    Ovulation
No stabilizing effect on cycle

TABLE 3. *Advantages of estriol over estrone and estradiol*

Application
    Oral, vulvo-vaginal and parenteral
Good effect on
    Cervix, vagina, vulva, urinary bladder, urethra, epidermis
Weak effect on endometrium
    No hyperproliferation
    Continuous use acceptable
    No cocarcinogenicity
Less/no untoward effects on
    Hormone-binding globulins, liver enzymes, coagulation, carbohydrate
    metabolism, blood pressure, weight
Weak antigonadotropic effect

TABLE 4. Clinical differences between the actions of commonly used estrogens

Estrogenic substances	Effects				Side effects of long-term use	
	Endometrial	Lower genital tract	Climacteric changes	Cocarcinogenicity[a]	Uterine bleeding	Others
Stilbenes	+ + +	+ + +	+ + +[b]	+	+ +	+ +
Ethinylestradiol (ethers)	+ + +	+ + +	+ + +	+	+ +	+ +
Estradiol esters	+ +	+ +	+ + +	(+)	+ +	(+)
Conjugated estrogens	+	+ +	+ +	+	+	(+)
Estriol	(+)	+ +	+ +	–	–	–
Esters/ethers	(+)	+ +	+ +	–	–	–

[a]Subject still controversial.
[b]No psychotropic effect (after 24).
(From ref. 24.)

SUMMARY

Knowledge of many actions of the natural human estrogen estriol and their relative potencies compared to those of other estrogens, is still incomplete. However, there is abundant evidence that estriol is biologically active and distinguishable from estrone and estradiol by quantitative and perhaps qualitative differences in the pharmacological profile.

Estriol is not bound to SHBG, hardly metabolized, to a certain extent an impeded estrogen, and can be antiestrogenic. Estriol binds to the nuclear estrogen receptor sites for too short a time to cause full biologic response when given in the usual dosage scheme, which makes it a short-acting estrogen. Estriol is a weak inhibitor of gonadotropins and of ovulation. It hardly stabilizes the cycle and may be less potent than other estrogens for the treatment of severe menopausal complaints, postmenopausal psychic disturbances, and postmenopausal calcium loss. On the other hand, estriol has some significant advantages above estradiol and estrone: excellent activity after oral administration and vulvo-vaginal application; good effect on cervix, vagina, vulva, urinary bladder, urethra, and epidermis; weak endometriotropic effect with no shedding-producing hyperproliferation upon continuous use; no evidence of cocarcinogenicity; less or no untoward effects on hormone-binding globulins, liver enzymes, coagulation factors, carbohydrate metabolism, blood pressure, and body weight. Thus estriol has a specific pharmacological profile determining its use in therapeutic practice.

REFERENCES

1. Al Turk, W. A., Stohs, S. J., and Roche, E. B. (1980): Effect of acute and chronic estrone, estradiol, and estriol treatment on hepatic, pulmonary, and intestinal mixed-function mono-oxygenase activities in female rats. *Drug Metab. Dispos.*, 8:143–146.

2. Bennett, N. B., Bennett, P. N., Fullerton, H. W., Ogston, C. M., and Ogston, D. (1966): Effect of oestriol on platelet adhesiveness and fibrinolysis in men. *Lancet*, 2:881–882.
3. Bergink, E. W. (1981): Estriol and estrogen receptor in the different target tissues. In: *Proceedings of the 1st Int. Symposium on Steroids and Endometrial Cancer*, Bologna. *(this volume)*
4. Bernutz, C. (1979): Isolation, characterization and radioimmunoassay of corticosteroid-binding globulin (CBG) in human serum—clinical significance and comparison to thyroxine-binding globulin (TBG). *Acta Endocrinol.*, 92:370–384.
5. Bonta, I. L., and de Vos, C. J. (1965): The effect of estriol-16,17-dihemisuccinate on vascular permeability as evaluated in the rat paw oedema test. *Acta Endocrinol.*, 49:403–411.
6. Bulbrook, R. D., Swain, M. C., Wang, D. Y., Hayward, J. L., Kumaoka, S., Takatani, O., Abe, O., and Utsunomiya, J. (1976): Breast cancer in Britain and Japan: Plasma oestradiol-17β, oestrone and progesterone, and their urinary metabolites in normal British and Japanese women. *Eur. J. Cancer*, 12:725–735.
7. Christiansen, C., Christensen, M. S., and Transbøl, I. (1981): Bone mass in postmenopausal women after withdrawal of oestrogen/gestagen replacement therapy. *Lancet*, 1:459–461.
8. Clark, J. H., and Peck, E. J., Jr. (1979): Female sex steroids. Receptors and function. In: *Monogr. Endocrinol. Vol. 14*, edited by F. Gross, M. M. Grumbach, A. Labhart, M. B. Lipsett, T. Mann, L. T. Samuels, and J. Zander. Springer-Verlag, Berlin, Heidelberg, New York.
9. Davies, T., Fieldhouse, G., and McNicol, G. P. (1976): The effects of therapy with oestriol succinate and ethinyl oestradiol on the haemostatic mechanism in post-menopausal women. *Thromb. Haemost.*, 35:403–414.
10. Eiff, A. W., von (1975): Blood pressure and estrogens. In: *Estrogens in the post-menopause. Front. Hormone Res. Vol. 3*, edited by P. A. van Keep and C. Lauritzen, pp. 177–184. Karger, Basel.
11. Englund, D., Axelsson, O., and Nilsson, O. (1980): An electron microscopic study on the stimulatory effect of estriol on the endometrium. *Acta Obstet. Gynecol. Scand. [Suppl.]*, 93:62.
12. Englund, D. E., and Johansson, E. D. B. (1979): A pharmacokinetic study on oestriol. Endometrial effect of oestriol treatment in postmenopausal women. *Acta Endocrinol. (Suppl.)*, 225:109.
13. Follingstad, A. H. (1978): Estriol, the forgotten estrogen? *J. Amer. Med. Assn.*, 239:29–30.
14. Gitsch, E., and Golob, E. (1962): Zur Frage der idealen Östriolkonzentration in Salben bei genitaler Anwendung. *Zentralbl. Gynäkol.*, 12:454–458.
15. Gordan, G. S. (1980): Estrogens, osteoporosis, cancer and public policy. *J. Med.*, 11:203–222.
16. Greenblatt, R. B., Natrajan, P. K., Aksu, M. F., and Tzingounis, V. A. (1979): The fate of a large bolus of exogenous estrogen administered to postmenopausal women. *Maturitas*, 2:29–35.
17. Heuser, H. P., and Staemmler, H.-J. (1973): Histological investigations into the effect of oestriol succinate on the corpus uteri in postmenopausal women. *Arzneim.-Forsch.*, 23:558–562.
18. Huggins, C., and Jensen, E. V. (1955): The depression of estrone-induced uterine growth by phenolic estrogens with oxygenated functions at positions 6 or 16; the impeded estrogens. *J. Exp. Med.*, 102:335–346.
19. Keller, P. J., Riedmann, R., Fischer, M., and Gerber, C. (1981): Oestrogens, gonadotropins, and prolactin after intra-vaginal administration of oestriol in post-menopausal women. *Maturitas*, 3:47–53.
20. Kicovic, P. M., Cortes-Prieto, J., Milojevic, S., Haspels, A. A., and Aljinovic, A. (1980): The treatment of postmenopausal vaginal atrophy with ovestin vaginal cream or suppositories: clinical, endocrinological and safety aspects. *Maturitas*, 2:275–282.
21. Klopper, A. (1980): The risk of endometrial carcinoma from oestrogen therapy of the menopause. *Acta Endocrin. (Suppl.)*, 233:29–35.
22. Kopera, H. (1979): Effects, side-effects and dosage schemes of various sex hormones in the peri- and post-menopause. In: *Female and Male Climacteric. Current Opinion 1978*, edited by P. A. van Keep, D. M. Serr, and R. B. Greenblatt, pp. 43–67. MTP Press, Lancaster.
23. Kopera, H. (1980): Die Pharmakotherapie klimakterischer Veränderungen. *Pharmakotherapie*, 3:24–34.
24. Kopera, H. (1980): The actions and relative potencies of oestrogens. *Pharmatherapeutica, (Suppl.)*, 2:16–28.
25. Kopera, H. (1980): Female hormones and brain function. In: *Hormones and the Brain*, edited by D. de Wied and P. A. van Keep, pp. 189–203. MTP Press, Lancaster.
26. Lagrelius, A., Johnson, P., Lunell, N.-O., and Samsioe, G. (1981): Treatment with oral estrone

sulphate in the female climacteric. I. Influence on lipids. *Acta Obstet. Gynecol. Scand.*, 60:27–31.

27. Lauritzen, C. (1973): *Östrogene in Theorie und Praxis.* Klinge GmbH & Co. München.
28. Lauritzen, C. (1973): The management of the pre-menopausal and the post-menopausal patient. In: *Ageing and Estrogens. Front. Hormone Res. Vol. 2*, edited by P. A. van Keep, and C. Lauritzen, pp. 2–21. Karger, Basel.
29. Lauritzen, C. (1979): Erfahrungen mit einer Östriol-Vaginalcreme. *Ther. Ggw.*, 118:567–577.
30. Lauritzen, C., and van Keep, P. A., editors (1978): *Estrogen Therapy. The Benefits and Risks. Front. Hormone Res. Vol. 5*, Karger, Basel.
31. Leis, D., and Braun, S. (1981): The effect of oral estrogen therapy on serum FSH and LH levels in young women with hypergonadotrophic ovarian failure. *Arch. Gynecol.*, 230:225–230.
32. Lemon, H. M. (1980): Pathophysiologic considerations in the treatment of menopausal patients with oestrogens; the role of oestriol in the prevention of mammary carcinoma. *Acta Endocrinol. (Suppl.)*, 233:17–27.
33. L'Hermite, M., Badawi, M. M., Michaux Duchene, A., and Robyn, C. (1979): Unaltered basal prolactin secretion during short-term oestriol treatment in post-menopausal women. *Clin. Endocrinol.*, 11:173–177.
34. Lindsay, R., Hart, D. M., MacLean, A., Garwood, J., Clark, A. C., and Kraszewski, A. (1979): Bone loss during oestriol therapy in postmenopausal women. *Maturitas*, 1:279–285.
35. Luisi, M., Franchi, F., and Kicovic, P. M. (1980): A group–comparative study of effects of ovestin cream versus premarin cream in post-menopausal women with vaginal atrophy. *Maturitas*, 2:311–319.
36. Martinez-Manautou, J. (1966): Antiovulatory activity of several synthetic and natural estrogens. In: *Ovulation*, edited by R. B. Greenblatt. Lippincott, Philadelphia.
37. Martius, G., and Horchler, H.-H. (1975): Experimentelle Darstellung der Wirkung von Östriol im Klimakterium. *Geburtshilfe Frauenheilkd.*, 35:938–943.
38. Nilsson, B. O., Knoth, M., and Nathan, E. (1980): Scanning electron microscopy of the responses of postmenopausal endometrium to treatment with estriol and estriol-progesterone. *Upsala J. Med. Sci.*, 85:1–6.
39. Pierer, H. (1966): Hämostyptischer Effekt von per os verabreichtem Östriolsukzinat. *Med. Klin.*, 61:1293–1296.
40. Puck, A., Korte, W., and Hübner, K. A. (1957): Die Wirkung des Oestriol auf Corpus uteri, Cervix uteri und Vagina der Frau. *Dtsch. Med. Wschr.*, 82:1864–1866.
41. Punnonen, R., Loevgren, T., and Kouvonen, I. (1980): Demonstration of estrogen receptors in the skin. *J. Endocrinol. Invest.*, 3:217–221.
42. Punnonen, R., and Rauramo, L. (1976): Effect of castration and long-term oral oestrogen therapy with oestriol succinate on serum lipids. *Ann. Chir. Gynaecol.*, 65:216–219.
43. Punnonen, R., Vilska, S., Grönroos, M., and Rauramo, L. (1980): The vaginal absorption of oestrogens in postmenopausal women. *Maturitas*, 2:321–326.
44. Quinn, M. A., Murphy, A. J., Kuhn, R. J. P., Robinson, H. P., and Brown, J. B. (1981): A double blind trial of extraamniotic oestriol and prostaglandin $F_{2\alpha}$ gels in cervical ripening. *Br. J. Obstet. Gynaecol.*, 88:644–649.
45. Rauramo, L., and Punnonen, R. (1973): The effect of castration and peroral estrogen therapy on a woman's skin. In: *Ageing and Estrogens. Front. Hormone Res. Vol. 2*, edited by P. A. van Keep and C. Lauritzen, pp. 48–54. Karger, Basel.
46. Richards, C. (1981): The assessment of the effect of Synapause in complex bladder symptoms at the menopause. *3rd International Congress on the Menopause*, Ostend, June 9–12.
47. Saarikoski, S., Niemela, A., Jokela, H., and Pystynen, P. (1980): Effect of estriol succinate on serum lipids. *Acta Obstet. Gynecol. Scand., (Suppl.)*, 93:60.
48. Salmi, T. (1980): Endometrial carcinoma risk factors, with special reference to the use of oestrogens. *Acta Endocrinol., (Suppl.)*, 233:37–43.
49. Samsioe, G., Jansson, I., Mellström, D., and Svanborg, A. (1981): Urinary incontinence in 70–75 year-old women, prevalence and effects of oestriol-treatment. *3rd Intern. Congr. on the Menopause*, Ostend, 9–12 June.
50. Schiff, I., Tulchinsky, D., Ryan, K. J., Kadner, S., and Levitz, M. (1980): Plasma estriol and its conjugates following oral and vaginal administration of estriol to postmenopausal women: correlations with gonadotropin levels. *Am. J. Obstet. Gynecol.*, 138:1137–1141.

51. Schmidt-Matthiesen, H., and Poliwoda, H. (1965): Östrogene, Gefäße und hämorrhagische Dia-
    thesen. *Arch. Gynäkol.*, 200:231–258.
52. Schoultz, B. von, Carlstrom, K., Damber, M. G., Helgasson, S., and Stigbrand, T. (1980):
    Estrogenic potency assayed by protein induction. *Acta Obstet. Gynecol. Scand.*, Suppl. 93, 59–
    60.
53. Speroff, L. (1977): The breast as an endocrine target organ. *Contemp. Obstet. Gynecol.*, 9:69–
    72.
54. Teller, M. N., Stock, C. C., Bowie, M., and McMahon, S. (1979): Resorcyclic acid lactones:
    new compounds active against DMBA-induced rat mammary carcinomas. *Proc. Am. Assoc. Cancer
    Res.*, 20:81.
55. Thueroff, J. W., Frohneberg, D., Petri, E., and Jonas, U. (1981): Therapie bei Reizblase und
    Harninkontinenz. *Dtsch. Med. Wschr.*, 106:215–217.
56. Toy, J. L., Davies, J. A., Hancock, K. W., and McNicol, G. P. (1978): The comparative effects
    of a synthetic and a "natural" oestrogen on the haemostatic mechanism in patients with primary
    amenorrhoea. *Br. J. Obstet. Gynaecol.*, 85:359–362.
57. Toy, J. L., Davies, J. A., and McNicol, G. P. (1978): The effects of long-term therapy with
    oestriol succinate on the haemostatic mechanism in postmenopausal women. *Br. J. Obstet. Gyn-
    aecol.*, 85:363–366.
58. Utian, W. H. (1980): The place of oestriol therapy after menopause. *Acta Endocrinol., (Suppl.)*,
    233:45–50.
59. Vikhljaeva, E., and Tscherevischnik, G. (1979): Oestriol und seine Anwendung in der gynäko-
    logischen Klinik. *Zentralbl. Gynäkol.*, 101:1133–1138.

Steroids and Endometrial Cancer,
edited by V. M. Jasonni, et al.
Raven Press, New York © 1983.

Use of the Progestogen Challenge Test to Detect Endometrial Proliferation in Postmenopausal Women

Carlo Campagnoli, Paola Belforte, Graziella Martoglio,
Alessandra Sandzi, Luisa Belforte, and Luisa Prelato Tousijn

*Department of Gynecological Endocrinology, St. Anna's Gynecological Hospital,
10126 Turin, Italy*

Postmenopausal bleedings frequently are related to endometrial cancer or its precursors (8,19). Therefore, every postmenopausal bleeding requires immediate and thorough evaluation. In skilled hands, an office biopsy can be an appropriate initial diagnostic procedure (8,19). However, fractional dilation and curettage is generally indicated (33).

Immediate investigation is required even if bleeding (particularly an unscheduled breakthrough bleeding) occurs during estrogen replacement therapy (8,33). Bleedings are especially frequent when estrogen preparations with strong endometriotrophic activity are used, e.g., conjugated equine estrogens (3,8,17,25). Actually, functional bleedings occur more easily when a proliferative effect on the endometrium is present (8,24). Anyway, a careful histopathological evaluation is essential either to remove the fear of cancer or to detect the frequent cases of endometrial hyperplasia (3,8,25), possible cancer precursors (11). A particular concern of this point for both patient and doctor is caused by the data showing an increased risk of malignancy in the menopausal women exposed to highly endometriotrophic exogenous estrogens (13,28,30,38). The anxiety caused by bleeding and urgent diagnostic surgery is usually high so that the patient is often ill-disposed toward carrying on replacement therapy (18). Furthermore, dilation and curettage involve a certain risk and high costs (36). So it is highly desirable to minimize the incidence of the unscheduled breakthrough bleedings.

When there is a proliferative endometrium as a consequence of estrogen activity, a progestogen treatment induces withdrawal bleeding (8,31). Actually, a progestogen withdrawal bleeding is considered a good index of endometrial proliferation (7,31) and estrogen activity (14,21). Thus the administration of progestogen is widely used in the endocrino–gynecological field for diagnostic purposes (so called "progestogen challenge test").

The unscheduled bleedings are far less frequent when the progestogen is sequentially added to highly endometriotrophic exogenous estrogens (17,37). In the

Gambrell's series, for instance, an irregular bleeding occurred in 21% of the women treated with conjugated equine estrogens alone; conversely, only 0.9% of the estrogen-progestogen users had irregular bleedings, whereas in 97% a regular withdrawal bleeding occurred (17). A progestogen induced bleeding generally occurs in association with a normal endometrium, even in the presence of a high estrogen activity (4,25). However, this does not eliminate the need of direct evaluations on the endometrium (4) that can be performed with scheduled office biopsies.

We present here data on the use of the progestogen test to detect endometrial proliferation in postmenopausal women without any treatment or treated with different estrogen preparations. In addition, the benefits and problems of cyclic progestogen treatment in women with endometriotrophic activity, either of endogenous or of exogenous origin, are discussed; and the usefulness of the progestogen test to better define the suitability of direct histopathological evaluations of the endometrium is pointed out.

PROGESTOGEN CHALLENGE TEST IN SUBJECTS WITH MENOPAUSAL AMENORRHEA

Endometrial proliferation in women in menopausal amenorrhea may be present independently of estrogen administration as a consequence of persisting endogenous estrogen activity. To detect endometrial proliferation, a progestogen challenge test was carried out in 55 women visiting the Menopause Unit of our hospital because of climacteric complaints. All had had their last menstrual period at least 6 months earlier (range: 6–120 months) and had not taken any hormonal medication since then. All of them had high gonadotropin values. These women were treated with medroxyprogesterone acetate (MPA) 10 mg daily for 10 days, a dose sufficient to achieve full secretory transformation and a complete shedding of the endometrium upon withdrawal. Of 55 women, 21 (38.2%) had a MPA induced bleeding (positive progestogen test), suggesting endometrial proliferation due to endogenous estrogen activity. Table 1 compares the main characteristics of these 21 women with those of the remaining 34 patients without MPA induced bleeding (negative progestogen test). The women with a positive progestogen test were rather younger and had a shorter menopausal amenorrhea; yet, these differences are not significant. These positive progestogen test women differed significantly from patients with a negative progestogen test for lower follicle stimulating hormone (FSH) levels and for less severe climacteric complaints; of these latter, we considered only the most specific ones, namely hot flushes and perspiration (2,15), assessing the severity by means of the Blatt's Menopausal Index scoring system (15). The difference is highly significant regarding the "degree of obesity" (difference in kg between the real and the ideal weight) (35): the women with a positive progestogen test had a degree of obesity higher than the negative ones.

An endometrial proliferation may take place in women in the earlier postmenopausal period, for a residual estrogen production by the ovary (34); or in overweight women, for a higher estrogen activity due to extraglandular production of estrone

TABLE 1. *Comparison of patients in menopausal amenorrhea with or without progestogen-induced bleeding*

| | Age (years) | Months of amenorrhea | Blood pressure | | FSH mIU/ml | LH mIU/ml | Score of main climacteric complaints[a] | Degree of obesity in Kg |
			Systolic mm Hg	Diastolic mm Hg				
Patients with progestogen-induced bleeding (N = 21) (28.2%)	49.5 ± 5.0	22.5 ± 31.2	144.1 ± 17.6	89.7 ± 10.9	41.2 ± 13.3[b]	27.0 ± 15.8	9.9 ± 4.6[c]	10.3 ± 4.9[d]
Patients without progestogen-induced bleeding (N = 34) (61.8%)	51.6 ± 3.6	26.9 ± 22.4	139.8 ± 13.8	89.3 ± 9.2	53.6 ± 17.9[b]	35.2 ± 11.8	14.8 ± 5.7[c]	4.6 ± 5.4[d]

[a]Severity was assessed by using the following scores. Hot flushes: absent = 0, slight = 4, moderate = 8, severe = 12; perspiration: absent = 0, slight = 2, moderate = 4, severe = 6.
[b]$p < 0.05$.
[c]$p < 0.01$.
[d]$p < 0.001$.
Mean ± SD.

(16,34) and to a higher concentration of free estradiol (23). Actually, in our series (Fig. 1) a positive progestogen challenge test, although more frequent in overweight women, also occurred in subjects with a low degree of obesity in the earlier post-menopausal period. Conversely, in the later postmenopausal period, a positive test occurred only in women with a higher "obesity degree." Among these, there was a 57-year-old women with a menopausal amenorrhea lasting 10 years who had been complaining for years of rather severe climacteric complaints (score = 14). On the other hand, a 54-year-old-subject in menopausal amenorrhea for 2 years with degree of obesity of +20 kg and complaining of slight climacteric symptoms (score = 4) did not respond to the progestogen challenge test. Therefore, the presence or absence of endometrial proliferation is difficult to foresee on the basis of individual char-

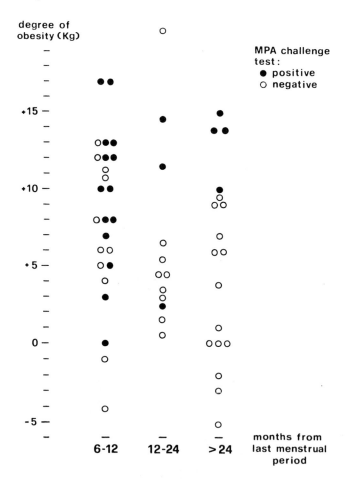

FIG. 1. Positive or negative response to medroxyprogesterone acetate (MPA) in women with menopausal amenorrhea, according to the degree of obesity and to the length of amenorrhea.

acteristics (body weight, length of amenorrhea, severity of climacteric complaints, etc.), possibly because there is an individual endometrial responsiveness to hormonal stimulation. So a simple clinical test such as the progestogen challenge test may be useful in the detection of those women in menopausal amenorrhea who are still having an endometrial proliferation.

In subjects with a shorter menopausal amenorrhea, the hypoestrogenic condition (and the consequent rise of plasmatic gonadotropins) can be in the beginning temporary because a renewal of follicular growth may take place with estrogen production (and a return to normalcy of gonadotropin levels) (1). In these circumstances, there may be a renewal of endometrial proliferation, and a previously negative progestogen challenge test may become positive (Fig. 2). Such a possibility should be considered when evaluating the effects of estrogen treatments. For instance, the progestogen challenge test becoming positive in the case shown in Fig. 3 might be related to a renewal of endogenous estrogen production rather than to the estriol therapy. Actually, estriol, especially if given in a single daily dose, has no significant proliferative effect on the endometrium (6,20,32).

PROGESTOGEN CHALLENGE TEST DURING TREATMENT WITH DIFFERENT ESTROGEN PREPARATIONS

Figure 4 shows the response to the progestogen challenge test after different estrogen treatments in four groups of selected postmenopausal women. The first three groups were treated with three peroral estrogen formulations in doses sufficient to relieve hot flushes in most patients (33). Group D was treated with an injectable long-acting estrogen–androgen preparation, used in European countries for treatment of the climacteric syndrome (26). All the selected patients were over 45 years old; they had had their last spontaneous menstrual period at least 6 months before; none had been on hormonal therapy for at least 3 months; none was severely overweight. In all cases, a pretreatment MPA challenge test had been negative. The four groups were not statistically different in each of the following parameters: age, length of amenorrhea, degree of obesity, severity of main climacteric complaints, and gonadotropin levels. The MPA was administered over a period of treatment exactly equivalent for each of the four groups. The results of the progestogen test were classified according to Hull et al. (14). As already pointed out, a negative or a positive progestogen test, respectively, signifies the absence or presence of endometrial proliferation. An impaired response suggests the presence of proliferation but in a very moderate degree.

The results obtained in the first two groups confirmed the value of the progestogen challenge test as an index of endometrial proliferation. In all patients treated with estriol continuously, the test remained negative. In fact, in the Tzingounis series (32), for instance, estriol in a single daily dose, even if much higher than that we used, did not induce endometrial proliferation. Conversely, in all patients treated cyclically with conjugated equine estrogens the progestogen test became positive. Actually, this preparation has a strong proliferative effect on endometrium, so that

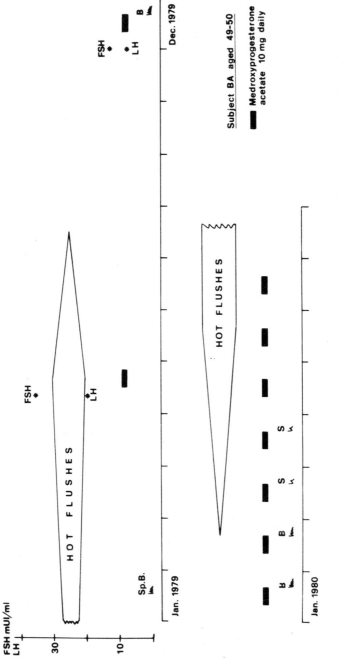

FIG. 2. Response to medroxyprogesterone acetate (MPA) in a woman in early postmenopause. The progestogen test detected a temporary renewal of endometrial proliferation, due to a renewal of endogenous estrogen production. Sp.B = spontaneous bleeding; B = bleeding; S = spotting.

even if the low dose of 0.625 mg daily is used, the progestogen produces withdrawal bleeding in 90% of cases (8).

In the last two groups, the number of patients was small, but data were sufficient to indicate an endometriotrophic effect for both preparations used, though not present in every case and weaker than the effect of conjugated equine estrogens. Injectable, long-acting estrogen–androgen preparations are still popular in Italy for climacteric women, mostly because androgens are believed to inhibit endometrial proliferation, despite the fact that androgens are suspected to play a role in the etiology of endometrial cancer (5). Particularly, dehydroepiandrosterone is believed to maintain the antiestrogenic effect on the endometrium without the virilizing activity of testosterone (22). In our small series, the progestogen challenge test detected a renewal of endometrial proliferation in all women (less important in some than in others) treated with long-acting estradiol valerate-dehydroepiandrosterone enanthate. The case shown in Fig. 5 points out the endometriotrophic effect of the estrogen–androgen preparation compared to estriol. Picha and Weghaupt (26), using long-acting estradiol valerate-dehydroepiandrosterone enanthate, observed a breakthrough bleeding in 4.8% of cases; in about half of these women, histological examination of the endometrium showed cystic hyperplasia. So, when estrogen–androgen preparations are used, all precautions to prevent or to detect endometrial pathology should be recommended as well as for the endometriotrophic estrogens.

CYCLIC PROGESTOGEN TREATMENT IN POSTMENOPAUSAL WOMEN. BENEFITS AND POSSIBLE PROBLEMS

Until a progestogen withdrawal bleeding shows endometrial proliferation as a consequence of either endogenous or exogenous estrogens, the prosecution of cyclic administration of progestogen has been suggested (8). If withdrawal bleeding does not occur after some months of such treatment, the progestogen can be administered at wider intervals, mostly in women at higher risk of endometrial pathology (e.g., the obese ones); finally, it can be discontinued (8,9).

Actually, cyclic use of adequate doses of progestogen in postmenopausal women exposed to endometriotrophic estrogens (either endogenous or exogenous) offers undeniable benefits. Prevention and reversal of endometrial hyperplasia (often, even of the atypical adenomatous type) has been proved (7,8,25,33,37); a possible prevention of endometrial cancer has even been suggested (9); and the incidence of irregular unscheduled bleedings is sharply reduced (17,33,37), thus avoiding the problems, especially psychological ones, produced by urgent diagnostic surgery.

Cyclic progestogen treatment also may cause some problems. Unpleasant minor side effects (fluid retention, tender breasts, reversal of estrogen mental tonic effect) may be produced (33); nevertheless, these are often transient complaints and generally beared well if the patient has been forewarned and informed about the aim of the treatment. A negative effect of progestogen on lipoproteins, particularly a decrease of high-density-lipoprotein (HDL) cholesterol, has been observed (12). HDL cholesterol levels are negatively correlated with higher risk of coronary heart

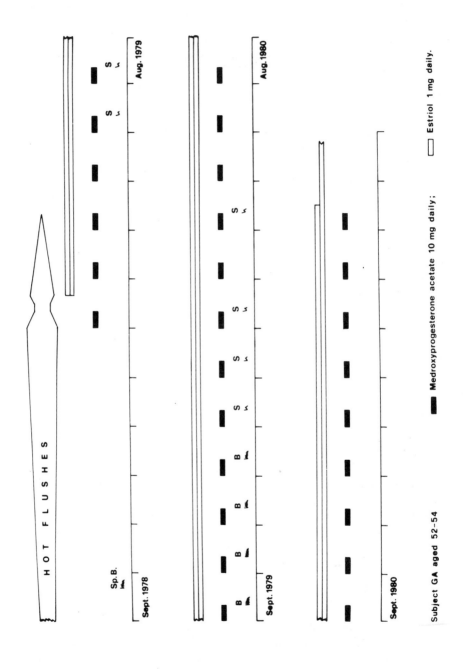

HOT FLUSHES

Sp.B.

Sept. 1978

Aug. 1979

B   B   B   B   S   S   S   S   S

Sept. 1979

Aug. 1980

Sept. 1980

Subject GA aged 52-54

■ Medroxyprogesterone acetate 10 mg daily;   ▢ Estriol 1 mg daily.

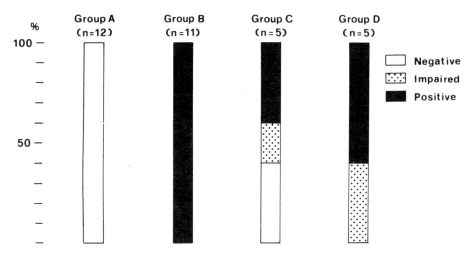

FIG. 4. Response to medroxyprogesterone acetate (MPA) challenge test after different estrogen treatment in postmenopausal women with negative pretreatment test. Type of treatment: Group A: estriol (oral), 2 mg once a day, continuously, MPA (10 mg daily) from day 124 to day 133 of treatment. Group B: conjugated equine estrogens (oral), 0.625 mg daily, for cycles of 21 days on and 7 days off; MPA from day 12 to day 21 of the fifth cycle of therapy. Group C: estradiol valerate (oral) 2 mg every second day, for cycles of 20 days on and 8 days off; MPA from day 11 to day 20 of the fifth cycle of treatment. Group D: estradiol valerate 4 mg + dehydroepiandrosterone enanthate 200 mg (intramuscular), 1 injection every fourth week; MPA from day 12 to day 21 from the fifth injection.

disease (10). The effect on lipoproteins is greatest when the androgenic progestogens of the 19-nortestosterone series are used, whereas it is less important with MPA (12). Obviously, such an effect should create few clinical problems when a weakly endometriotrophic estrogen for treatment of climacteric complaints is used; in this case, the need of a cyclic progestogen treatment generally is limited to a brief period until the residual endogenous estrogen production stops. Possibly, the above-mentioned benefits will exceed the problems also for the women in which cyclic progestogens have to be prolonged because an endogenous estrogen activity persists, or, mainly, highly endometriotrophic estrogens are used. Nevertheless, the clinical consequences of a prolonged administration of progestogens, mainly the possible interferences with the beneficial effects of estrogens on the cardiovascular system (27), await clarification.

FIG. 3. Response to medroxyprogesterone acetate (MPA) in a woman in early postmenopause treated with estriol (2 mg in single daily dose, continuously). The temporary renewal of endometrial proliferation, detected by the progestogen test, seems to be related to a renewal of endogenous estrogen production, rather than to estriol. In a subsequent phase, the test turned negative again in spite of treatment. Sp.B. = spontaneous bleeding; S = spotting; B = bleeding.

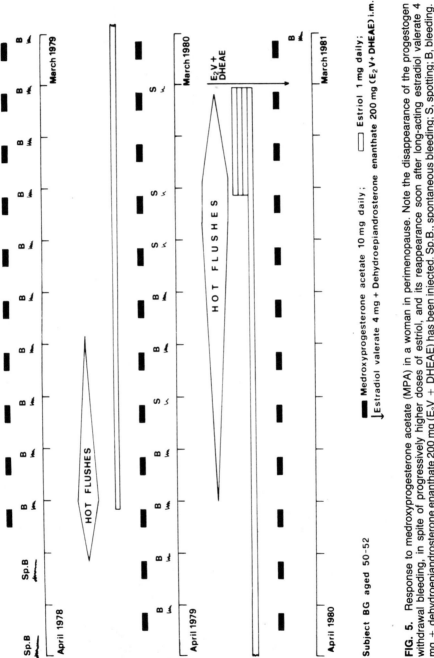

FIG. 5. Response to medroxyprogesterone acetate (MPA) in a woman in perimenopause. Note the disappearance of the progestogen withdrawal bleeding, in spite of progressively higher doses of estriol, and its reappearance soon after long-acting estradiol valerate 4 mg + dehydroepiandrosterone enanthate 200 mg (E₂V + DHEAE) has been injected. Sp.B., spontaneous bleeding; S, spotting; B, bleeding.

SCREENING FOR ENDOMETRIAL CANCER AND ITS PRECURSORS

As already stated, progestogen withdrawal bleeding usually occurs in association with a normal endometrium (4,25). Yet, this does not avoid performing a minimum of direct endometrial evaluations (4) using an outpatient screening method, e.g., the aspiration curettage (11).

If the patient continues to present with progestogen withdrawal bleeding as a consequence of endometriotrophic effect of exogenous or endogenous origin, a biopsy should be performed periodically; an interval of 12 to 18 months is enough (4)[1].

The possibility that the absence of progestogen withdrawal bleeding could be related to an endometrial pathology causing unresponsiveness to hormonal effect rather than to absence of proliferation must be considered. For instance, a 24-year-old amenorrheic women with a history of primary oligoamenorrhea, a hormonal pattern of anovulation, and clinical signs of estrogen production had no withdrawal bleeding after progestogen or after sequential estrogen–progestogen treatment; a histological examination revealed an atypical adenomatous hyperplasia. The histopathological pattern did not change even after a subsequent prolonged progestogen treatment, suggesting unresponsiveness to hormonal action. Therefore, an endometrial biopsy should be performed occasionally and also in patients with negative response to the progestogen, mostly in subjects with a risk factor (11).

Once an eventual preliminary biopsy has been performed and a repeatedly negative response to the progestogen has excluded endometrial proliferation due to residual endogenous estrogens, a weakly endometriotrophic preparation as estriol can be used without need of further endometrial evaluation.

CONCLUSIONS

The progestogen challenge test in postmenopausal women may detect endometrial proliferation due to persisting endogenous estrogen activity; it checks the endometriotrophic effect of estrogen replacement therapies; a positive result suggests prosecution of cyclic progestogen treatment in order to prevent endometrial pathologic changes due to unopposed estrogen stimulation and to minimize irregular bleedings and unnecessary diagnostic surgery; it provides data useful to define the suitability of biopsies for screening of the endometrial cancer and its precursors.

ACKNOWLEDGMENTS

We wish to thank Mrs. S. Battaglia for her secretarial assistance.

REFERENCES

1. Ben-David, M., and van Look, P. F. A. (1979): Hypothalamic-pituitary-ovarian relationships

---

[1]Due emphasis must be given to the fact that in women exposed to highly endometriotrophic estrogens without progestogen, endometrial evaluations should be performed at yearly intervals at the very minimum (25,29,37).

around the menopause. In: *Female and Male Climacteric*, edited by P. A. Van Keep and R. B. Greenblatt, pp. 35–41. MTP Press, Lancaster.

2. Bungay, G. T., Vessey, M. R., and McPherson, C. K. (1980): Study of symptoms in middle life with special reference to the menopause. *Br. Med. J.*, 281:181–183.

3. Campbell, S., and Whitehead, M. (1977): Oestrogen therapy and the menopausal syndrome. *Clin. Obstet. Gynaecol.*, 4:31–47.

4. Campbell, S., and Whitehead, M. I. (1979): The endometrium in the menopause. In: *Female and Male Climacteric*, edited by P. A. van Keep, D. M. Serr, and R. B. Greenblatt, pp. 111–120. MTP Press, Lancaster.

5. Carlström, K., Damber, M. G., Furujhelm, M., Joelsson, I., Lunell, N. O., and von Schoultz, B. (1979): Serum levels of total dehydroepiandrosterone and total estrone in postmenopausal women with special regard to carcinoma of the uterine corpus. *Acta Obstet. Gynecol. Scand.*, 58:179–181.

6. Englund, D. E., and Johansson, E. D. B. (1980): Endometrial effect of oral estriol treatment in postmenopausal women. *Acta Obstet. Gynecol. Scand.*, 59:449–451.

7. Gambrell, R. D., Jr. (1976): Estrogens, progestogens and endometrial cancer. In: *Consensus on Menopause Research*, edited by P. A. Van Keep, R. B. Greenblatt, and M. Albeaux-Fernet, pp. 152–163. MTP Press, Lancaster.

8. Gambrell, R. D., Jr. (1977): Postmenopausal bleeding. *Clin. Obstet. Gynaecol.*, 4:129–143.

9. Gambrell, R. D., Jr. (1978): The prevention of endometrial cancer in postmenopausal women with progestogens. *Maturitas*, 1:107–112.

10. Gordon, T., Castelli, W. P., Hjortland, M. C., Kannel, W. B., and Dawber, D. R. (1977): High density lipoprotein as a protective factor against coronary heart disease: the Framingham study. *Am. J. Med.*, 62:707–714.

11. Gusberg, S. B., and Milano, C. (1981): Detection of endometrial cancer and its precursors. *Cancer*, 47:1173–1175.

12. Hirvonen, E., Mälkönen, M., and Manninen, V. (1981): Effects of different progestogens on lipoproteins during postmenopausal replacement therapy. *N. Engl. J. Med.*, 304:560–563.

13. Hulka, B. S. (1980): Effect of exogenous estrogen on postmenopausal women: The epidemiologic evidence. *Obstet. Gynecol. Survey* (Suppl.), 35:389–399.

14. Hull, M. G. R., Knuth, U. A., Murray, M. A. F., and Jacobs, H. S. (1979): The practical value of the progestogen challenge test, serum oestradiol estimation or clinical examination in assessment of the oestrogen state and response to clomiphene in amenorrhoea. *Br. J. Obstet. Gynaecol.*, 86:799–805.

15. Jaszmann, L. J. B. (1976): Epidemiology of the climacteric syndrome. In: *The Management of the Menopause and Post-Menopausal Years*, edited by S. Campbell, pp. 11–23. MTP Press, Lancaster.

16. Judd, H. I., Davidson, B. J., Fumar, A. M., Shamonki, I. M., Lagasse, L. D., and Ballon, S. C. (1980): Serum androgens and estrogens in postmenopausal women with and without endometrial cancer. *Am. J. Obstet. Gynecol.*, 136:859–866.

17. Kopera, H. (1979): Effects, side-effects, and dosage schemes of various sex hormones in the peri- and post-menopause. In: *Female and Male Climacteric*, edited by P. A. van Keep, D. M. Serr, and R. B. Greenblatt, pp. 43–67. MTP Press, Lancaster.

18. Lauritzen, C. (1979): Management of the patient, including the high-risk patient. In: *Female and Male Climacteric*, edited by P. A. van Keep, D. M. Serr, and R. B. Greenblatt, pp. 121–132. MTP Press, Lancaster.

19. Merril, J. A. (1981): Management of postmenopausal bleeding. *Clin. Obstet. Gynecol.*, 24:285–299.

20. Myhre, E. (1978): Endometrial response to different estrogens. In: *Estrogen Therapy. The Benefits and Risks. Frontiers of Hormone Research*, edited by C. Lauritzen, and P. A. van Keep, pp. 126–144. Karger, Basel.

21. Nakano, R., Hashiba, N., Washio, M., and Tojo, S. (1979): Diagnostic evaluation of progesterone challenge test in amenorrheic patients. *Acta Obstet. Gynecol. Scand.*, 58:59–64.

22. Nyholm, H., and Plesner, R. (1979): Serum testosterone, FSH/LH and urinary excretion of estrogens and corticoids during treatment with an injectable, longacting estrogen-DHEA preparation. *Acta Obstet. Gynecol. Scand.*, 58:385–388.

23. Nisker, J. A., Hammond, G. L., Davidson, B. J., Frumar, A. M., Takaki, N. K., Judd, H. L., and Siiteri, P. H. (1980): Serum sex hormone-binding globulin capacity and the percentage of

free estradiol in postmenopausal women with and without endometrial carcinoma. A new biochemical basis for the association between obesity and endometrial carcinoma. *Am. J. Obstet. Gynecol.*, 138:637–642.

24. Pacheo, J. C., and Kempers, R. D. (1968): Etiology of postmenopausal bleeding. *Obstet. Gynecol.*, 32:46–51.

25. Paterson, M., Wase-Evans, T., Sturdee, D. W., Thom, M., and Studd, J. W. W. (1980): Endometrial disease after treatment with oestrogens and progestogens in the climacteric. *Br. Med. J.*, 1:822–824.

26. Picha, E., and Weghaupt, K. (1972): Erfahrungen mit einer nuen Hormonkombination bei klimakterishen Beschwerden. *Med. Klin.*, 67:382–386.

27. Ross, R. K., Paganini-Hill, A., Mack, T. M., Arthur, M., and Henderson, B. E. (1981): Menopausal oestrogen therapy and protection from death from ischaemic heart disease. *Lancet*, 18:858–860.

28. Schwarz, B. E. (1981): Does estrogen cause adenocarcinoma of the endometrium? *Clin. Obstet. Gynecol.*, 24:243–251.

29. Simsen, D. A., Shirts, S., Howard, F. M., Sims, J., and Hill, J. M. (1981): Endometrial findings in asymptomatic postmenopausal women on exogenous estrogens. A preliminary report. *Gynecol. Oncol.*, 11:56–63.

30. Smith, D. C., Prentice, R., Thompson, D. D., and Herman, W. L. (1975): Association of exogenous estrogen and endometrial carcinoma. *N. Engl. J. Med.*, 293:1164–1167.

31. Speroff, L., Glass, R. H., and Kase, N. G. (1978): *Clinical gynecologic endocrinology and infertility.* Williams and Wilkins, Baltimore.

32. Tzingounis, V. A., Aksu, M. F., and Greenblatt, R. B. (1978): Estriol in the management of the menopause. *J.A.M.A.*, 239:1638–1641.

33. Utian, W. H. (1980): *Menopause in modern perspective. A guide to clinical practice.* Appleton-Century Crofts, New York.

34. Vermeulen, A. (1980): Sex hormone status of the postmenopausal woman. *Maturitas*, 2:81–89.

35. Vermeulen, A., and Verdonck, L. (1978): Sex hormone concentrations in post-menopausal women. Relation to obesity, fat mass, age and years post-menopause. *Clin. Endocrinol.*, 9:59–66.

36. Weinstein, M. C. (1980): Estrogen use in postmenopausal women—costs, risks, and benefits. *N. Engl. J. Med.*, 303:308–316.

37. Whitehead, M. I., McQueen, J., Beard, R. J., Minardi, J., and Campbell, S. (1977): The effects of cyclical oestrogen therapy and sequential oestrogen/progestogen therapy on the endometrium of post-menopausal women. *Acta Obstet. Gynecol. Scand.*, (Suppl.) 65:91–101.

38. Ziel, H. K., and Finkle, W. D. (1975): Increased risk of endometrial carcinoma among users of conjugated estrogens. *N. Engl. J. Med.*, 293:1167–1170.

Steroids and Endometrial Cancer,
edited by V. M. Jasonni, et al.
Raven Press, New York © 1983.

Androstenedione Metabolism in Normal and Neoplastic Human Endometrium

*V. M. Jasonni, *M. Bonavia, *S. Lodi, *S. Preti, *C. Bulletti,
**G. Pelusi, and **C. Flamigni

*Departments of *Reproductive Pathophysiology and **Obstetrics and Gynecology,
St. Orsola's General Hospital, University of Bologna, 40138 Bologna, Italy*

Previous studies have shown that uterine tissues are able to metabolize many steroid hormones (1) and possess the enzyme Δ^4-3 ketosteroid-5α-oxidoreductase which is required to reduce testosterone to DHT (5,6). A possible role of androgens in the etiology of endometrial cancer has been suggested by Poortman and Thijssen (4); in addition, the presence of a discrete androgen receptor and DHT binding proteins in uterus of human, rat, and calf (2,3,7) suggested that androgen activation may be important in the uterotrophic action of androgens in these tissues. This report compares the metabolism of androstenedione by human normal endometrium with that of endometrial cancer.

RESULTS

Incubations of normal endometrium ($N = 6$) and endometrial cancer ($N = 7$) were carried out using Δ^4-androstenedione-4-^{14}C as substrate. In all instances, the following radiometabolites were found: 5α-androstanedione, androsterone, testosterone, DHT, 3α,5α-androstanediol; whereas 19-OH androstenedione was identified only once in normal endometrium. There was no evidence of formation of phenolic steroids.

The experiments carried out with normal endometrium showed that 5α-androstanedione was the compound formed in higher yields, and a significant difference was found between 5α-androstanedione and testosterone ($p < 0.05$), but no significant difference was found between these two metabolites in endometrial cancer.

DISCUSSION

In this study, we demonstrate that the endometrium is able to convert androstenedione to 5α-reduced metabolites as androgen target tissues. It is not known whether androgen metabolism is affected in any neoplastic disorder of the uterus; however, when we compared normal and neoplastic endometrium, we observed the formation of 5α-androstanedione in higher yields in normal endometrium ($p = 0.02$),

TABLE 1. *In vitro conversion of 4-^{14}C-androstenedione by human endometrial tissue and endometrial cancer (pmole/g tissue/4 hr)*

Stage of endometrium	5α-A	Androsterone	T	DHT	3α-diol	19 OH-dione
Normal	919 ± 80	124.5 ± 52	54.3 ± 21	51.4 ± 21.4	3.34 ± 0.7	
Neoplastic	422.5 ± 156.3	685 ± 268.1	309.7 ± 98	48.94 ± 14	12.2 ± 0.3	3.3

Mean ± SE.

whereas testosterone was mainly produced in the endometrial cancer ($p = 0.04$). These results seem to support the hypothesis that an altered androgen metabolism may be involved in the pathophysiology of uterine tissues.

REFERENCES

1. Collins, W. P., Mansfield, M. D., Bridges, C. E., Sommerville, I. F. (1969): Studies on steroid metabolism in human endometrial tissue. *Biochem. J.*, 399–407.
2. Giannopoulos, G. (1971): Binding of Testosterone to cytoplasmic components of the immature rat uterus. *Biochem. Biophys. Res. Commun.*, 44:943–946.
3. Poortman, J., Prenen, J. A. C., Schwarz, F., and Thijssen, M. M. (1975): Interaction of Δ^4-Androstene-3 17-diol with Estradiol and dihydrotestosterone receptors in human myometrium and mammary cancer tissue. *J. Clin. Endocrinol. Metab.*, 40:373–377.
4. Poortman, J., Thijssen, M. M. (1978): The role of androgens in the aethiology of endometrial cancer: a hypothesis. In: *Endometrial cancer*, edited by Brush, King, Taylor, p. 375. Baillère Tindall, London.
5. Reddy, V. V., and Rose, L. I. (1979): Δ^4-3-ketosteroid-5α-oxidoreductase in human uterine leiomyoma *Am. J. Obstet. Gynecol.*, 135:4185–4188.
6. Rose, L. I., Reddy, V. V., and Biondi, R. (1978): Reduction of Testosterone to 5α-dihydrotestosterone by human and rat uterine tissues. *J. Clin. Endocrinol. Metab.*, 46:766–769.
7. Wagner, R. K., Gorlich, L., and Junglunt, P. W. (1972): Multiple steroid hormone receptors in calf uterus binding Specificities and distribution. *Hoppe Seylers Z. Physiol. Chem.*, 353:1654–1660.

Steroids and Endometrial Cancer,
edited by V. M. Jasonni, et al.
Raven Press, New York © 1983.

Rapid Method for the Determination of 17β-Hydroxysteroid Dehydrogenase in Normal and Neoplastic Endometrium

F. De Cicco Nardone, G. D'Aurizio, N. Russo, M. Benedetto, and A. Montemurro

Department of Obstetrics and Gynecology, Catholic University, 00168 Rome, Italy

Human endometrial tissue contains a 17β-hydroxy steroid dehydrogenase (17β-HSD) that catalyzes the oxidation of the 17β-hydroxy group of both C_{18} and C_{19} steroids. Previous studies on normal human endometrium have revealed that 17β-HSD activity is about 10 times higher in secretory than in proliferative phase of the menstrual cycle (4,5).

It is known that progesterone has an inductive effect upon endometrial 17β-HSD activity and that the responsiveness of endometrial carcinoma to progestin therapy may be evaluated by testing for the ability of progestins to induce 17β-HSD *in vivo* or *in vitro* (1,2,6). Since 17β-HSD is important for its clinical applications in endometrial carcinoma, a rapid and easy method to evaluate this activity has been set up.

MATERIALS AND METHODS

All radioactive steroids were purchased from the Radiochemical Centre Amersham, England and were used after purification; unlabeled steroids were a gift from Sigma; NAD^+ was purchased from Boehringer; organic solvents and other chemicals were products of E. Merck. The specimens of normal and neoplastic endometrium were obtained by curettage or after hysterectomy.

ASSAY OF 17β-HSD ACTIVITY

Tissue is homogenized at 4°C using an Ultra-turrax in buffer 50mM Tris/HCL pH 8.6 to obtain a final protein concentration in the homogenate of about 1 mg/ml. The estimation of 17β-HSD activity was performed by incubation of the 800 g supernatant of human endometrial adenocarcinoma with ^3HE and NAD^+ (total volume, 1 ml). The incubation was made at 37°C for 30 min. An aliquot (0.1 ml) was taken and immediately mixed with 2 ml of methanol containing $^{14}CE_1$, unlabeled E_1, and unlabeled E_2. An aliquot (0.1 ml) of the methanolic solution, containing the radioactive steroid extracted was chromatographed on a thin layer plate I.T.L.C. type serum globulin purchased from Gelman Instrument. With this plate, the time of the run was 30 min, using the system cyclohexsane, ethyil acetate, 96:4 (Rf estrone 0.50 and Rf estradiol 0.26). Reference steroids were located by exposing the thin layer plate to iodine vapors; spots corresponding to estrone and estradiol were cut out and counted. Activity of 17β-HSD was expressed as nmole of E_1 formed per mg protein in 30 min. Protein concentration was estimated by Lowry's method (3) using bovine serum albumin as standard.

RESULTS

The reliability of this method was examined in terms of specifity, accuracy, and precision. The specifity of 17β-HSD was studied by incubating ^{3}H-testosterone and ^{3}H-estradiol as substrates. Thin layer chromatography showed nonformation of androstenedione and all the radioactivity was found in the zone with the same mobility as testosterone.

The estrone-^{3}H formed during the assay procedure from the incubated estradiol-^{3}H was acetylated and chromatographed on silica gel thin layer plates. In both conditions of normal and neoplastic endometrium the mobility of the radioactivity of the estrone acetate like material was identical with that of pure estrone acetate.

The Km for 17β-HSD at pH 8.6 was 3.1×10^{-6} M. The recovery of the radioactivity in estrone and estradiol fractions after chromatography on I.T.L.C. type serum globulin was 88.4% ± 3.2%.

CONCLUSION

Because the assay of 17β-HSD is very important for its clinical applications, the standard method has been made easier and more rapid. The exemplification of the standard method can give us in a shorter time precise information about the hormone sensitivity of each endometrial adenocarcinoma.

REFERENCES

1. Bevan, B. J., and Roland, H. (1975): Metabolism of estradiol-17β in human endometrium during the menstrual cycle. *J. Steroid Biochem.*, 6:1489–1494.
2. De Cicco Nardone, F., Iansiti, A., Randina, G. M., and Bompiani, A. (1980): Induction of human endometrial carcinoma dehydrogenase by progestins. Raven Press, New York *(in press)*.
3. Lowry, O. H., Rosebrough, N. J., Farr, A. L., and Randall, R. J. (1951): Protein measurement with the polin phenal reagent. *J. Biol. Chem.*, 193:265–275.
4. Pollow, K., Lubbert, H., Boquoi, E., Kreutzer, G., Jeske, R., and Pollow, B. (1975): Studies on 17β-hydroxysteroid dehydrogenase human endometrium and endometrial carcinoma. *Acta Endocrinol.*, 79:134.
5. Tseng, L., and Gurpide, E. (1974): Estradiol and 20-dihidroprogesterone dehydrogenase activities in human endometrium during the menstrual cycle. *Endocrinology*, 94:419.
6. Tseng, L., and Gurpide, E. (1975): Induction of human endometrial dehydrogenase by progestins. *Endocrinology*, 97:825.

Steroids and Endometrial Cancer,
edited by V. M. Jasonni, et al.
Raven Press, New York © 1983.

Therapeutic Use of Intrauterine Progesterone in Preneoplastic and Dysfunctional Endometrium's Pathology

*U. Leone, *A. D'Angelo, **G. Tanara, and †M. Messeni Leone

*Department of Obstetrical and Gynecological Pathology, University of Sassari, 07100 Sassari, Italy; **The National Center for Research on Cancer and †Department of Histology and Embryology, University of Genoa, 16100 Genoa, Italy*

Glandulocystic hyperplasia of the endometrium in preneoplastic lesion is being taken into consideration. There are many situations in which demolitive surgery is neither desired by the patient nor advisable otherwise. On the other hand, in many cases parentheral or oral hormonal therapy is equally inadvisable because of the inevitable alteration of the normal endocrinological equilibrium.

The use of progesterone therapy in preneoplastic endometrial lesions avoids the inconveniences of radical surgery and has as another advantage the noninhibition of future fertility of the patient.

In the present study, progesterone was administered topically by means of intrauterine devices in the form of a T made up of a biocompatible polymer outer membrane containing an inner core of 52 mg progesterone suspension, intrauterine release of 65 microgramma/die. The treatment was performed for 12 to 24 months in the case of glandulocystic hyperplasia and for 6 to 12 months in the cases of initial adenomatous hyperplasia of the endometrium. The latter were submitted to total hysterectomy, and the endometrium was examined histologically. All procedures were performed in 1979 and 1980.

In the six cases of glandulocystic hyperplasia and in two cases of initial adematous hyperplasia in women whose ages ranged from 17 to 50, control histological examinations were carried out after 4, 6, 12, and 24 months of treatment. In all cases, the control histological preparations demonstrated uniformity.

After treatment with topical progesterone, released from an intrauterine system, advanced glandulocystic hyperplasia and the initial adenomatous hyperplasia disappeared and gave way to athrophic endometrium with some decidual reaction.

Steroids and Endometrial Cancer,
edited by V. M. Jasonni, et al.
Raven Press, New York © 1983.

Cytoplasmic Estradiol and Progesterone Receptors in Normal Endometrium: Changes after Tamoxifen Treatment

P. Biondani, C. Costanzo, G. Cerruti, and A. Ros

Department of Obstetrics and Gynecology, University of Padua—Verona Branch, 37100 Verona, Italy

We have assayed changes of cytoplasmic estradiol (ER) and progesterone (PR) receptors in normal endometrium, using two different doses of tamoxifen (20–40 mg/day).

MATERIALS AND METHODS

We used dextran coated charcoal technique [this method has been described in detail elsewhere (1,2)]. Endometrial samples were obtained by diagnostic curettage or hysterectomy performed for medical indications. After removal of part of the endometrial sample for histology, the remainder was washed in phosphate buffer (pH 7.5), frozen in liquid nitrogen, and transported to the laboratory where it was stored at $-80°C$ until assayed.

CONCLUSIONS

The concentrations of cytoplasmic ER and PR before and after tamoxifen treatment are shown in Fig. 1. All the endometria were in middle proliferative phase according to histological appearance of the tissue samples. In our opinion, tamoxifen has a similar estrogenic action when employed at the 20 mg daily dose. In fact, an ex novo PR synthesis and reduction at the lowest levels of cytoplasmic ER can be seen in three of four cases. Using a double dose (40 mg/day) the ex novo synthesis of PR is detected in only one of three cases, whereas in the other two cases, there is a complete antiestrogenic action and even the cytoplasmic PR is suppressed. We suggested that a better comprehension of the surprising behavior of the drug at these two different doses could be achieved studying ER nuclear translocation.

ACKNOWLEDGMENTS

The authors thank ICI—PHARMA, Italian Division of Imperial Chemical Industries, for technical and scientific support.

207

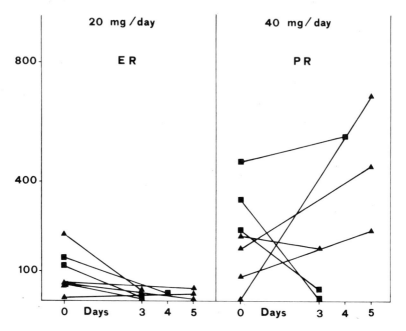

FIG. 1. Changes in cytoplasmic ER and PR in four patients after 3–5 days treatment with tamoxifene 20 mg/day (▲) and in three patients after 3–4 days treatment with tamoxifen 40 mg/day (■).

REFERENCES

1. E.O.R.T.C. Breast Cancer Cooperative Group (1980): Revision of the standards for the assessment of hormone receptors in human breast cancer. *Eur. J. Cancer*, 16:1513–1515.
2. Ros, A., Cappelletto, T., Cerruti, G., Adami, L., and Merz, R. (1980): Aspetti metodologici del dosaggio dei recettori dell'estradiolo e del progesterone. *Attual Ost. Gin.*, 26:159–177.

Steroids and Endometrial Cancer,
edited by V. M. Jasonni, et al.
Raven Press, New York © 1983.

Endometrial Cancer: Steroid Receptors and Medroxyprogesterone Acetate Treatment

P. Biondani, C. Costanzo, G. Cerruti, and A. Ros

Department of Obstetrics and Gynecology, University of Padua—Verona Branch, 37100 Verona, Italy

PURPOSE OF THE WORK

We have studied estradiol (ER) and progesterone (PR) receptor values in endometrial cancer, the relationship between neoplastic grading versus receptor concentration, and changes of cytoplasmic ER and PR concentration during medroxyprogesterone acetate (MPA) administration.

MATERIALS AND METHODS

We collected nine endometrial carcinoma specimens before and after MPA treatment (1 g/day for 10–12 days). After removal of part of the endometrial samples for histology, the remainder was washed in phosphate buffer (pH 7.5), frozen in liquid nitrogen, and transported to the laboratory where it was stored at $-80°C$ until assayed. We used the dextran coated charcoal technique, which has been described in detail elsewhere (1,3).

CONCLUSIONS

We have measured cytoplasmic ER and PR in nine endometrial cancer specimens before and after MPA treatment. The majority (8/9 = 88%) of the tissues contained both receptors; one of nine samples had measurable ER without progestin receptors (Fig. 1). Progestin receptor concentrations in the adenocarcinoma specimens were lower than those in the normal or hyperplastic endometria, whereas there was no major difference in the estrogen receptor values. According to the degree of the differentiation, tissues which were more differentiated contained a higher receptor concentration than those less differentiated. After MPA treatment, oral or parentheral, both receptor values were lower than before progestin therapy. The mean cytoplasmic PR levels dropped to about one-fourth of the pretreatment values when two consecutive samples of neoplastic tissue were studied. It is possible that not only the presence but also the concentration of the receptors is important for the therapeutic response (2).

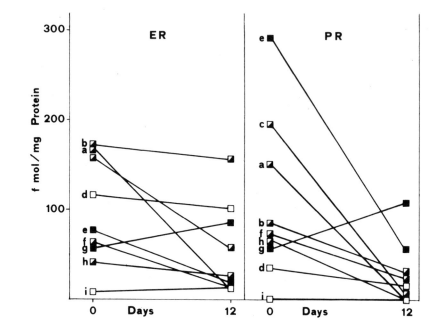

FIG. 1. Changes in cytoplasmic estradiol (ER) and progesterone (PR) in nine patients with endometrial cancer after 10 to 12 days treatment with medroxyprogesterone acetate (1 g/day). (■): well-differentiated cancer; (◪): medium-differentiated cancer; (□): poorly-differentiated cancer.

REFERENCES

1. E.O.R.T.C. Breast Cooperative Group (1980): Revision of the standard for the assessment of hormone receptors in human breast cancer. *Eur. J. Cancer,* 16:1513–1515.
2. Gurpide, E. (1981): Hormone receptors in endometrial cancer. *Cancer,* 48:638.
3. Ros, A., Cappelletto, T., Cerruti, G., Adami, L., and Merz, R. (1980): Aspetti metodologici del dosaggio dei recettori dell'estradiolo e del progesterone. *Attual. Ost. Gin.,* 26:159–177.

Steroids and Endometrial Cancer,
edited by V. M. Jasonni, et al.
Raven Press, New York © 1983.

Effects of a Progestin on the Ultrastructural Morphology of Endometrial Cancer Cells

*Antonio Rigano and **Clemente Pullè

*Department of Oncology and **Department of Obstetrics and Gynecology,
University of Messina, 98100 Messina, Italy

In this chapter, the major findings were changes observed in the ultrastructure of endometrial cancer cells, as compared with untreated carcinoma, after brief but intensive treatment with medroxyprogesterone acetate (MPA) (altogether 20 g in 4 weeks) before surgery.

By the transmission electron microscope (TEM), the secretory tendency of nearly all the superficial cells was evident. This was shown by the presence of numerous rounded granules, strongly osmiophilic, at the apical supranuclear part of the cell or by a marked vacuolization of cytoplasm and frequently with a picture of apocrine secretion.

There are three changes in the plasma membrane of the cell: the disappearance of cytoplasmatic counter, more numerous but short and large microvilli, and the appearance of intercellular bridges without desmosomal apparatus due to phenomenon of acantomatic metaplasia.

By the scanning electron microscope (SEM), a considerable reduction of hypertrophy and cellular dysmorphism was well shown; moreover, the apex of the cells became less prominent and often even bent inwards with an actual hole in it; in addition, we have seen numerous and swollen microvilli of considerable size.

It is evident from our studies that in most endometrial cancer cells it is possible to induce secretory changes with MPA that are similar to normal endometrial ones. However, it is our opinion that in cancer cells, MPA effects are not only hormonal, but also directly toxic, due presumably to the plasmatic membrane changes produced by contact with a great deal of tessutal hormone.

These changes occur when steroid receptors are low, as reported by others (2,3,5,7,8); furthermore, these changes become evident when hormonal plasmatic levels are over 90 ng/ml, namely when doses are very large, and therefore not physiological (1,4,7). Whatever is the mechanism involved, our experience demonstrates that for good results, MPA must be used in very large doses (6).

REFERENCES

1. Bonte, J., Decoster, J. M., Ide, P., and Billiet, G. (1978): Hormonoprophylaxis and hormonotherapy in the treatment of endometrial carcinoma by means of Medroxyprogesterone Acetate. *Gynecol. Oncol.*, 6:60.
2. Brush, M. G., Taylor, R. W., and King R. J. B. (1967): The uptake of oestradiol by the normal human female reproductive tract. *J. Endocrinol.*, 39:599.
3. Gurpide, E., and Tseng, L. (1974): Factors controlling intracellular levels of estrogens in human endometrium. *Gynecol. Oncol.*, 2:221.
4. Kokorn, E. I., and Tchao, B. (1968): The effect of hormones on endometrial carcinoma in organ culture. *J. Obstet. Gynaecol. Br. Comnw.*, 75:1262.
5. MacLaughlin, D. T., and Richardson, G. S. (1976): Progesterone binding by normal and abnormal human endometrium. *J. Clin. Endocrinol. Metab.*, 42:667.
6. Pullè, C., and Rigano, A. (1980): Azione del MAP nell'adenocarcinoma dell'endometrio. Risultati clinici e studio ultrastrutturale ed istochimico. *Min. Gin.*, 32:1.
7. Tseng, L., Gusberg, S. B., and Gurpide, E. (1977): ref. by Ferenczy et alii (1978): *Ann. N.Y. Acad. Sci.*, 286:190.
8. Young, P. C. M., Ehrlich, C. E., and Cleary, R. E. (1976): Progesterone binding in human endometrial carcinoma. *Am. J. Obstet. Gynecol.*, 125:353.

Steroids and Endometrial Cancer,
edited by V. M. Jasonni, et al.
Raven Press, New York © 1983.

Further Suggestions in the Detection and Control of Hormone-Related Risk for Endometrial Cancer

D. Marchesoni, B. Mozzanega, T. Maggino,
D. Paternoster, and M. Gangemi

Obstetric and Gynecological Clinic, University of Padua, 35100 Padua, Italy

Plasma levels of E_2 in postmenopausal patients affected with endometrial cancer (FIGO Stage 1 & 2) are higher than in the controls; the hormone-assay, however, does not seem useful in the screening of patients at risk for this malignancy, since its values appear connected to the higher amount of fat tissue present in affected patients compared to control patients and independent of the presence of the neoplastic disease (2).

What seems to render the woman at risk is the presence of estrogen-induced E_2 receptors through which the active hormone might express its action, and which probably depend on the E_2 impregnation to which the target tissues have been exposed in their life. This is in accordance with Geller (1) in a work carried out on postmenopausal patients affected with breast cancer or other pathologies considered to be estrogen-dependent. Geller found in these patients a preferential postclimateric luteinizing hormone (LH) release after GnRH 100 mcg i.v., associated with a higher concentration of E_2 receptors in the target tissues removed at

TABLE 1. *Plasma levels before and after GnRH 100 mcg i.v. and their response area integrals*

	Control (mU/ml)		Cancer (mU/ml)	
	FSH	LH	FSH	LH
Base	22.18 ± 3.81	38.12 ± 5.13	13.53 ± 3.16	31.91 ± 5.06
15'	74.62 ± 10.23	60.06 ± 11.52	69.81 ± 17.76	55.78 ± 12.81
30'	136.21 ± 17.12	96.23 ± 8.61	89.71 ± 11.93	128.73 ± 5.31
45'	68.15 ± 16.81	79.90 ± 9.42	83.28 ± 13.01	232.49 ± 3.71
60'	92.41 ± 18.89	50.16 ± 12.61	69.12 ± 15.29	91.07 ± 9.96
	$\int$FSH = 5,720.62	> $\int$LH = 4,367.42	$\int$FSH = 4,425.75	< $\int$LH = 7,734.97

Mean ± SE.
FSH = follicle stimulating hormone; LH = luteinizing hormone.

surgery, in spite of the patients' low E_2 plasma levels: thus, the same receptors at the hypophyseal level might determine the preferential LH release.

In our attempt to better identify the subjects at risk for endometrial cancer, we tested through GnRH 100 mcg i.v. 20 patients affected with this neoplasm (independently from their actual E_2 plasma levels and their percentage of the ideal weight).

MATERIAL AND METHODS

Follicle stimulating hormone (FSH) and LH levels were determined through radioimmunoassay (RIA) (Serono-Biodata kit) in plasma samples from 20 patients affected with endometrial cancer whose mean age was 60.42 ± 1.94 (SE) years and who had been postmenopausal for 131.12 ± 18.43 (SE) months, and 20 controls free from any endometrial pathology whose mean age was 57.05 ± 1.75 (SE) years and who had been postmenopausal for 86.65 ± 17.78 (SE) months. Samples were drawn from their cubital veins before the injection of GnRH 100 mcg (Relisorm, Serono) i.v., and after 15, 30, 45, 60 min.

RESULTS

The results are shown in Table 1. In the controls, FSH response area integral was greater than LH response area integral as expected in normal menopause. A preferential LH release was noted in the affected patients, probably due to a higher concentration of hypophyseal E_2 receptors.

An increased hypophyseal endowment with E_2 receptors in endometrial cancer-affected patients may be deduced also through the analysis of PRL-plasma level-drop in them, after a 5-day assumption of 20 mg of tamoxifen, which probably works by displacing the active hormone from E_2 receptors (3).

The authors consider the results reason to suggest the use of the GnRH test in screening patients with hormone-dependent risk for endometrial cancer and to suggest for this malignancy an eventual endocrine therapy, based on a reliable supposition that working E_2 receptors are present.

REFERENCES

1. Judd, H. L., Davidson, B. J., Frumar, A. M., Shamonki, I. M., Lagasse, L. D., and Ballon, S. C. (1980): Serum androgens and estrogens in postmenopausal women with and without endometrial cancer. *Am. J. Obstet. Gynecol.*, 136:859–871.
2. Geller, S., Ayme, Y., Balozet, J., Lemasson, C., Defosse, J. N., Pasqualini, J. R., and Scholler, R. (1979): Liberation preferentielle postclimaterique de LH. In: *Peri et postmenopause*, edited by R. Scholler, pp. 213–241. Sepe Ed., Paris.
3. Marchesoni, D., Mozzanega, B., Gangemi, M., and Enrichi, M. (1980): Tamoxifen in the therapy of post-menopausal endometrial cancer: variations in some hormonal parameters. *Eur. J. Gynaecol. Oncol.*, 1:116–121.

Steroids and Endometrial Cancer,
edited by V. M. Jasonni, et al.
Raven Press, New York © 1983.

Plasma Androstenedione, Estrone, and 17β-Estradiol Levels in Glandular Hyperplasia and Adenocarcinoma of Endometrium

P. Scirpa, D. Mango, A. Montemurro, S. Scirpa,
F. Battaglia, and L. Cantafio

Department of Obstetrics and Gynecology, Catholic University, 00168 Rome, Italy

The possible role of the estrogen production and peripheral conversion of androstenedione to estrone in the development of glandular hyperplasia and adenocarcinoma of endometrium is not yet well known.

This chapter is concerned with androstenedione (A), estrone (E_1), and 17β-estradiol (E_2) plasma levels as determined by specific radioimmunoassays in healthy women and patients affected by glandular hyperplasia and adenocarcinoma of endometrium before and after the menopause. The mean body weight of healthy subjects (63 ± 9 kg, mean $\pm$ SD) was similar to the mean weight of patients affected by glandular hyperplasia (66 ± 7 kg) and adenocarcinoma of endometrium (69 ± 8 kg).

Figure 1 shows the mean plasma levels ($\pm$SD) of A, E_1, and E_2 in a group of healthy women before (A = 0.90 ± 0.33 ng/ml; E_1 = 160 ± 90 pg/ml; E_2 = 65 ± 55 pg/ml) and after the menopause (A = 0.53 ± 0.17 ng/ml; E_1 = 68 ± 35 pg/ml; E_2 = 18 ± 6 pg/ml). Plasma levels of A, E_1, and E_2 fall significantly after the menopause.

Figure 2 shows that in tumor patients the mean plasma levels ($\pm$SD) of A (0.56 ± 0.27 ng/ml), E_1 (70 ± 46 pg/ml), and E_2 (22 ± 15 pg/ml) are not significantly different from those obtained in normal women of similar weight after the menopause. On the other hand, in patients affected by glandular hyperplasia of the endometrium (Fig. 3), the mean plasma levels ($\pm$SD) of A and E_2 before (A = 1.32 ± 0.59 ng/ml; E_2 = 108 ± 106 pg/ml) and after the menopause (A = 1.19 ± 0.53 ng/ml; E_2 = 27 ± 24 pg/ml) are significantly higher than those obtained in normal women of similar weight, whereas E_1 levels are in normal range before (146 ± 123 pg/ml) and after the menopause (70 ± 55 pg/ml).

On the basis of these results, it seems likely that a different endocrine plasma situation is present in glandular hyperplasia and in adenocarcinoma of endometrium.

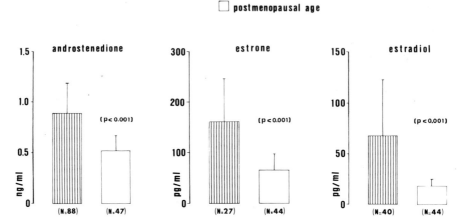

FIG. 1. Concentrations of androstenedione, estrone, and 17β-estradiol (mean ± SD) in peripheral plasma of healthy women before and after the menopause.

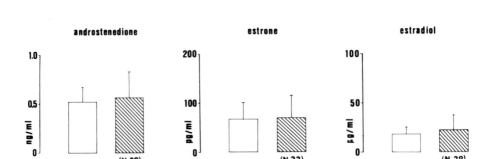

FIG. 2. Concentrations of androstenedione, estrone, and 17β-estradiol (mean ± SD) in peripheral plasma of patients affected by endometrial adenocarcinoma, after the menopause.

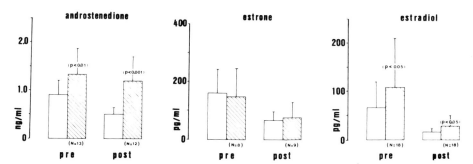

FIG. 3. Concentrations of androstenedione, estrone, and 17β-estradiol (mean ± SD) in peripheral plasma of patients affected by endometrial hyperplasia before and after the menopause.

Steroids and Endometrial Cancer,
edited by V. M. Jasonni, et al.
Raven Press, New York © 1983.

Adjuvant Progestin Therapy in Endometrial Carcinoma

*Antti Kauppila, **Matti Grönroos, and †Usko Nieminen

Departments of Obstetrics and Gynecology, *University of Oulu, **University of Turku,
and †University of Helsinki, Finland

Surgery and radiotherapy do not always yeild curative results in endometrial carcinoma. Hence, systemic therapy with progestin has gained wide acceptance in cases of advanced malignancy, and it has resulted in an objective response in about one-third of the patients treated. The value of adjuvant progestin therapy, on the other hand, is still unclear. For this reason, we evaluated our results in the treatment of endometrial carcinoma confined to the uterus obtained with a combination of surgery, radiotherapy, and adjuvant medroxyprogesterone acetate (MPA).

MATERIALS AND METHODS

From 1970 to 1974, conventional therapy with surgery and irradiation in cases of endometrial carcinoma was complemented with the use of MPA (Lutopolar®, Medipolar, Oulu, Finland) for 2 years in every patient. The daily oral dose of MPA was 100 mg. All patients were followed up for a minimum of 5 years. Patients with inadequate therapy and those who died of intercurrent disease have been excluded from the analysis.

TABLE 1. Corrected 2- and 5-year survival rates of patients treated with surgery, radiotherapy, and MPA with different histological grades of endometrial adenocarcinoma in clinical stages I and II

Stage	Grade	No. of patients	Survival rate 2 years	(%) at 5 years
I	1	421	97.1	93.8
I	2	143	97.2	89.5
I	3	83	86.7	69.9
II	1	51	94.1	88.2
II	2	35	94.3	85.7
II	3	27	63.0	55.6

MPA = medroxyprogesterone acetate.

219

RESULTS

The corrected 5-year survival figures for patients with different grades in his-topathological differentiation in stages I and II are presented in Table 1. In spite of the use of adjuvant MPA, there were deaths from endometrial carcinoma during the first 2 years after the primary therapy. In clinical stage I, the 2-year death rates from endometrial carcinoma of patients with grade 1, 2, or 3 adenocarcinoma were 2.9, 2.8, and 13.3% respectively. The corresponding results were 3.9, 5.7, and 37.0% in clinical stage II. The relative frequency of recurrences during the MPA period was much lower in patients with grade 1 or 2 carcinoma than in patients with anaplastic carcinoma (Table 2).

DISCUSSION

Opinions of the value of adjuvant progestin therapy in endometrial carcinoma are controversial. The results of some studies have not confirmed any benefit from this kind of therapy (3,4), whereas other investigators have obtained a 5-year survival figure of 100% with the combination of surgery, radiotherapy, and adjuvant MPA (1). In our hands, this combination did not totally prevent recurrences of early carcinomas. This was also the case for grade 1 carcinomas, which are known to very often possess receptors for progestin in rich concentrations (2), and as advanced malignancies to respond favorably to hormonal chemotherapy (5). How-ever, our results corroborate recent observations showing that some well-differ-entiated carcinomas have no, or a very low concentration, of female steroid hormone receptors (2). The difference in the development of recurrences between various histopathological grades of endometrial malignancy in the conditions described may be due to the aggressive behavior of anaplastic carcinoma or to the intracellular growth suppressing action of MPA in grades 1 and 2 endometrial carcinoma. In view of what is presently known, receptor status, rather than the degree of histo-logical differentiation of carcinomatous tissue of the endometrium, might be the best indicator in selection of patients suitable for treatment with progestin.

TABLE 2. *Appearance of recurrences in relation to MPA administration for 2 years*

| | | Frequency of recurrences | |
| | | During MPA (%) | After MPA (%) |
Stage	Grade		
I	1	50	50
I	2	43	57
I	3	74	26
II	1	50	50
II	2	25	75
II	3	89	11

MPA = medroxyprogesterone acetate.

SUMMARY

Medroxyprogesterone acetate (MPA; 100 mg per os daily) was administered for 2 years to 799 patients with stage I ($N = 677$) or II ($N = 122$) disease. All were operated on and irradiated. The corrected 5-year survival rates in clinical stages I and II were 89.8 and 80.3%, respectively. The death rates from endometrial carcinoma at the end of the MPA period for patients with grade 1, 2, or 3 lesions were 2.9, 2.8, and 13.3% respectively in clinical stage I and 3.9, 5.7, and 37.0% respectively in stage II. Thus, adjuvant MPA at the doses used could not totally prevent recurrences of even differentiated adenocarcinomas. The relatively rare and delayed appearance of grade 1 and 2 recurrences in comparison with anaplastic recurrences may be at least partly related to the intracellular growth suppressing action of MPA.

REFERENCES

1. Bonte, J., Decoster, J. M., Ide, P., and Billiet, G. (1978): Hormonoprophylaxis and hormonotherapy in the treatment of endometrial adenocarcinoma by means of medroxyprogesterone acetate. *Gynecol. Oncol.*, 6:60–75.
2. Kauppila, A., Kujansuu, E., and Vihko, R. (1982): Cytosol estrogen and progestin receptors in endometrial carcinoma of patients treated with surgery, radiotherapy, and progestin; Clinical correlates. *Cancer*, 50:2157–2162.
3. Lewis, G. C., Slack, N. G., Mortel, L., and Bross, D. J. (1974): Adjuvant progestogen therapy in the primary definitive treatment of endometrial cancer. *Gynecol. Oncol.*, 2:368–376.
4. Malkasian, Jr, G. D., and Decker, D. G. (1978): Adjuvant progesterone therapy for stage I endometrial carcinoma. *Int. J. Gynecol. Obstet.*, 16:48–49.
5. UICC Technical Report Series, vol. 42 (1978): Hormonal biology and endometrial cancer, edited by G. S. Richardson and D. T. MacLaughlin, International Union Against Cancer, Geneva.

Steroids and Endometrial Cancer,
edited by V. M. Jasonni, et al.
Raven Press, New York © 1983.

Endocrinological Aspects and *In Vitro* Prolactin Secretion of Endometrial Adenocarcinoma

A. Volpe, E. Dalla Vecchia, V. Mazza, A. M. Previdi, A. Grasso, and G. C. Di Renzo

Department of Obstetrics and Gynecology, University of Modena, 41100 Modena, Italy

Basal levels of follicle stimulating hormone (FSH), luteinizing hormone (LH), prolactin (PRL), growth hormone (GH), estrone (E_1), estradiol (E_2), testosterone (T), androstenedione (Δ^4), progesterone (Pg), 17-Idrossiprogesterone (17-OH-PG) and dynamic tests with GnRH, thyrotropin releasing hormone (TRH) and sulpiride were evaluated in 40 patients affected by endometrial adenocarcinoma (EA) and were compared with controls matched for age, glicometabolism, arterial tension and years after menopause. E_1 and PRL levels were significantly ($p < 0.01$) higher in EA group than in controls. In the EA group, E_1 and PRL levels were 68.2 ± 15.4 ng/ml and 15.3 ± 7.6 ng/ml respectively, whereas in controls hormone levels were 46.4 ± 19.8 and 9.7 ± 3.4 ng/ml, respectively. No significant difference in gonadotropins response to GnRH and PRL response to TRH and sulpiride tests was observed between the two groups examined.

We also examined *in vitro* PRL and GH secretion of five endometrial adenocarcinomas compared with five normal endometria from similarly aged women. All tissues were obtained after abdominal hysterectomy and were available in amounts enough to provide duplicate flasks for incubation. In these instances, *de novo* protein synthesis was inhibited in the second flasks by the addition of 100 mcg/ml of cycloheximide to the incubation medium (1). The samples from culture medium were taken every 3 days for 24 days. The levels of GH resulted not measurable either in the medium of neoplastic tissue or in the medium of normal endometrium. Mean levels of PRL in endometrial adenocarcinoma culture were 6.1 ± 3.9 ng/ 100 mg wet tissue, whereas in controls mean values were not detectable. The addition of 100 mcg/ml of cycloheximide to the medium prevented the increase in PRL content during incubation (Table 1). From these findings, we can speculate that in patients affected by endometrial adenocarcinoma at least some PRL results from neoplastic tissue.

REFERENCES

1. Maslar, I. A., and Riddick, D. H. (1978): Prolactin production by human endometrium during the normal menstrual cycle. *Am. J. Obstet. Gynecol.*, 15:751–754.

TABLE 1. *Prolactin production (ng/100 mg wet tissue: mean ± SD) by endometrial adenocarcinoma and controls*

	Day							
	3° Day	6° Day	9° Day	12° Day	15° Day	18° Day	21° Day	24° Day
Endometrial adenocarcinoma	ND	ND	ND	3.2 ± 1.3	7.4 ± 3.2	8.1 ± 4.1	6.9 ± 3.7	8.6 ± 4.6
Endometrial adenocarcinoma + cycloheximide (100 mcg/ml)	ND	ND	ND	ND	ND	ND	ND	ND
Controls	ND	ND	ND	ND	ND	ND	ND	ND

ND = not detectable; $N = 5$ in each group.

Steroids and Endometrial Cancer,
edited by V. M. Jasonni, et al.
Raven Press, New York © 1983.

A Model of Intracellular Recycling of Steroid Receptors

Gian Paolo Rossini

*Department of Biological Chemistry, University of Modena,
41100 Modena, Italy*

The fate of steroid-receptor complexes after their nuclear retention in target cells has not been firmly established. In glucocorticoid (9) and androgen (5,6) responsive tissues, nuclear steroid-receptor complexes can be recycled back to the cytoplasm, whereas in progesterone and estrogen responsive tissues it is not clear whether receptor complexes are degraded (2,3,8) or can be recycled (3,4).

In the hypothetical model of androgen and glucocorticoid receptor recycling (6,9), steroid-receptor complexes are released from nuclei into the cytoplasm (Fig. 1). Loss of steroid (H) is then followed by inactivation of receptor proteins to a form unable to bind the steroid (R°), receptor reactivation to a steroid binding form (R), further steroid binding (R-H), and nuclear retention of transformed receptor complexes (R-H*).

The data supporting steroid receptor recycling are still very fragmentary, and more research should be done to establish whether this model could represent intracellular dynamics of steroid receptors in every responsive system. Moreover, the many steps involved in this hypothetical model should be investigated together with factor(s) that can control them (Fig. 1). For instance, steroid-receptor complex release from chromatin could be caused by RNA molecules carrying specific sequences committed to binding of steroid-receptor complexes (7). Whereas translocation of steroid-receptor complexes from the nucleus into the cytoplasm might involve interaction between receptor complexes and ribonucleoprotein particles (5).

Other factors, however, could control the inactivation-reactivation process (1,6,9,10). In fact, androgen and glucocorticoid receptor activation requires a constant energy supply (6,9).

An activation process that can control very rapidly the steroid binding capacity of receptor proteins can be a good candidate as a modulator of steroid hormone action.

Small environmental changes as well as internal stimuli could affect the factors involved in the activation process leading in a very short time to a control of intracellular levels of receptors available for steroid binding.

Because steroid binding to its receptor protein is the parameter used to quantitate the cellular receptor pools, whose levels play a major role in the development of

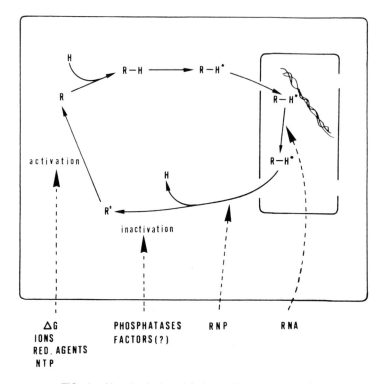

FIG. 1. Hypothetical model of steroid receptor recycling.

basic as well as clinical research, a complete understanding of inactivation–reactivation process(es) is required. A process that modulates the levels of receptor available for steroid binding would then control the amount of receptor complexes translocatable into nuclei, and then it could determine the magnitude of cellular responses to the hormone under those specific physiological conditions.

REFERENCES

1. Auricchio, F., Migliaccio, A., and Rotondi, A. (1981): *Biochem. J.*, 194:569–574.
2. Horwitz, K. B., and McGuire, W. L. (1978): *J. Biol. Chem.*, 253:6319–6322.
3. Isotalo, J., Isomaa, V., and Jänne, O. (1981): *Endocrinology*, 108:868–873.
4. Kassis, J. A., and Gorski, J. (1981): *J. Biol. Chem.*, 256:7378–7382.
5. Liao, S., Liang, T., and Tymoczko, J. L. (1973): *Nature New Biology*, 241:211–213.
6. Liao, S., Rossini, G. P., Hiipakka, R. A., and Chen, C. (1980): In: *Perspectives in Steroid Receptor Research*, edited by F. Bresciani, pp. 99–112. Raven Press, New York.
7. Liao, S., Smithe, S., Tymoczko, J. L., Rossini, G. P., Chen, C., and Hiipakka, R. A. (1980): *J. Biol. Chem.*, 255:5545–5551.
8. Little, M., Szendro, P., Teran, C., Huges, A., and Jungblut, P. W. (1975): *J. Steroid Biochem.*, 6:493–500.
9. Munck, A., Wira, C., Young, D. A., Mosher, K. M., Hallahan, C., and Bell, P. A. (1972): *J. Steroid Biochem.*, 3:567–578.
10. Nielsen, C. J., Sando, J. J., and Pratt, W. B. (1977): *Proc. Natl. Acad. Sci. U.S.A.*, 74:1398–1402.

Steroids and Endometrial Cancer,
edited by V. M. Jasonni, et al.
Raven Press, New York © 1983.

Ovarian and Peripheral Plasma Levels of C_{21}, C_{19}, and C_{18} Steroids in Postmenopausal Women with and without Endometrial Cancer

S. Dell'Acqua, A. Lucisano, M. G. Acampora, E. Parlati, B. Cinque, E. Maniccia, A. Montemurro, and A. Bompiani

Department of Obstetrics and Gynecology, Catholic University San Cuore, 00168 Rome, Italy

In postmenopausal women, the role of estrogens and their precursors' production in the genesis of adenocarcinoma of the endometrium is discussed still. Moreover, the ovarian steroids' production in the postmenopausal women is not defined completely yet.

This work was undertaken to compare the peripheral and ovarian vein plasma levels of C_{21}, C_{19}, and C_{18} steroids in 15 postmenopausal women with endometrial cancer and in corresponding appropriately matched control subjects. We matched each control to a specific cancer patient for percentage of ideal weight, calculated by dividing the subject's actual weight by her ideal weight, and multiplying by 100. Ideal weights were obtained from tables supplied by the Metropolitan Life Insurance Co., USA. The mean of percentage of ideal weight for women with endometrial cancer was 124 (± 18.4 SD) and for control subjects 124.5 (± 19 SD).

Ovarian blood was obtained by insertion into the vessel isolated from the infundibulopelvic ligament of a microneedle connected to a small tube. Steroids determination was carried out by radioimmunoassays using highly specific antisera obtained in our laboratory. Before radioimmunoassays, the material was purified through a small column of Sephadex LH 20.

Figure 1 presents plasma estrone and estradiol levels in peripheral and ovarian veins in postmenopausal women with and without endometrial cancer. No significant difference between the two groups for both estrone and estradiol has been found, but for both groups, highly significant differences between ovarian and peripheral levels of estrone and estradiol were found.

For androstenedione and testosterone there was no difference between the two groups (Fig. 2). At laparotomy, peripheral level of androstenedione increases, indicating that androstenedione adrenal contribution increases because of surgical stress. Also for progesterone and 17α-hydroxy-progesterone, no difference between

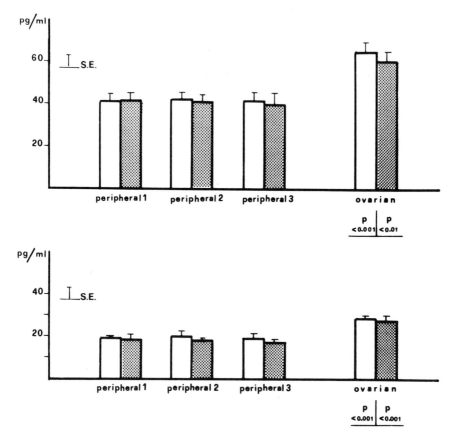

FIG. 1. Plasma estrone **(top)** and estradiol **(bottom)** levels in peripheral and ovarian veins in 15 postmenopausal women with endometrial adenocarcinoma (*open columns*) and in 15 control subjects (*hatched columns*). Peripheral 1: before anesthesia; 2: after anesthesia; 3: at laparotomy.

the two groups was found (Fig. 3). The surgical stress provokes a conspicuous increase of peripheral levels of progesterone and especially of 17α-hydroxy-progesterone. The difference between peripheral and ovarian levels of progesterone was significant, indicating that ovarian postmenopausal tissue produces and secretes C_{21} steroids.

Figure 4 shows the significant correlation of estrone and estradiol peripheral levels with percentage of ideal weight in patients with and without endometrial cancer. In the two groups, the slopes of regression are in very close agreement. No significant correlations were found between the percentage of ideal weight and the peripheral C_{19} and C_{21} steroids considered and between age of the patients or years since menopause in all steroids considered.

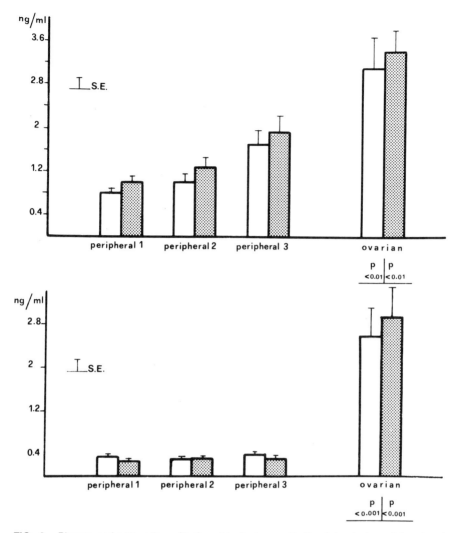

FIG. 2. Plasma androstenedione **(top)** and testosterone **(bottom)** levels in peripheral and ovarian veins in 15 postmenopausal women with endometrial adenocarcinoma (*open columns*) and in 15 control subjects (*dotted columns*). Peripheral 1: before anesthesia; 2: after anesthesia; 3: at laparotomy.

A significant correlation of circulating estrone to androstenedione levels with the percentage of ideal weight was found in patients with and without endometrial cancer. Moreover, analysis of possible relationships among the peripheral levels of the six steroids considered revealed a significant correlation between estrone and estradiol with a very close agreement of the slopes of the regressions in the cancer patients and in the control subjects (Fig. 5). In both groups, the ovarian levels of

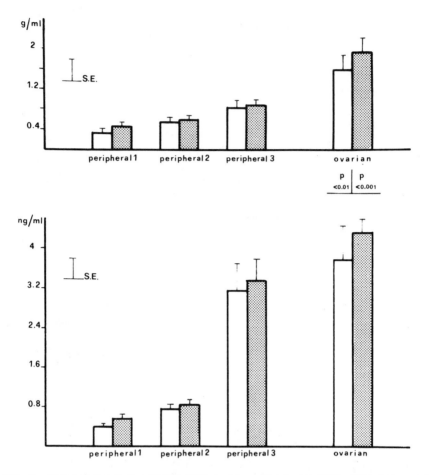

FIG. 3. Plasma progesterone **(top)** and 17α-hydroxy-progesterone **(bottom)** levels in peripheral and ovarian veins in 15 postmenopausal women with endometrial adenocarcinoma (*open columns*) and in 15 control subjects (*hatched columns*). Peripheral 1: before anesthesia; 2: after anesthesia; 3: at laparotomy.

the six steroids considered did not correlate with each other or with peripheral ones or with percentage of ideal weight and age of the patients.

Our results confirm that there is no difference in the ovarian and peripheral plasma levels of C_{21}, C_{19}, and C_{18} steroids in cancer patients and in control subjects, at least in patients with excess body weight, and that estrogens in postmenopausal women are produced mainly from androstenedione in peripheral tissue.

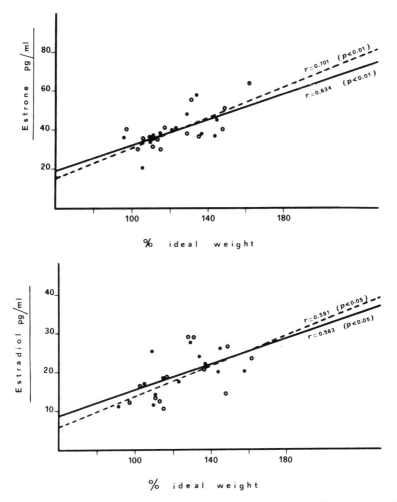

FIG. 4. Correlations of estrone and estradiol peripheral plasma levels with percentage of ideal weight in 15 patients with endometrial adenocarcinoma (●, *solid regression line*) and in 15 control subjects (○, *broken regression line*).

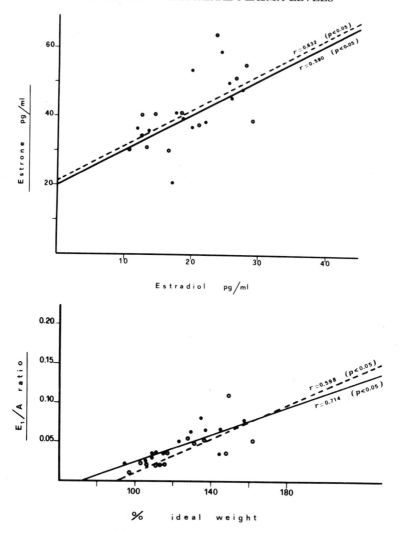

FIG. 5. Correlation of estrone with estradiol peripheral plasma levels and correlation of circulating estrone to androstenedione level (E₁/A ratio) with percentage of ideal weight in 15 patients with endometrial adenocarcinoma (●, *solid regression line*) and in 15 control subjects (○, *broken regression line*).

Steroids and Endometrial Cancer,
edited by V. M. Jasonni, et al.
Raven Press, New York © 1983.

Studies on Estrogen Status and Estrogen Hormone Sensitivity in Advanced Endometrial Cancer

*L. Castagnetta, *G. D'Agostino, *O. M. Granata, **A. Traina, and †R. E. Leake

*Institute of Biochemistry, Faculty of Medicine—Policlinico, 90127 Palermo, Italy; **Cancer Hospital Center "M. Ascoli", Palermo, Italy; and †Department of Biochemistry, Glasgow University, G. 12-8QQ, Glasgow, United Kingdom

The characterization of the steroid status in hormone-sensitive human tumors was first carried out many years ago and has produced a vast amount of data, i.e., the discriminant function (1), the estriol quotient (2), and the generally accepted conclusion that an abnormal steroid metabolism is often associated with these tumors. Approximately 40 to 50% of patients with endometrial cancer have higher estrogen values than the controls; this estrogen is not of ovarian origin (Brown, J. B. et al., *unpublished data*). Attention recently has been directed to the need to conduct further more detailed studies in this field (3).

This study was carried out on 33 patients with the object of comparing estrogen hormone-sensitivity (HS) with estrogen status in postmenopausal ($N = 28$ of 33) advanced endometrial cancer. Most of these tumors could be clinically defined as advanced and were marked by a high percentage (21.4%) of poorly differentiated tumors.

The hormone-sensitive status was evaluated by the estrogen receptor (ER) status, which was considered positive when both the soluble and the nuclear fractions were positive (i.e., they exhibited an unimpaired function) (4). Furthermore, to obtain a better definition of the HS status, studies were carried out on the intratumoral

TABLE 1. *Distribution of hormone sensitive (HS) status of postmenopausal endometrial cancer*

HS Status	+ +	+	−
% Patients	53.5	23.5	21.4
	($N = 15$)	($N = 7$)	($N = 6$)
Postmenopause age (Mean ± SD)	12.5 ± 6.8	8.6 ± 4.7	6.6 ± 4.5
Age (Mean ± SD)	62.1 ± 5.6	59.1 ± 4.5	56.6 ± 3.4

variations of the ER status in at least two different portions of the same tumor. It was, therefore, possible to subdivide the patients into three groups (Table 1) with differing hormone-sensitivity: group a: broad hormone-sensitive status, when both ER determinations turned out positive ($+ + $HS); group b: narrow hormone-sensitive status, when only one determination was positive ($+$HS); group c: negative hormone-sensitive status, when both determinations turned out negative ($-$HS).

The hormone status was studied through gas liquid chromatography and, when necessary, mass spectrometry, by considering the three classical estrogens, both individually and as a whole, the minor estrogens (including the catecholestrogens), and the total estrogens, as well as some of their ratios (2,5).

RESULTS AND COMMENTS

The estrogen excretion levels in relation to menopausal groups (Table 2) do not exhibit any significant variations according to the age of menopause except the excretion levels of estrone, which show a significant increase in postmenopause. Nevertheless, there was a surprising increase in the levels of estriol and the classical estrogens in the advanced postmenopausal group.

Minor estrogens, the so-called unusual metabolites, display roughly the same excretion levels in all three postmenopausal groups (although they show a slight increase in the advanced postmenopausal group).

Regarding the ratios between suitably selected metabolites, the estriol ratio (E_3R) shows a reduction (though a nonsignificant one) from 6.2, median value of premenopausal group (I.R. values = 1.2–9.8), to 2.5 (I.R. values = 0.7–7.1) in the postmenopause group greater than 6 years, as was expected.

On the contrary, the ratio between classical estrogens and unusual metabolites turns out to be constant and well above the discriminant values obtained from a reanalysis study of the clinical response of patients with breast cancer (6). In fact, median values vary from 3.5 in premenopausal group (I.R. values = 2.9–4.4) to 5.0 in postmenopausal group (I.R. values = 1.3–13.1) (6).

If we divide the patients with endometrial cancer on the basis of HS status, there emerges an impressive association between the negative HS status of endometrial

TABLE 2. *Estrogen excretion levels in different menopausal groups of endometrial cancer (median and IR values)*

	E_1	E_2	E_3	Classical estrogen	Unusual metabolites
Premenopause	1.7	1.5	12.8	15.8	3.0
	(1.0–2.8)	(1.0–3.0)	(1.5–27.6)	(3.5–30.5)	(1.0–9.5)
Postmenopause	5.4	1.2	15.6	21.2	5.1
	(3.6–9.3)	(1.0–2.0)	(2.9–24.6)	(9.1–28.2)	(2.0–46.2)
Wilcoxon's test	$p < 0.01$	NSD	NSD	NSD	NSD

NSD = not significantly different.

tumors and several expressions of abnormality in the estrogen excretion profiles as shown in Table 3.

In fact, estrone and estrone-sulfate (the two fractions were not considered separately) can be seen to increase in a significantly abnormal manner in group c, as compared with the group a, which was composed for the most part of advanced postmenopause.

The unusual metabolites of estrogens also exhibited a considerable and significant increase in both groups b and c in comparison with group a. At the same time, we can observe a slight though not significant increase both in the classical estrogens and the total estrogens in the same way.

The C/U ratio drops from 5.8 to 0.8 median values, and with the respective I.R. values clearly separated (i.e., in the first with a minimum I.R. value of 3.8, in the second with a maximum I.R. value of 1.94). This appears connected strictly with the negative HS status; but it also seems to be related, though to a lesser extent, with the narrow HS group.

In both cases, this connection turns out to be highly significant, as evidenced by Wilcoxon's test. On the contrary, the estriol ratio exhibits more or less the same median values not significantly different in all three groups.

A concluding comment to these studies would suggest yet again that an abnormal increase in the estrone levels (and those of estrone-sulfate) is connected with a defective estradiol receptor function in endometrial cancer, as recently observed in breast tumors (7).

Our studies also indicate that abnormally increased amounts of the unusual metabolites are also associated with tumors with negative HS status.

Conversely, these experimental results indicate that a normal estrogen metabolism, at least at the level of estrogen excretion profiles, is significantly related to an unimpaired ER function.

These data do not lend any support to the hypothesis previously put forward (7) that the 17β-estradiol reduction pathway may be responsible for a higher degree of blockade of hormone binding sites, accompanied by increased nuclear receptor levels, because a similar increase in the estradiol nuclear receptor concentrations

TABLE 3. *Estrogen excretion patterns in endometrial tumors with different receptor function (median and IR values)*

Hormone Status	E_1	E_2	E_3	Classical estrogen	Unusual metabolites
(a) + +HS	2.8	2.0	9.8	16.8	2.0
	(1.0–4.0)	(1.0–2.0)	(2.0–22.9)	(5.0–24.9)	(1.0–3.0)
(b) +HS	4.3	1.0	20.5	28.6	12.2
	(0.5–19.2)	(0.5–3.8)	(3.6–40.1)	(11.6–56.6)	(1.5–67.7)
(c) −HS	11.2	2.0	7.1	25.5	43.3
	(5.7–17.8)	(1.5–3.0)	(3.2–25.9)	(19.7–33.5)	(16.5–82.5)
Wilcoxon's test (a–c)	$p < 0.0001$	NSD	NSD	NSD	$p = 2 \times 10^{-7}$

HS = hormone-sensitive status; NSD = not significantly different.

was not observed in the cases with narrow hormone-sensitivity nor in cases with an impaired ER function (O/+ tissues).

This therefore disproves the hypothesis that the relationship between ER status and certain aspects of estrogen metabolism might be a simple consequence of quantitative modulation by the hormone on the estrogen receptor mechanism.

ACKNOWLEDGMENTS

We are very pleased to acknowledge essential financial support from the British Council (R.E.L. and L.C.) and the Ciba foundation (L.C.). This study was part of a special project supported by CNR contract No. 80.01506.96 (L.C.).

REFERENCES

1. Bulbroock, R. D., Greenwood, F. C., and Hayward, J. L. (1960): *Lancet*, 1:1154–1157.
2. Lemon, H. M., Wotiz, H. H., Pearsons, L., and Mozden, P. J. (1966): *JAMA*, 196:1128–1136.
3. Dao, T. L. (1979): *Biochem. Biophys. Acta*, 560:397–426.
4. Leake, R. E., Laing, L., and Smith, D. C. (1979): In: *Steroid Receptor Assays in Human Breast Tumours: Methodological and Clinical Aspects*, edited by R. J. B. King, pp. 73–85. Alpha Omega Alpha Publishing, Cardiff.
5. Castagnetta, L. (1979): *Bladder tumours and other topics in urological oncology*, edited by M. Pavone-Macaluso, P. H. Smith, and F. Edsmyr. pp. 431–441. Plenum Press, New York.
6. Castagnetta, L., D'Agostino, G., Lo Casto, M., Traina, A., and Leake, R. E. (1981): *Br. J. Cancer (in press)*.
7. Wilking, M., Carlström, K., Gustafssön, S. A., Skölferfors, H., and Tollbom, O. (1980): *Eur. J. Cancer*, 16:1339–1344.

Steroids and Endometrial Cancer,
edited by V. M. Jasonni, et al.
Raven Press, New York © 1983.

Immunohistochemical Method for Estrogen and Progesterone Receptors

*G. Pelusi, **A. D'Errico, *R. Cavallina, †A. Cunsolo,
‡V. M. Jasonni, and **V. Eusebi

*Departments of *Obstetrics and Gynecology, ‡Reproductive Endocrinology, †General
Surgery, and **Institute of Histopathology, University of Bologna, 40138 Bologna, Italy*

The study of estrogen receptors (ER) and progesterone receptors (PR) is very useful in the prognosis and management of therapy of breast and endometrial carcinoma. An immunohistochemical method is proposed that stains saturated ERs and PRs (2,3).

METHOD

Five consecutive 5 μ sections are cut in a cryostat at $-32°C$. The first section is stained with hematoxylin-eosin (H-E), and the second and third are studied with the immunohistochemical methods. The other sections are used as controls without prior incubation with the respective hormonal substrate. All the reactions are carried out at a temperature of 4°C.

ER analysis	PgR analysis
1. Washing in PBS pH 7.2	1. Same
2. Incubation with 17β-estradiol-6CMO-BSA 7 × 10^{-5} M	2. Incubation with 11-α-hydroxyprogesterone hemisuccinate-BSA 7 × 10^{-6} M
3. Washing in PBS 10′	3. Same
4. Fixation in Carson's solution (1) 30′	4. Same
5. Immunoperoxidase method according to Sternberger (5)	5. Same
6. The anti 17-β-estradiol-6CMO-BSA antiserum (4) was diluted 1:150	6. The anti-11-α-hydroxyprogesterone-hemisuccinate-BSA antiserum (4) was diluted 1:1000

CONTROLS

Tissues. Rat uterus is used as a positive control and human stomach as negative control.

Methods. Prior incubation of sections with diethylstilbestrol (7×10^{-5} moles) and with medroxyprogesterone acetate. The specific antisera also were previously absorbed with 17-β-estradiol-6CMO-BSA and 11-α-hydroxyprogesterone-hemisuccinate-BSA.

With this method, it is possible to assess cytoplasmic and nuclear positivity. It is also possible to demonstrate the percentage of positive cells. The stain is permanent and this is an advantage over immunofluorescence methods.

ACKNOWLEDGMENTS

Work supported by Grant n. 81.01.360.96 from C.N.R. "Progetto Finalizzato Controllo della Crescita Neoplastica," Rome, Italy.

REFERENCES

1. Carson, F. L., Martin, J. H., and Lynn, J. A. (1973): Formalin fixation for electron microscopy: a re-evaluation. *Am. J. Clin. Pathol.*, 49:365–373.
2. Eusebi, V., Cerasoli, P. T., Guidelli Guidi, S., Grilli, S., Bussolati, G., and Azzopardi, J. G. (1981): A two stage immunocytochemical method for oestrogen receptor analysis: correlation with morphological parameters of breast carcinoma. *Tumori*, 67:315–323.
3. Eusebi, V., Grilli, S., Papotti, M., Fedeli, F., Caruso, F., Bussolati, G. (1982): An immunocytochemical method for progesterone receptor determination in human breast carcinoma. *Appl. Pathol. (in press).*
4. Roda, A., and Bolelli, G. F. (1980): Production of a high-titre antibody to bile acids. *J. Steroid Biochem.*, 13:449–454.
5. Sternberger, L. A. (1979): *Immunochemistry*, 2nd ed. Wiley and Sons, New York.

Subject Index